Progress in Inflammation Research

Series Editor

Prof. Dr. Michael J. Parnham
PLIVA
Research Institute
Prilaz baruna Filipovica 25
10000 Zagreb
Croatia

Published titles:

T Cells in Arthritis, P. Miossec, W. van den Berg, G. Firestein (Editors), 1998
Chemokines and Skin, E. Kownatzki, J. Norgauer (Editors), 1998
Medicinal Fatty Acids, J. Kremer (Editor), 1998
Inducible Enzymes in the Inflammatory Response, D.A. Willoughby, A. Tomlinson (Editors), 1999
Cytokines in Severe Sepsis and Septic Shock, H. Redl, G. Schlag (Editors), 1999
Fatty Acids and Inflammatory Skin Diseases, J.-M. Schröder (Editor), 1999
Immunomodulatory Agents from Plants, H. Wagner (Editor), 1999
Cytokines and Pain, L. Watkins, S. Maier (Editors), 1999
In Vivo *Models of Inflammation*, D. Morgan, L. Marshall (Editors), 1999
Pain and Neurogenic Inflammation, S.D. Brain, P. Moore (Editors), 1999
Anti-Inflammatory Drugs in Asthma, A.P. Sampson, M.K. Church (Editors), 1999
Novel Inhibitors of Leukotrienes, G. Folco, B. Samuelsson, R.C. Murphy (Editors), 1999
Vascular Adhesion Molecules and Inflammation, J.D. Pearson (Editor), 1999
Metalloproteinases as Targets for Anti-Inflammatory Drugs, K.M.K. Bottomley, D. Bradshaw, J.S. Nixon (Editors), 1999
Free Radicals and Inflammation, P.G. Winyard, D.R. Blake, C.H. Evans (Editors), 1999
Gene Therapy in Inflammatory Diseases, C.H. Evans, P. Robbins (Editors), 2000
New Cytokines as Potential Drugs, S. K. Narula, R. Coffmann (Editors), 2000
High Throughput Screening for Novel Anti-inflammatories, M. Kahn (Editor), 2000
Immunology and Drug Therapy of Atopic Skin Diseases, C.A.F. Bruijnzeel-Komen, E.F. Knol (Editors), 2000
Inflammatory Processes. Molecular Mechanisms and Therapeutic Opportunities, L.G. Letts, D.W. Morgan (Editors), 2000
Novel Cytokine Inhibitors, G.A. Higgs, B. Henderson (Editors), 2000

Forthcoming titles:

Inflammatory and Infectious Basis of Atherosclerosis, J.L. Mehta (Editor), 2001

Cellular Mechanisms in Airways Inflammation

Clive P. Page
Katharine H. Banner
Domenico Spina

Editors

Springer Basel AG

Editors

Prof. Dr. Clive P. Page
The Sackler Institute of
Pulmonary Pharmacology
King's College
GKT School of Biomedical Sciences
Guy's Campus
London SE1 9RT
UK

Dr. Katharine H. Banner
Pfizer Central Research
Postcode 826
Ramsgate Road
Sandwich
Kent CT13 9NJ
UK

Dr. Domenico Spina
The Sackler Institute of
Pulmonary Pharmacology
Department of Respiratory Medicine and Allergy
GKT School of Medicine
King's College
Bessemer Road
London SE5 9PJ
UK

Deutsche Bibliothek Cataloging-in-Publication Data
Cellular mechanism in airways inflammation / Clive P. Page ..., ed. - Basel ; Boston ; Berlin :
Birkhäuser, 2000
(Progress in inflammation research)
ISBN 978-3-0348-9583-5 ISBN 978-3-0348-8476-1 (eBook)
DOI 10.1007/978-3-0348-8476-1

ISBN 978-3-0348-9583-5

Originally published by Birkhäuser Verlag, Basel, Switzerland in 2000
Softcover reprint of the hardcover 1st edition
Printed on acid-free paper produced from chlorine-free pulp. TCF ∞
Cover design: Markus Etterich, Basel
Cover illustration: Bronchial biopsy from an asthmatic subject. With the friendly permission of Dr. Paul J. Sullivan, Hope Hospital, Manchester, UK

ISBN 978-3-0348-9583-5

9 8 7 6 5 4 3 2 1

Contents

List of contributors ... vii

Preface ... xi

Peter K. Jeffery
Pathological spectrum of airway inflammation ... 1

Gianni Marone, Massimo Triggiani, Giuseppe Spadaro, Anna Maria Onorati and Arturo Genovese
Role of basophils in airways inflammation ... 53

Paolo Gresele and Roberta Vezza
Platelets ... 79

Moira Whyte
Neutrophils ... 125

Anthony J. Coyle, Jose Carlos Gutierrez-Ramos
Eosinophils in asthma ... 147

Ian A. Akers, Robin J. McAnulty and Geoffrey J. Laurent
Fibroblasts and myofibroblasts ... 159

Elaine Lee and Stephen A. Kilfeather
Airway macrophages and dendritic cells ... 199

Anne Burke-Gaffney and Paul G. Hellewell
Contribution of endothelial cells to airway inflammation ... 223

Jagdish Laxman Devalia, Jia Hua Wang and Robert James Davies
Airway epithelial cells 245

Alastair G. Stewart, Darren J. Fernandes, Valentina Koutsoubos, Aurora Messina, Claire E. Ravenhall, Ross Vlahos and Kai-Feng Xu
Airway smooth muscle cells 263

Katherine H. Banner, Domenico Spina and Clive P. Page
Drugs that reduce airways inflammation 303

David M. Kemeny and Brian J. O'Connor
T cells in the lung 333

Index 357

List of contributors

Ian A. Akers, The Centre for Cardiopulmonary Biochemistry and Respiratory Medicine, Royal Free and University College London Medical School, The Rayne Institute, 5, University Street, London WC1E 6JJ, UK; e-mail: ian.akers@ucl.ac.uk

Katharine H. Banner, Pfizer Central Research, Ramsgate Rd, Sandwich CT13 9NJ, UK

Anne Burke-Gaffney, Unit of Critical Care, Imperial College School of Medicine at the National Heart and Lung Institute, Dovehouse St., London SW3 6LY, UK

Anthony J. Coyle, Department of Biology, Inflammation Division, Millennium Pharmaceuticals, Inc., 45-75 Sidney St., Cambridge, MA 02139, USA; e-mail: coyle@mpi.com

Robert James Davies, Academic Department of Respiratory Medicine, St. Bartholomew's and The Royal London School of Medicine and Dentistry, The London Chest Hospital, Bonner Road, London E2 9JX, UK

Jagdish Laxman Devalia, JD Scientific and Medical Communications Ltd, 305 Norwood Road, Norwood Green, Southall, Middlesex UB2 4JJ, UK

Darren J. Fernandes, Department of Pharmacology, University of Melbourne, Parkville, Victoria 3052, Australia

Arturo Genovese, Division of Clinical Immunology and Allergy, University of Naples Federico II, Via S. Pansini, 80131 Napoli, Italy

Paolo Gresele, Institute of Internal and Vascular Medicine, University of Perugia, Via Enrico Dal Pozzo, I-06126 Perugia, Italy; e-mail: grespa@unipg.it

Jose Carlos Gutierrez-Ramos, Department of Biology, Inflammation Division, Millennium Pharmaceuticals, Inc., 45-75 Sidney St., Cambridge, MA 02139, USA; e-mail: gutierrez@mpi.com

Paul G. Hellewell, Section of Vascular Biology, University of Sheffield, Cardiovascular Research Group, Northern General Hospital, Herries Rd, Sheffield S5 7AU, UK

Peter K. Jeffery, Lung Pathology Unit, Histopathology, Royal Brompton Hospital, National Heart and Lung Institute, Imperial College, London SW3 6NP, UK; e-mail: p.jeffery@ic.ac.uk

Valentina Koutsoubos, Department of Pharmacology, University of Melbourne, Parkville, Victoria 3052, Australia

David M. Kemeny, Department of Immunology, Guys, King's and St. Thomas's School of Medicine and Dentistry, Rayne Institute, 123 Coldharbour Lane, London SE5 9NU, UK; e-mail: david.kemeny@kcl.ac.uk

Stephen A. Kilfeather, School of Health Sciences, University of Sunderland, Sunderland SR1 3SD, UK; e-mail: stephen.kilfeather@sunderland.ac.uk

Geoffrey J. Laurent, The Centre for Cardiopulmonary Biochemistry and Respiratory Medicine, Royal Free and University College London Medical School, The Rayne Institute, 5, University Street, London WC1E 6JJ, UK

Elaine Lee, School of Health Sciences, University of Sunderland, Sunderland SR1 3SD, UK

Gianni Marone, Division of Clinical Immunology and Allergy, University of Naples Federico II, Via S. Pansini 5, 80131 Napoli, Italy; e-mail: marone@unina.it

Robin J. McAnulty, The Centre for Cardiopulmonary Biochemistry and Respiratory Medicine, Royal Free and University College London Medical School, The Rayne Institute, 5, University Street, London WC1E 6JJ, UK

Aurora Messina, Bernard O'Brien Institute of Microsurgery, St Vincent's Hospital, Fitzroy, Victoria 3065, Australia

Brian J. O'Connor, Department of Respiratory Medicine, Guys, King's and St. Thomas's School of Medicine and Dentistry, Rayne Institute, 123 Coldharbour Lane, London SE5 9NU, UK

Anna Maria Onorati, Division of Clinical Immunology and Allergy, University of Naples Federico II, Via S. Pansini 5, 80131 Napoli, Italy

Clive P. Page, The Sackler Institute of Pulmonary Pharmacology, King's College London, GKT School of Biomedical Sciences, Guy's Campus, London SE1 9RT, UK

Claire E. Ravenhall, Department of Pharmacology, University of Melbourne, Parkville, Victoria 3052, Australia

Giuseppe Spadaro, Division of Clinical Immunology and Allergy, University of Naples Federico II, Via S. Pansini 5, 80131 Napoli, Italy

Domenico Spina, The Sackler Institute of Pulmonary Pharmacology, King's College London, Bessemer Rd, London SE5 9PJ, UK

Alastair G. Stewart, Department of Pharmacology, University of Melbourne, Parkville, Victoria 3052, Australia;
e-mail: a.stewart@pharmacology.unimelb.edu.au

Massimo Triggiani, Division of Clinical Immunology and Allergy, University of Naples Federico II, Via S. Pansini 5, 80131 Napoli, Italy

Roberta Vezza, Center for Experimental Therapeutics, University of Pennsylvania, School of Medicine, 809 BRB II/III, 421 Curie Blvd., Philadelphia, PA 19104, USA

Ross Vlahos, Department of Pharmacology, University of Melbourne, Parkville, Victoria 3052, Australia

Jia Hua Wang, Academic Department of Respiratory Medicine, St. Bartholomew's and The Royal London School of Medicine and Dentistry, The London Chest Hospital, Bonner Road, London E2 9JX, UK

Moira Whyte, Respiratory Medicine, Division of Molecular and Genetic Medicine, Royal Hallamshire Hospital, Sheffield S10 2JF, UK;
e-mail: m.k.whyte@sheffield.ac.uk

Kai-Feng Xu, Peking Union Medical College Hospital, Beijing, China

Preface

Airways disease encompasses a broad range of pathologies including bronchial asthma, rhinitis, chronic obstructive pulmonary disease, bronchitis, acute bronchiolitis, emphysema and fibrosing alveolitis. A characteristic feature of these diseases is the recruitment and activation of inflammatory cells and resident cells. The general consensus is that alterations in the function of these cells contribute to airways disease. A greater understanding of the mechanisms which lead to altered cell responsiveness in disease will hopefully enhance the development of new anti-inflammatory modalities for the treatment of airways disease.

In the first chapter, an exhaustive review of the composition and integrity of pulmonary cells in various pathophysiological conditions is given and is accompanied by an excellent selection of electron photomicrographs of various cell types thought to be important in the disease process. This is followed by individual chapters devoted to an in-depth analysis of the contribution of various cell types to airways inflammation and focus on the cellular structure, mechanism of activation, biological activity and pharmacological modulation of the major cells that can contribute to airways disease. It is evident that no single cell type can explain airways disease, but rather, cell to cell communication at various levels is a characteristic feature of these diseases and highlights the complex and chaotic nature that underlies the inflammatory process.

The last chapter is devoted to summarizing the state of play with regard to the current anti-inflammatory drugs that are available to clinicians, including providing an up to date review of emerging therapies.

We thank Katrin Serries, Janine Kern and Hans Detlef Klüber of Birkhäuser Verlag AG for their extreme patience and expert assistance in the preparation of this volume. We are also deeply indebted to the authors who have helped contribute to this volume which we believe will provide an important compendium for those interested in airways disease.

February 2000

Katharine H. Banner
Domenico Spina
Clive Page

Pathological spectrum of airway inflammation

Peter K. Jeffery

Lung Pathology Unit, Histopathology, Royal Brompton Hospital: National Heart and Lung Institute, Imperial College, London, SW3 6NP, UK

Introduction

In man and other mammalian species, the upper (nasal passages) and lower airways are lined by a continuous moist mucosal layer. The mucosa forms the border between the external environment and host tissue where irritants, infection and allergens are first deposited. It is the site at which immune responses are initiated by immuno-competent cells in association with resident antigen presenting cells (APC). In humans, subsequent exposure to the relevant allergen initiates immune reactions, which may become chronic. These reactions are designed as defence mechanisms that normally protect the body; however, when they are inappropriate or misdirected they may injure host tissue. At rest, approximately 10,000 to 15,000 L of air, containing pollutants and allergens, moves daily over the human nasal and tracheobronchial airway mucosa. In the nasal passages and proximal conducting airways of the lung the air is sampled, conditioned, and rendered free of irritants and allergens before it reaches the respiratory portion of the lung. The cleansing function of the conducting airways depends upon its branching pattern and the dynamic interactions of structural cells, immuno-competent cells, and neural elements. Changes in the composition and integrity of airway-wall structural components may alter its effectiveness and predispose the respiratory portion of the lung to injury.

A prerequisite to understanding the pathogenesis of allergic inflammatory disorders is an appreciation of normal airway structure and function. The present chapter first outlines briefly the normal structure of the airways and the lining mucosa, considers the role and salient features of inflammation and then focuses on the structural changes and inflammatory events of several selected inflammatory conditions including rhinitis, bronchial asthma, acute bronchitis and bronchiolitis (particularly that due to respiratory infections), chronic bronchitis and chronic obstructive pulmonary disease (henceforth referred to as COPD) and briefly fibrosing alveolitis.

Cellular Mechanisms in Airways Inflammation, edited by Clive P. Page, Katharine H. Banner and Domenico Spina

Normal micro-structure

Airway divisions

The larynx is conventionally considered to mark the boundary between upper and lower respiratory tracts (henceforth referred to as URT and LRT): the upper extends from the external nares to the larynx, and the lower from the larynx to the visceral pleura. The upper respiratory tract consists of the nose and the pharynx; the former is divided into two nostrils by a median septum. The superior part of the nose is surrounded entirely by bone, and posteriorly it opens into the nasopharynx which continues into the oro- and laryngopharynx. Each nasal cavity is wider anteriorly than posteriorly. On each latcral wall thcrc arc thrcc turbinatcs. A system of air sinuses also drains into the upper respiratory tract. Lymphoid tissue in the upper respiratory tract comprises the nasopharyngeal and palatine tonsils. The former, termed adenoids, are a diffuse aggregate of lymphoid cells in the mucosa lining of the nasopharynx, covered by folds of predominantly pseudostratified epithelium. Two palatine tonsils are situated in the lateral walls of the oropharynx, covered by a stratified, squamous, non-keratinizing epithelium invaginated to form deep crypts. Posterior to the pharynx are the larynx, the organ of speech, and the glottis, through which air enters into the lower respiratory tract and its tree of successively branching airways.

The larynx opens into the trachea, which enters the thorax and divides to form two main bronchi, one leading to each lung. The right and left lungs are lobed, occupy most of the thorax, are enclosed within the rib cage, and are enveloped by pleural membranes. Medially the lungs abut the mediastinum (which includes the pericardium) and posteriorly they rest on the diaphragm. Airways and vessels meet at the hilum of the lung at a point where it connects to the mediastinum. The pattern of airway branching is described as one of asymmetrical dichotomy, and from trachea to alveolus there are between 8–23 generations of airways, depending on the distance from the hilum to the pleural surface.

The summed cross-sectional area for each generation of airways increases logarithmically; thus, at the periphery, the resistance to air flow is negligible [1]. With inspiration, the velocity of air entering the lungs falls rapidly due to the marked increase in total cross-sectional area of the more peripheral airways. The surface of the alveolar walls available to gas transfer is about 60–70 m [2], i.e., about half the area of a singles tennis court. The respiratory zone is kept free of allergens, pollutants, and infection by airway defence mechanisms that include nervous reflexes leading to bronchoconstriction and/or cough, ciliary activity, secretion of mucus, lysozyme, lactoferrin, and secretory immunoglobulin A (IgA), and cellular immune response and reactions.

Mucosal structure

The airway wall is comprised of a surface epithelium supported by a reticular basement membrane (Fig. 1) and a poorly defined subepithelial zone consisting of bronchial vessels, connective tissue (Fig. 2), and lymphatics that merges with a submucosal zone of mucus-secreting glands, cartilage, and/or bronchial smooth muscle; external to this there is a thin adventitial coat (Fig 3). Tracheo-bronchial airways, by definition, have cartilage support whereas bronchioli do not. Mucus-secreting glands occur in the cartilagenous airways.

Surface epithelium

Upper respiratory tract epithelium is comprised mainly of ciliated, pseudostratified, columnar cells, interspersed with mucus-secreting cells. However, the anterior nares are lined by stratified keratinizing squamous epithelium. Areas of non-keratinizing squamous epithelium are found in the pharynx, whereas in the larynx, epithelium of this type is present on the epiglottis and the vocal chords. The stratified squamous epithelium covering the vocal chords gives way to one that is ciliated, pseudostratified, and columnar when the trachea is reached. The term "pseudostratified" refers to the appearance of more than one layer of cells and implies that all cells rest on the basement membrane but not all reach the airway lumen (see Figs. 1 and 2). However, basal cells also play a role in attachment of superficial cells to the basal lamina by acting as a bridge between columnar cells and the epithelial basement membrane. In humans, the appearance to the epithelium persists throughout the major bronchi, thereafter becoming simple cuboidal distally. Mucus-secreting cells are found regularly in the tracheo-bronchial tree in humans but are normally sparse in bronchioli less than 1 mm in diameter [2].

A variety of cell types are recognized in airway surface epithelium [3, 4]. There are at least eight morphologically distinct epithelial-cell types in the surface epithelium, determined by transmission electron microscopy (TEM): many of these have overlapping functions. The functions are many and are now known to include expression of cell surface adhesion molecules [5, 6] and synthesis and release of cytokines [7] which together may induce the selective recruitment of inflammatory cells from bronchial vessels and their tissue retention and accummulation. The terminal processes of nerve fibres whose cell bodies are present external to the epithelium also cross the epithelial reticular basement membrane to lie between and be enclosed by epithelial cells. Here they are thought to initiate airway reflexes such as bronchoconstriction and cough and also may initiate neurogenic inflammation [8, 9].

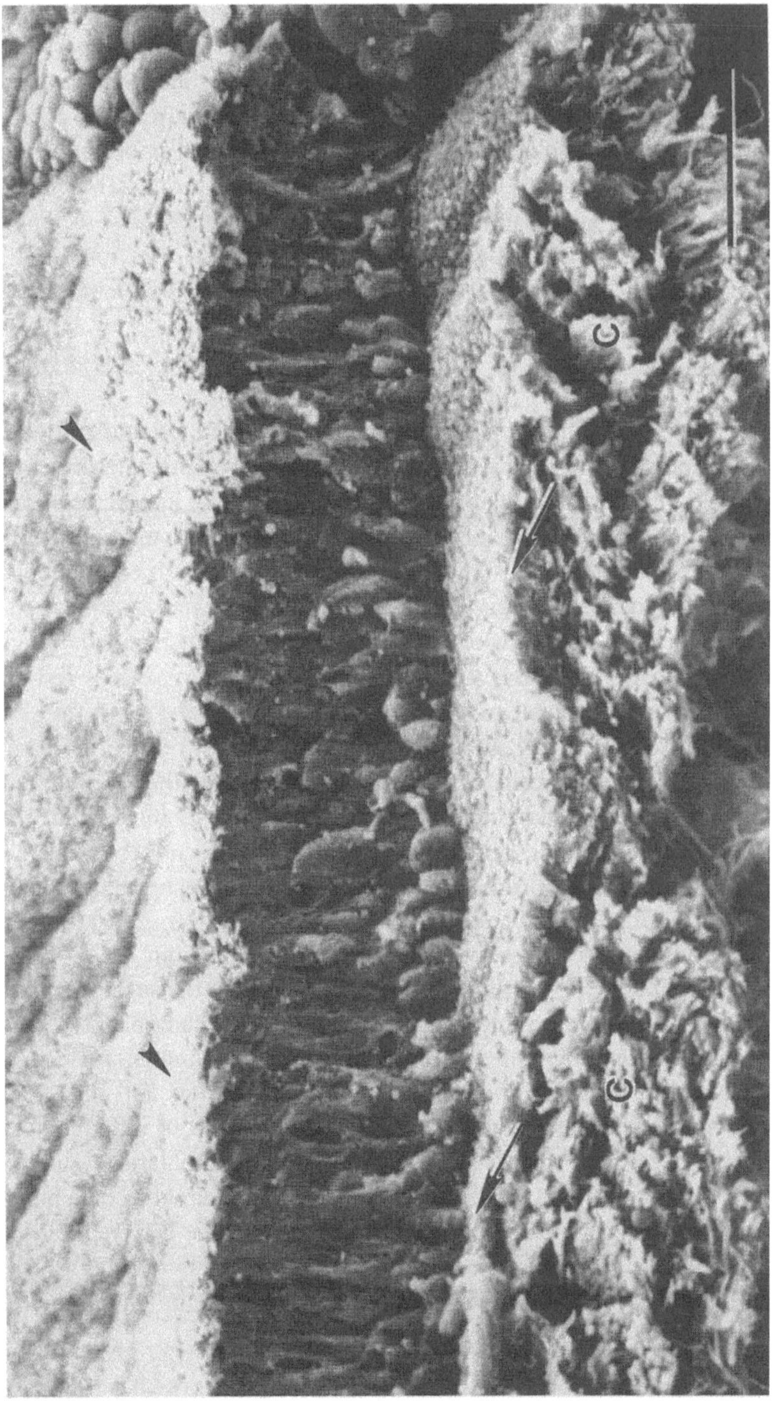

Figure 1
Scanning electron micrograph (SEM) of human bronchial epithelium which has been fractured to show the lateral surfaces of its cells. Cilia are abundant at the lumenal edge (arrowheads). All cells attach to the reticular basement membrane (arrows) but not all reach the airway lumen. Interstitial collagen (C) is present beneath the reticular basement membrane. Scale bar = 40 µm.

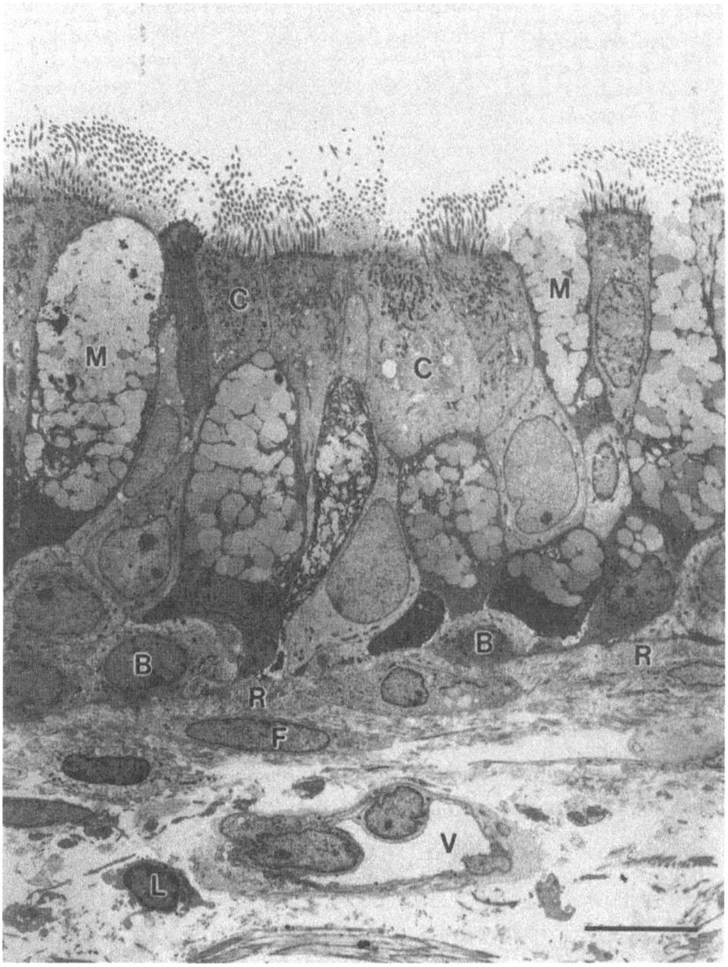

Figure 2
Transmission electron micrograph (TEM) of human bronchial mucosa in a biopsy demonstrating ciliated (C), mucous (M) and basal (B) cells which are the main cells of the surface epithelium. The subepithelial zone consists of a fibrillary layer referred to as the reticular basement membrane (R) beneath which there are fibroblasts (F), mast cells, lymphomononuclear cells (L) and a bronchial (systemic) capillary. Scale bar = 10 μm.

Inflammation

Inflammation is "the response of vascularized tissue to injury" and its purpose is to repair, restore and, if necessary, remodel the injured tissue. The key signs of acute

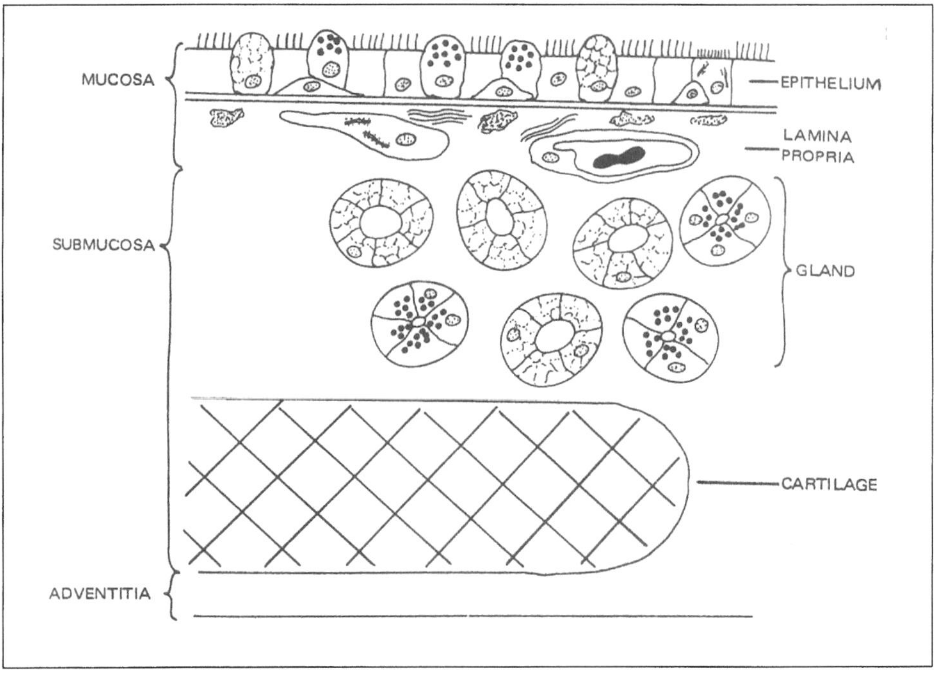

Figure 3
Diagrammatic representation of the airway wall showing surface epithelium supported by a subepithelial zone referred to as the lamina propria. The epithelium and lamina propria make up the mucosa. The underlying zone made up mainly of mucus-secreting glands, muscle and cartilage is often referred to as the submucosa. External to this there is an ill-defined adventitia.

inflammation, recognized by Celsus (30 BC–20 AD) are redness, swelling, heat and pain and loss or altered function, the last described by Galen (130–200 AD). In addition, Lord Florey recognized that acute inflammation at moist mucosal surfaces, such as the gut and airways, included injury (and sloughing) of surface epithelium and hypersecretion of mucus.

Apart from the reddening and swelling which may be observed macroscopically the microscopic changes of inflammation include changes in vascular calibre and blood flow, of tissue oedema (as a result of alterations of vascular permeability) and leukocyte emigration, referred to as "white cell events". If acute, there is oedema, the inflammatory cell infiltrate is predominantly of polymorphonuclear cells (mainly neutrophils) and the response to injury, infection or allergen is of short duration leading to resolution, healing and repair as in, for example, bacterial pneumonitis and viral induced bronchiolitis in children (Figs. 4 and 5). However, if the injury is repeated (low grade) or severe then there may be a switch to persistent or chronic

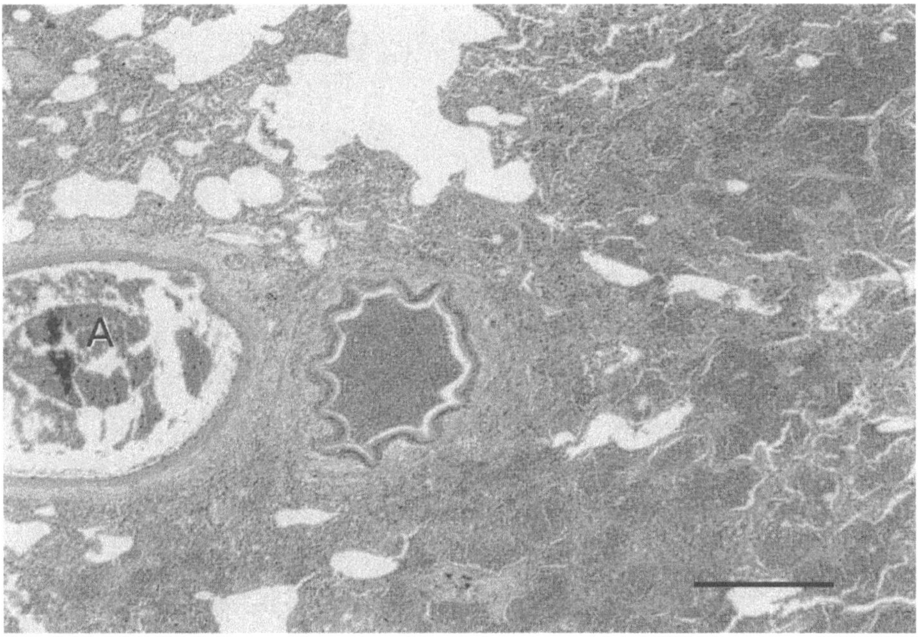

Figure 4
Haematoxylin and eosin (H&E) stained section through human lung of a patient with bronchopneumonia showing pulmonary artery (A) adjacent to a conducting airway whose lumen is filled with pus (neutrophils). The surrounding alveolar lumena show a similar copious neutrophilic exudation. Scale bar = 500 μm.
(reproduced with kind permission of Prof. B. Corrin)

inflammation which may lead to an abnormal tissue remodelling (i.e., enlargement or destruction) such that there is altered function or failure to function normally as in bronchiolitis obliterans (Fig. 6), pulmonary fibrosis or emphysema (see below). The reasons and mechanism(s) involved in the switch to chronicity are, as yet, unclear: an understanding of this process is critical to the future effective treatment/prevention of several persistent inflammation conditions of the conducting airways and lung.

To examine and characterize the structural and inflammatory changes at distinct anatomical sites, nasal, bronchial, transbronchial and open lung biopsies provide a way of directly sampling the tissues *in vivo*: biopsy is a powerful technique, and it provides information which is distinct and complementary to that obtained by bronchoalveolar lavage and other indirect methods of assessment of lung inflammation (e.g., exhaled NO) [10]. In addition, studies of airway tissues obtained *post mortem* are invaluable but interpretation may be difficult due to the effects on tissues of less

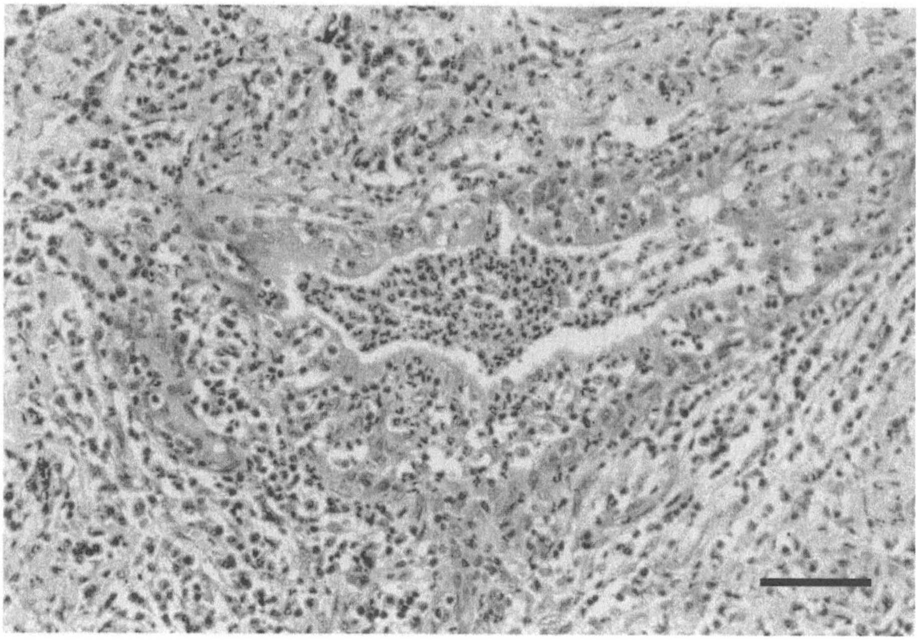

Figure 5
H&E stained section of a small airway (bronchiole) showing the changes of acute bronchiolitis: i.e. partial necrosis of the lining epithelium, airway lumen and wall extensively infiltrated by neutrophils. Scale bar = 100 µm.
(reproduced with kind permission of Prof. B. Corrin)

specific changes associated with end-stage disease such as terminal infection, vascular events and *post mortem* artefact. With these caveats in mind, examination of tissues obtained *post mortem*, during flexible fibre-optic bronchoscopy or at open lung biopsy, is the basis for the descriptions which follow.

Common inflammatory conditions of the airways

Rhinitis

The upper (URT) and lower respiratory tracts (LRT) share similar cellular and humoral defence mechanisms and it is common to find that diseases of the nose and paranasal sinuses (e.g. rhinosinusitis), pharynx, larynx and LRT occur in association. For example, there is some evidence that active allergic rhinitis may induce in an unexplained way a remodelling process (i.e. thickening of the reticular basement

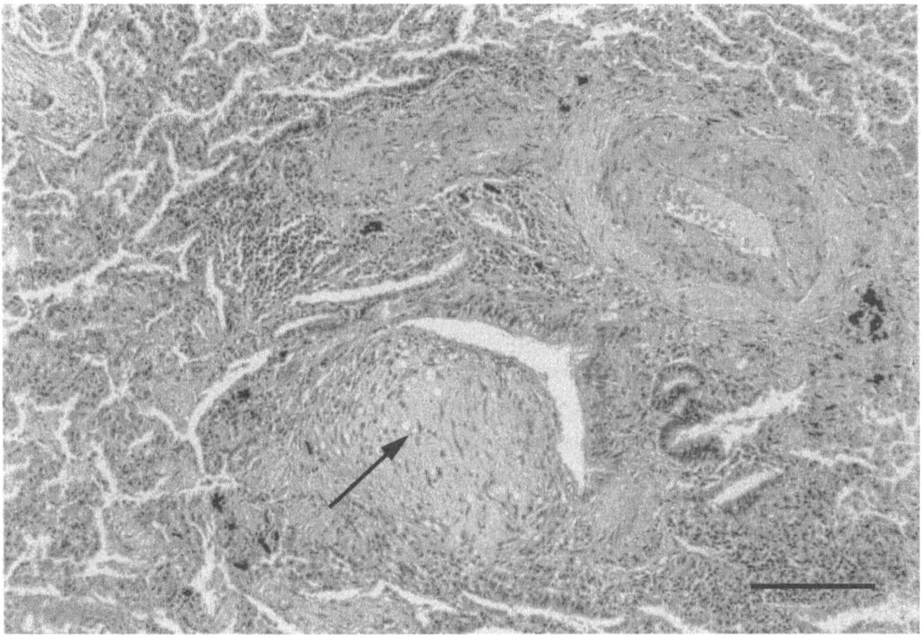

Figure 6
H&E of the remains of a small airway showing the alterations of bronchiolitis obliterans: pale staining granulation tissue severely compromises the airway lumen (arrow). Scale bar = 1000 μm.
(reproduced with kind permission of Prof. B. Corrin)

membrane) in the lower airways in subjects who are otherwise non-asthmatic [11]. The hallmark of allergic rhinitis is sneezing and underlying this there is an inflammatory process in which there is oedema, production of mucus and increased vascular permeability.

Infections of the URT may induce acute or chronic inflammation and seasonal, perennial or occupational allergy may contribute to allergic inflammation involving similar mechanisms as these which occur in the LRT. In addition, intrinsic rhinitis (also referred to as vasomotor rhinitis) may be present in the absence of infection or allergy. The common cold is probably the most frequent viral infection and as with the LRT a variety of viruses and serotypes may cause it. At the earliest stage of infection there is transient vasoconstriction, this is then followed by vasodilation, oedema and an increase of sero-mucous secretions. Leucocytic (lympho-mononuclear) infiltration of the nasal mucosa is accompanied by swelling and desquamation of surface epithelial cells. The secretions, at first clear, watery and sterile, later become coloured and viscid as bacteria invade and neutrophils are recruited to the tissues and lumen. Complications may include nasopharyngitis, pharyngitis, sinusitis, tonsillitis and on occasion, bronchitis and/or pneumonia. Importantly, such infections may also precipitate attacks of asthma or result in exacerbations of bronchitis in patients already compromised by chronic obstructive pulmonary disease (COPD).

There are many similarities between allergic rhinitis and asthma and there are important differences. Rhinitis, like asthma, has an increasing prevalence [12]. It occurs in 75% of patients with allergic asthma whereas the prevalence of asthma in those with rhinitis is only 20% [13]. The allergic manifestations and inflammation of allergic rhinitis and asthma are similar (both are IgE-mediated conditions of hypersensitivity) but the resultant effect of the allergic reaction may be altered by the differing anatomy and histology of the upper and lower airways. Accordingly, as in asthma, during seasonal exposure there is local accumulation of CD4 positive T lymphocytes, mast cells, eosinophils, basophils and neutrophils [14, 15] (Fig. 7). The inflammation is also present in chronic (perennial) rhinitis [16]. There are also increases in the numbers of circulating mast cells/basophil progenitors and seasonal epithelial mast cell migration [17]. The tissue eosinophilia associated particularly with the "late" nasal response is regulated by the presence of activated ($CD25^+$) T helper lymphocytes and the production of Th2-like cytokines, particularly interleukin (IL)-4 and IL-5 [18]: the majority are produced by T lymphocytes but mast cells and even eosinophils *per se* may participate.

Whilst the pattern of allergic inflammation is similar in allergic rhinitis and atopic asthma the thickening of the reticular basement seen in the bronchi in asthma is not as prominent in rhinitis and the increase in smooth muscle mass is a particular feature of asthma and is restricted to the lower airways by its airway distribution. In addition, the anatomic features of the URT prohibit the closure of nasal passage due to constriction but blockage instead depends on swelling of the nasal mucosa due to smooth muscle vascular changes and oedema.

There is mast cell and eosinophil accummulation and "activation" in both seasonal and perennial rhinitis and in the former there may be increases of antigen presenting cells (cells of Langerhan) also. The recruitment of these cells to the mucosa in rhinitis is as the result of increased expression of endothelial cell surface adhesion molecules and IL-4 following natural exposure to allergen or increased gene expression of IL-4, IL-5, GM-CSF and tumour necrosis factor α (TNFα) after experimental allergen challenge [19]. Of the many pro-inflammatory mediators produced during the allergic reactions of airways in both upper and lower respiratory tracts, products of eosinophil degranulation appear to be the most injurious to the mucosa. Gleich and colleagues have developed methods to study this using nasal epithelia [20]. They have demonstrated that the combined addition of eosinophil peroxidase (EPO), glucose/glucose oxidase (but neither acting alone) and bromide produce marked target cell lysis: the effect is time and EPO dose-dependent. Longer incubation periods of nasal mucosal with human eosinophil major basic protein also cause time and dose-dependent epithelial cell lysis.

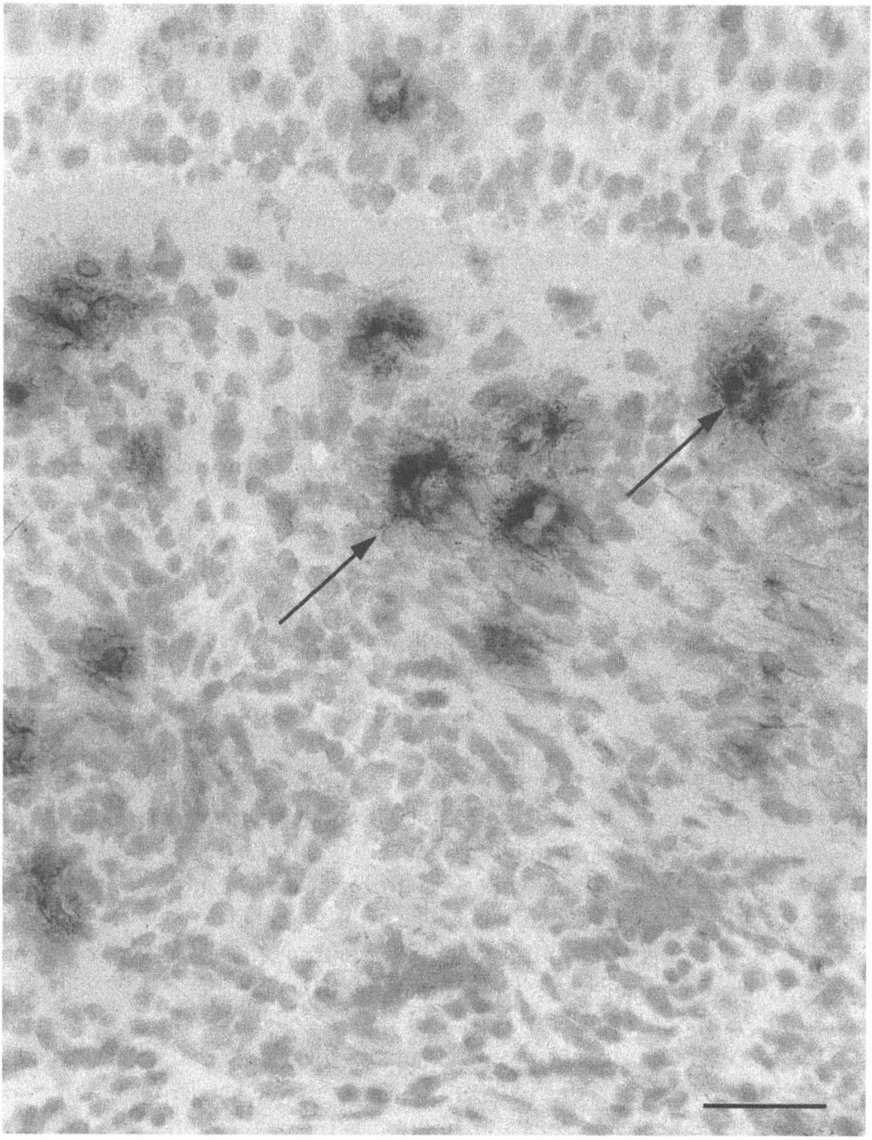

Figure 7
An immunostained (by the APAAP technique) section of the nasal mucosa of a patient with allergic rhinitis using an antibody directed against major basic protein, a characteristic constituent of eosinophils. The stained eosinophils (arrows) have accumulated beneath the pale staining reticular basement membrane and there is a single eosinophil within the surface epithelium. Scale bar = 25 µm.
(Reproduced with kind permission of Drs. M. Jacobson and S. Durham)

The role and importance of chemoattractant molecules (chemokines) in the selective recruitment of eosinophils and other inflammatory cells to the airway mucosa following allergen challenge to the nose and lower airways has recently been demonstrated in man and experimentally in the guinea pig [21, 22]. In this regard eotaxin, a selective chemoattractant for eosinophils was shown to be expressed by nasal epithelium and in man and guinea pigs in both large (proximal) and small (distal) airway surface epithelial cells, bronchial smooth muscle and airway and alveolar macrophages (Fig. 8). RANTES and MIP-1α are chemoattractants for lymphocytes, monocytes and eosinophils whereas MCP-1 is chemoattractant for monocytes, lymphocytes and basophils and these are also increased in both nasal and bronchial secretions/washes in response to allergen [22–25].

Acute inhalation of toxic chemicals (irritants) can also elicit an inflammation which may become chronic, referred to as "reactive airways dysfunction syndrome" [26]: the mechanisms involved in this interesting condition are, as yet, unclear.

Bronchial asthma

To date the pathologist recognizes only one form of asthma yet clinically the condition is clearly heterogeneous.

Appearances post mortem

Examination, post-mortem, of cases of fatal asthma has shown that the lungs are hyperinflated and remain so on opening the pleural cavities due to the widespread presence of markedly tenacious plugs in intrapulmonary bronchi. On intrabronchial inflation with fixative even a 1.5 m head fails to move these airway plugs [27, 28]. Histologically the airway plugs in asthma are a mixture of inflammatory exudate and mucus in which lie desquamated surface epithelial cells, lymphocytes and eosinophils. The arrangement of the cellular elements of the plug often takes the form of several concentric lamella suggesting that several episodes of inflammation have led to their formation rather than a single (terminal) event. The non-mucinous, proteinaceous contribution is the result of increased vascular permeability and includes a fibrinous component. Interaction of constituents of serum and mucin is likely to lead to increased viscosity of the airway plug [29]. The combination of tissue, blood and BAL/sputum eosinophilia is strongly associated with asthma but there may also be marked heterogeneity in the numbers of tissue eosinophils identified in fatal asthma [30]. This may be due, in part, to eosinophil degranulation, which makes cell identification difficult, or to the reported variation in the numbers and relative proportions of neutrophils and eosinophils with progressive duration of the terminal episode [31, 32]. Unlike chronic obstructive pulmonary disease (COPD) there is little evidence of destruc-

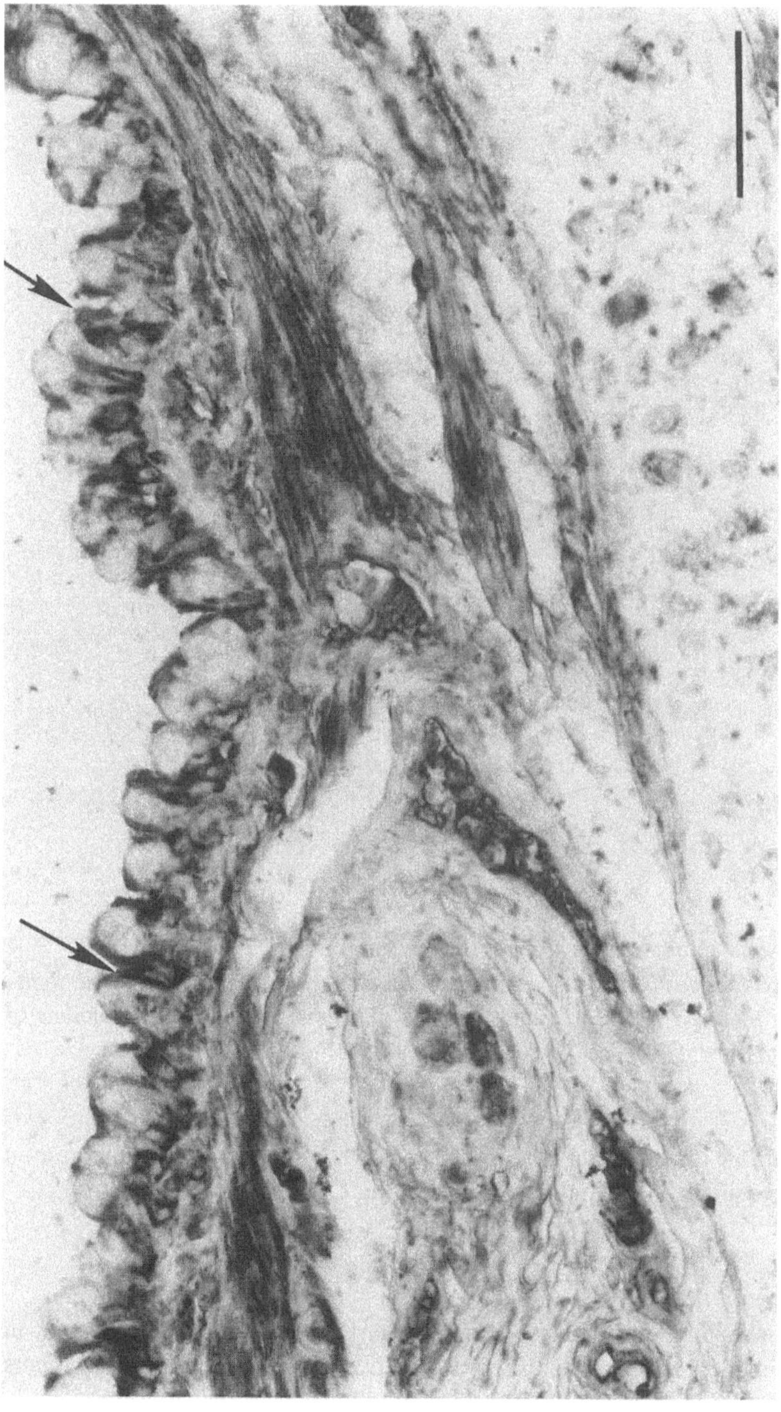

Figure 8
Bronchial mucosa in a guinea pig sensitised and then challenged with ovalbumin. The section which is immunostained with a polyclonal antibody to guinea pig eotaxin shows marked up-regulation of eotaxin protein present, as densely stained areas, in the surface epithelium (arrows). Scale bar = 40 μm.

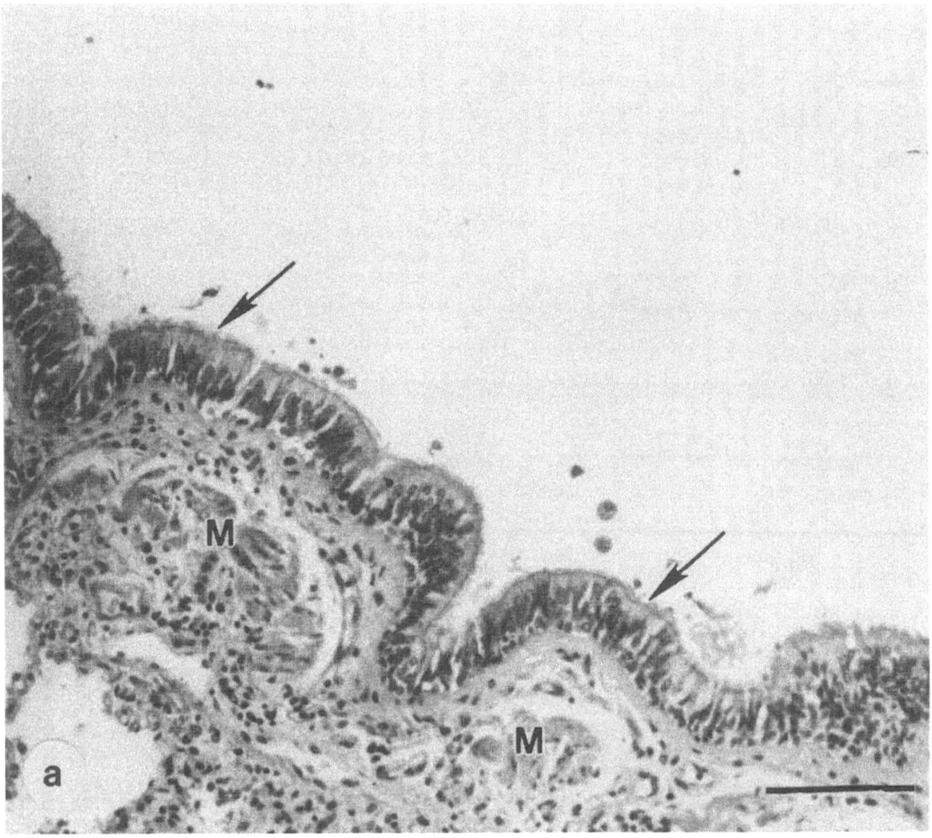

Figure 9a
H&E sections of human intrapulmonary bronchial mucosa:
A road traffic accident death showing intact ciliated surface epithelium (arrows) with indistinct underlying reticular basement membrane, few inflammatory cells, small amounts of bronchial smooth muscle (M). Scale bar = 120 μm.

tive emphysema in fatal asthma and right ventricular hypertrophy is uncommon when the diagnosis of asthma is uncomplicated by COPD.

Loss of surface epithelium

Histologically, shedding and damage of airway surface epithelium is prominent in asthma, both in fatal asthma (Fig. 9a and b) and in biopsy specimens of patients with mild disease [33–35]. Loss of epithelium is followed by areas of mitotic activity (see [36]), secretion of fibronectin [37, 38] and epithelial regeneration which first

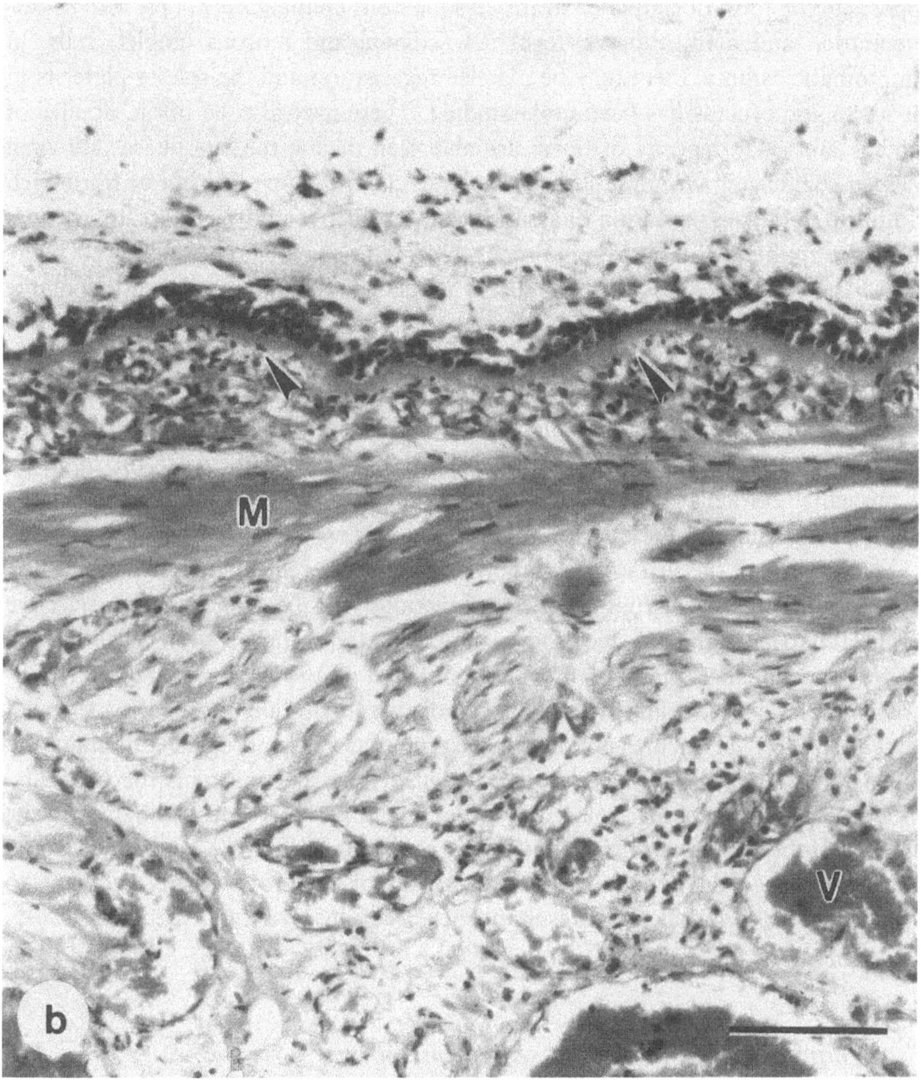

Figure 9b

By comparison, in the airway of a patient who died in status asthmaticus *there is sloughing of the surface epithelium with cells and exudate in the lumen. The reticular basement membrane (arrowheads) is now prominent due to homogeneous thickening. There is increased infiltration of the mucosa by affording an increased mass of bronchial smooth muscle (M) and dilatation and congestion of mucosal vessels (V). Scale bar = 120 µm.*

appears in the form of simple or stratified squamous epithelium [27] prior to its differentiation and maturation to form new ciliated and mucous (goblet) cells. In symptomatic asthma, there may be platelet aggregation and the role of platelets in the asthmatic process has been understudied. There may also be fibrin, at sites of damage and such deposits of fibrin are also seen during the late phase following allergen challenge (own unpublished results). Again, the involvement of fibrinogen and fibrin in the inflammation of asthma requires further study. The greater the loss of surface epithelium in biopsy specimens the greater appears to be the degree of airways hyperresponsiveness (AHR) [33]. It is recognised that there is an inevitable artefactual loss of surface epithelium during the taking and processing of these small (2 mm diameter) biopsy pieces, even in normal, healthy subjects, which makes interpretation of the extent of epithelial sloughing controversial [39]. The suggested fragility of the epithelium in asthma *in vivo* is supported by the frequent reports of Creola bodies in the sputa [40] and the reported association between the numbers of bronchial epithelial cells recovered by bronchoalveolar lavage (BAL) and the degree of AHR in asthmatics with mild disease [34].

The fragility of the surface may involve alteration of cell-cell adhesive molecules, such as cadherin, and disruption of tight junctions [41, 42] which act as a selective epithelial barrier to the passage of ions, molecules and water between cells: this disruption may enhance stimulation of intraepithelial nerves leading to axonal reflexes, stimulation of secretion by mucous glands, vasodilatation and oedema through the release of sensory neuropeptides, the last referred to as neurogenic inflammation [9, 43]. Experimentally there is also evidence that the sensitivity of bronchial smooth muscle to substances placed in the airway lumen correlates strongly with the integrity of the surface epithelium [44]. Loss or damage of surface epithelium would thus lead to a reduction in the concentration of factors normally relaxant to bronchial smooth muscle with resultant increased sensitivity and "reactivity" [45, 46].

Thickening of the epithelial "basement membrane"

Observed by light microscopy, thickening of the reticular basement membrane (i.e. lamina reticularis), has long been recognised as a consistent change in all forms of asthma [27, 33, 47–51] (see Fig. 9b). Whilst there may also be focal and variable thickening in COPD, and other inflammatory chronic diseases of the lung such as bronchiectasis and tuberculosis [51], the lesion, when homogenous and particularly when it is hyaline in appearance, is highly characteristic and present in both fatal and mild asthma and in patients with a long history of asthma but who have not died of their asthma. The thickening of the reticular layer which is immuno-positive for collagen types III and V together with fibronectin but not laminin has been referred to as "subepithelial fibrosis" [48]. However, its thickening is distinct from the fibrosis associated with scar formation as ultrastructurally it does not resemble the underlying interstitial collagen or a scar. The reticular layer is comprised of thinner fibres of reticulin linked to a matrix rich in sugars together with entrapped exogenous molecules such as tenascin, heparin sulphate and serum-derived components. In the author's opinion, swelling of this layer may also contribute to its thickening and it is curious that its thickening is maximal early on in the course of the disease and it does not appear to thicken further as the condition worsens or becomes fatal. In contrast, the "true" epithelial basement membrane (i.e. the basal lamina) which consists mainly of type IV collagen, glycosaminoglycans and laminin is not thickened, either in mild or severe disease.

Adjacent subepithelial fibroblasts may, of course, contribute to the thickening of the reticular layer (Fig. 10). In this regard, an association between the numbers of myofibroblasts underlying the reticular layer and thickening of the reticular layer has been demonstrated in asthma [52]. Gizycki and colleagues [53] have also observed that myofibroblast-like cells appear in substantial numbers during the late phase reaction following allergen challenge: these may contribute, *via* secretion of additional reticulin, to the thickening of the reticular basement membrane.

Increased numbers of mucus-secreting cells

Bronchial goblet cell hyperplasia and submucosal gland enlargement have been reported as the histological hallmarks and the correlate of hypersecretion of mucus in chronic bronchitis [54]. There is also significant submucosal gland enlargement seen in fatal asthma [28] and this may contribute to excessive production of mucus which thickens as it mixes with plasma-derived molecules and induces the plugging of airways usually associated with a fatal attack [55]. Dilatation of gland ducts, referred to as bronchial gland ectasia is also described [56].

Enlargement of bronchial smooth muscle mass

The percentage of bronchial wall occupied by bronchial smooth muscle shows a marked increase in fatal asthma [28] (Fig. 11). Importantly, the increase in muscle mass is reported to be in larger rather than in smaller intrapulmonary bronchi of lungs obtained following a fatal attack as compared with those of asthmatic subjects dying of other causes [57]: it is likely a major contributor to the thickening of the airway wall and hence to the increased resistance to airflow [58–61].

Whether the increase in muscle mass is due to muscle fibre hyperplasia [62] or hypertrophy is at present unclear. Interestingly, recent observations of the late phase response to allergen have demonstrated the increased presence of cell forms which share ultrastructural features of fibroblast, myofibroblast and bronchial smooth muscle [53]. In particular they contain bundles of filaments with electron-dense condensations identical to those found in the contractile apparatus of

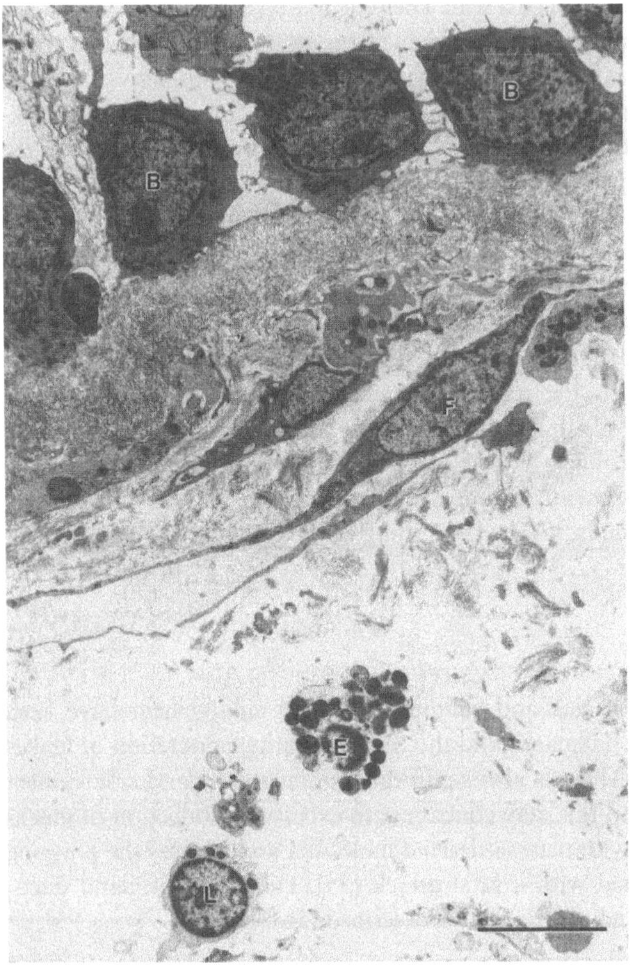

Figure 10
Transmission electron micrograph (TEM) of a biopsy of a subject with mild atopic (allergic) asthma showing a fibroblast (F) with long extensions beneath the reticular basement membrane to which are attached epithelial basal cells (B). An eosinophil (E) is in the process of "cytolytic" degranulation and there is a lymphomononuclear cell (L) nearby.
Scale bar = 5 µm.

bronchial smooth muscle (Fig. 12). These cells may represent the precursors of the additional blocks of bronchial smooth muscle reported in fatal asthma. Such remodelling in asthma [63] shows much similarity to that seen in vascular disease (i.e. atheroma) [64]. These new discoveries in the mucosal responsive to allergen

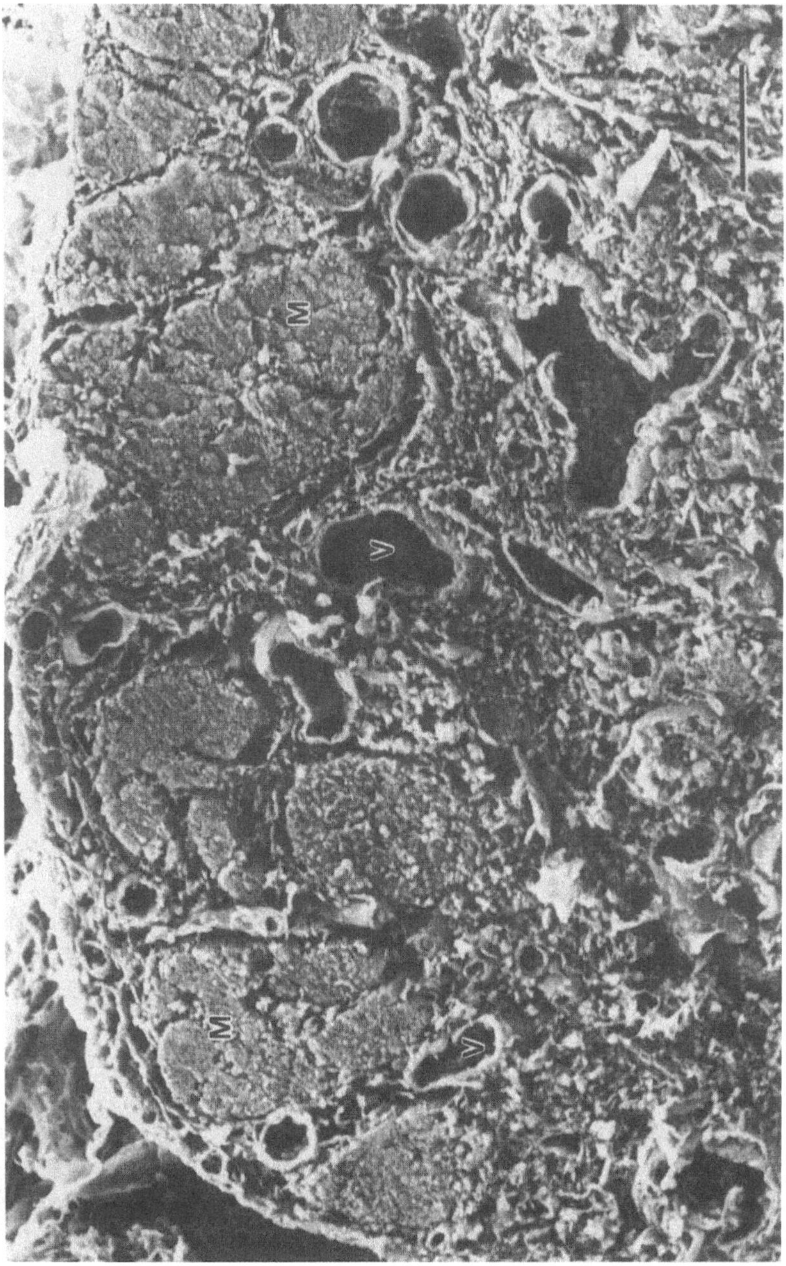

Figure 11
SEM of part of the airway wall in a case of fatal asthma. The surface epithelium has been completely lost. The airway wall is thickened due to vasodilatation (V) and to the blocks of bronchial smooth muscle (M) which are increased in size and number and appear to lie close to the surface. Scale bar = 60 μm.

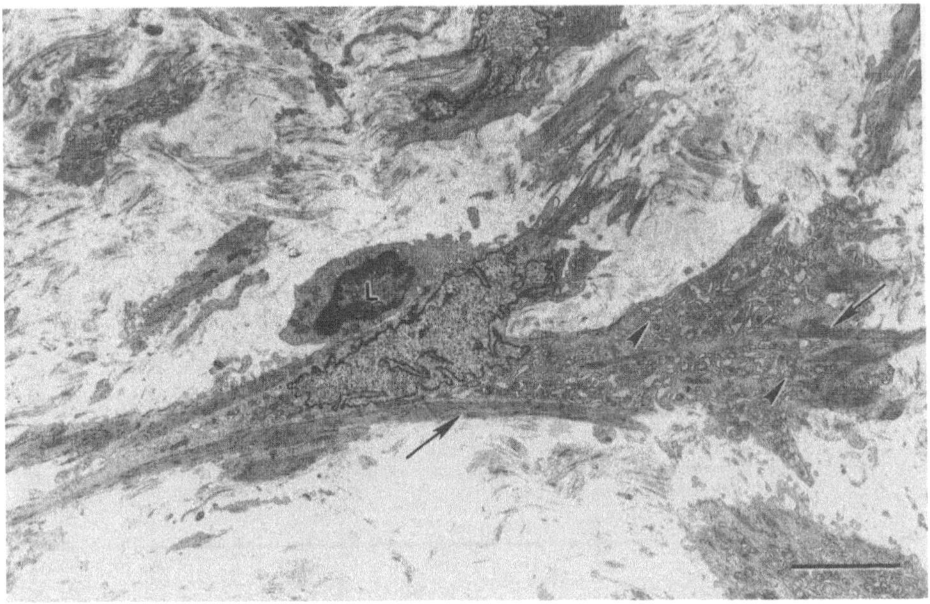

Figure 12
TEM of a myofibroblast from a bronchial biopsy of a subject with allergic asthma, taken during the late response 24 h after allergen challenge. In contrast to the fibroblast shown in Figure 10, this cell, referred to as a myofibroblast or "synthetic smooth muscle cell" is about twice the size, has an irregular outline, contains much dilated rough endoplasmic reticulum (arrowheads) and elongate bundles of myofilaments (arrows) with electron-dense condensations identical to those of smooth muscle. The cell has made contact with a lymphomononuclear cell (L). Scale bar = 5.0 μm.

are exciting and indicate that myofibroblast/myocyte differentiation and their role in bronchial smooth muscle mass enlargement may become a novel target for anti-asthma treatment in the future [63, 65].

Bronchial vasculature, congestion and oedema

The increase in thickness of the bronchial wall in asthma is unlikely accounted for by the increase in bronchial smooth muscle and mucous gland mass alone. Dilatation of the mucosal bronchial vasculature, congestion of its vessels, new vessel growth and wall oedema are also features of fatal asthma (see Fig. 11). Subepithelial oedema has been suggested to be responsible for lifting and sloughing of the surface epithelium [27]. The onset of vasodilatation, congestion and mucosal oedema in response to a variety of mediators of inflammation [66] and perhaps that which occurs in response to exercise can be rapid and, equally, should be relatively rapidly reversed by appropriate treatment.

James and colleagues have shown that airway wall thickening (due to one or more of the above changes) need only be relatively minor to have dramatic consequences on airflow limitation [58]. The association of structure and function is an interesting and important area requiring much further study.

Recruitment of inflammatory cells

In fatal asthma there is a marked inflammatory cell infiltrate throughout the airway wall (see Fig. 9b) and also in the occluding plug: lymphocytes are abundant [27, 31, 67], eosinophils are characteristic and neutrophils are usually absent or retained within vessels. The inflammation may spread to surrounding alveolar septae and affect adjacent arteries [67]. There is an association of tissue eosinophilia and the airways hyperresponsiveness of asthma: the extent of tissue eosinophilia varies with each case and, interestingly, with the duration of the terminal episode [30–32]. The longer the terminal episode the higher the concentration of eosinophils [31]; these are particularly abundant in the large (central) airways [68]. In contrast acute sudden death in asthma is associated with high numbers of neutrophils and plugging of the airways [32, 69].

As with allergic rhinitis, atopic asthma is now recognized as an inflammatory condition of the airways in which there is tissue eosinophilia and a predominance of T lymphocytes of the CD4 (T helper) subset [70]. The activation of the T helper (Th) cells results in the release of cytokines, particularly IL-4, -5 and -10 which characterize an "allergic" profile of inflammation (Fig. 13). Release of these pro-inflammatory cytokines together with chemokines specific for eosinophils (see Figs. 8 and 14) [71] leads to the recruitment of eosinophils (not neutrophils) from bronchial vessels (Fig. 15) their activation and the release of a range of highly charged molecules which damages mucosal tissue. Extensive eosinophil degranulation (Fig. 16) and cytolysis with the release of clusters of free eosinophil granules (cfegs) may make cell identification difficult [72, 73] (see Fig. 10). Whilst there are increased numbers of T cells in fatal asthma this is not unique to asthma as it occurs also and to a similar extent in cystic fibrosis [31].

Studies of biopsies obtained by flexible fibreoptic bronchoscopy or at open lung biopsy in asthma demonstrate the very early involvement of inflammatory cells [74] and this includes the presence and an interaction between (T) lymphocytes, eosinophils and plasma cells (Fig. 16) [33–35, 75]. The increase in leucocytes, including lymphocytes and eosinophils, occurs similarly in relatively mild atopic, occupational and intrinsic asthma and it is associated with an increase in "activation" markers for both lymphocytes ($CD25^+$ cells) and eosinophils ($EG2^+$ cells) [33, 70, 75–77]. EG2 is a marker for the cleaved ("secreted") form of eosinophil cation-

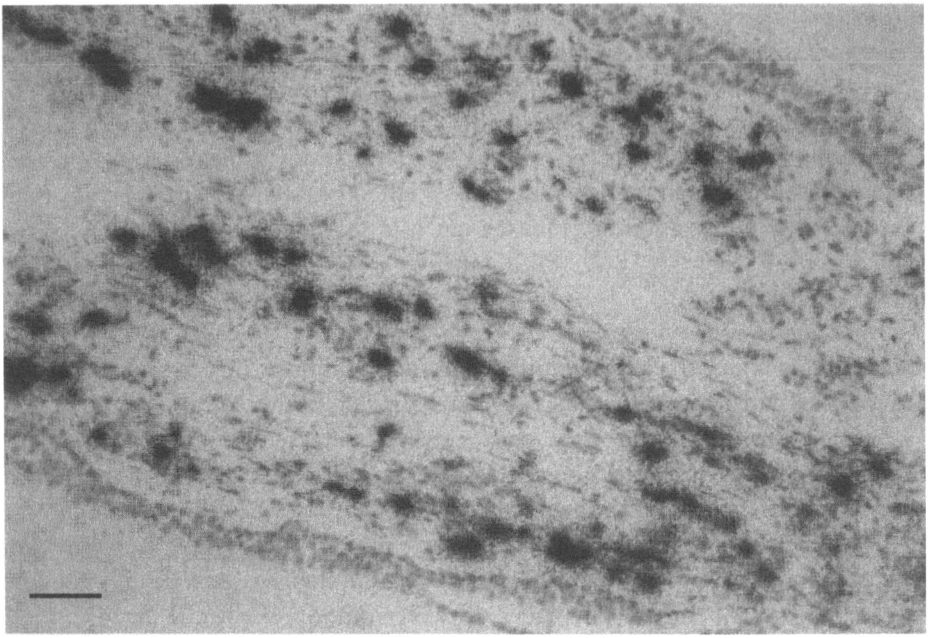

Figure 13
An autoradiogram of a section through a bronchial biopsy of an (intubated) patient with severe asthma. The section has been hybridised with a radiolabelled (^{35}S) probe for IL5 mRNA (a TH2 cytokine) which is strongly and frequently expressed in the sub-epithelial zone (demonstrated by intense and frequent labelling of cells). Scale bar = 30 µm.

ic protein which can be found both within eosinophils and diffusely in the wall, often in association with the reticular layer beneath the epithelium [70] (see also Fig. 10). Eosinophil-derived products such as major basic protein [78] together with toxic oxygen radicals and proteases probably all contribute to epithelial fragility: release of granules and of pro-fibrotic cytokines such as IL-4 and tumour grwoth factor β (TGFβ) may also stimulate nearby fibroblasts to produce additional reticulin and thicken the reticular basement membrane. Studies of bronchoalveolar lavage show increased numbers of eosinophils and T helper cells with evidence of mast cell and eosinophil degranulation [79–81]. Macrophages may also increase in number, particularly in the more severe intrinsic form of asthma [77]. Mast cells initiate the immediate response to allergen exposure. Mast cells may also be an important source of IL-4 and other pro-inflammatory cytokines whose secretion may act as a trigger to the induction of subsequent persistent production of IL-4 and IL-5 by

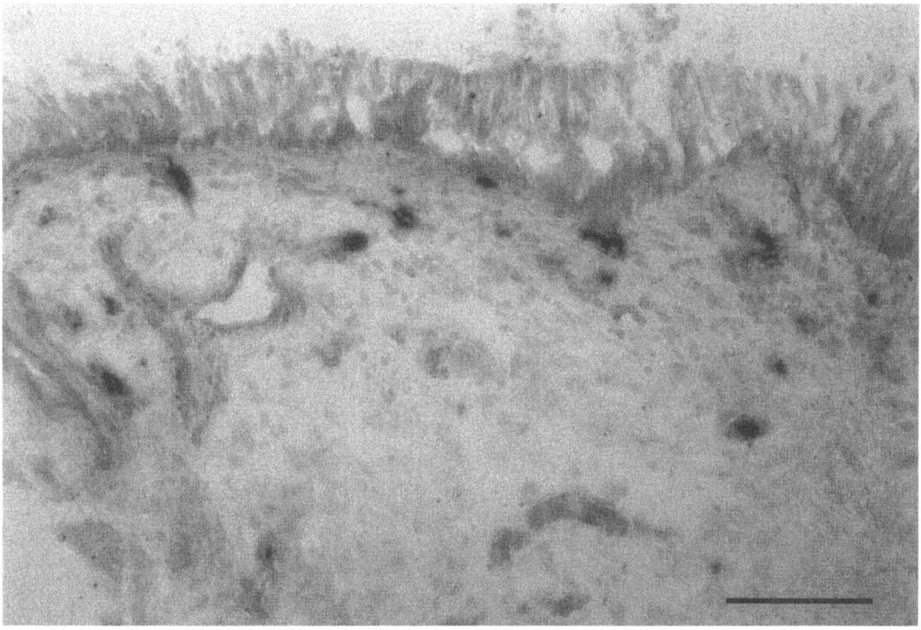

Figure 14
In situ *hybridisation using a digoxigenin-labelled ribo-probe for the C-C chemokine MCP-4 in a biopsy from a patient with atopic asthma. Mononuclear cells beneath the surface epithelium are heavily labelled for this eosinophil chemoattractant. Scale bar = 100 μm. (Produced by Dr. D. Li)*

lymphocytes [16, 82]. Little is known of the role of basophils in asthma albeit there is evidence for increased recruitment of basophils and their precursors to sites of allergic reaction in atopic patients [83].

Airway wall nerves

The topic of airway wall innervation and its relationship with asthma is a large one [9, 43]. There are data showing that in fatal asthma there is an absence of (relaxant) vasoactive intestinal polypeptide-containing nerve fibres and an increase in the numbers of substance P-containing fibres (stimulatory to bronchial smooth muscle) contrasting markedly with the innervation of the control lungs taken at resection from chronic smokers [84, 85]. The reduction has not, however, been confirmed in examination of bronchial biopsies in mild asthma [86]. Whilst Sharma and col-

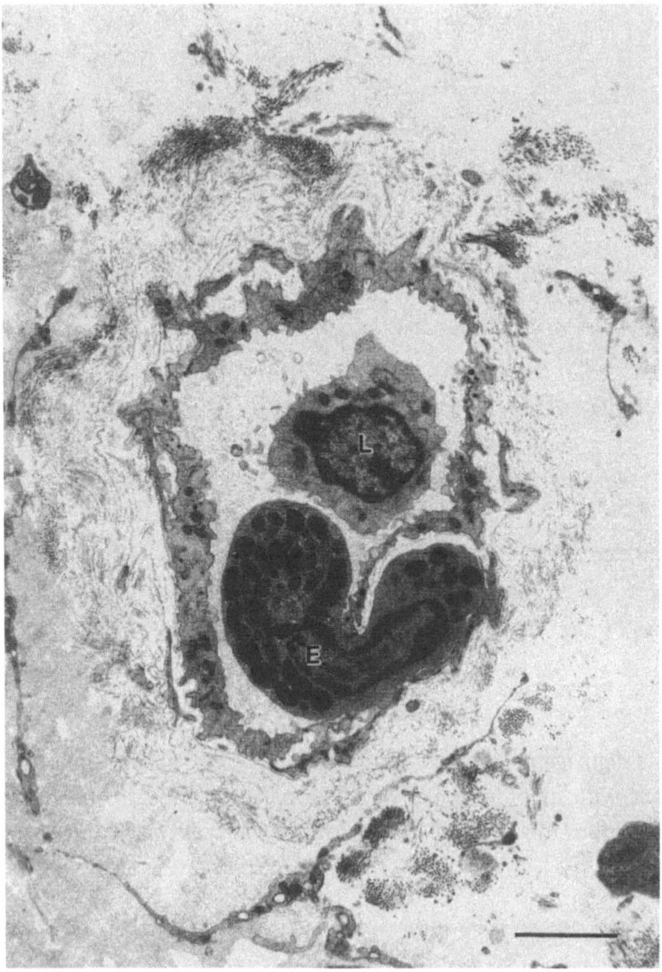

Figure 15
TEM of a biopsy showing a bronchial vessel in which there is both an eosinophil (E) and lymphomononuclear (L) cell. In this case of atopic asthma the eosinophil has adhered to the endothelial surface and is in the process of migrating between two endothelial cells to enter the interstitium. The eosinophil granules are intact and contain an electron-dense core. Scale bar = 2.0 μm.

leagues have described a reduction of airway VIP and β-adrenoreceptors in cystic fibrosis, the densities of both VIP receptors and β-adrenoreceptors are reported to be similar in asthma to those of grossly normal tissue of lungs resected for carcinoma [87, 88].

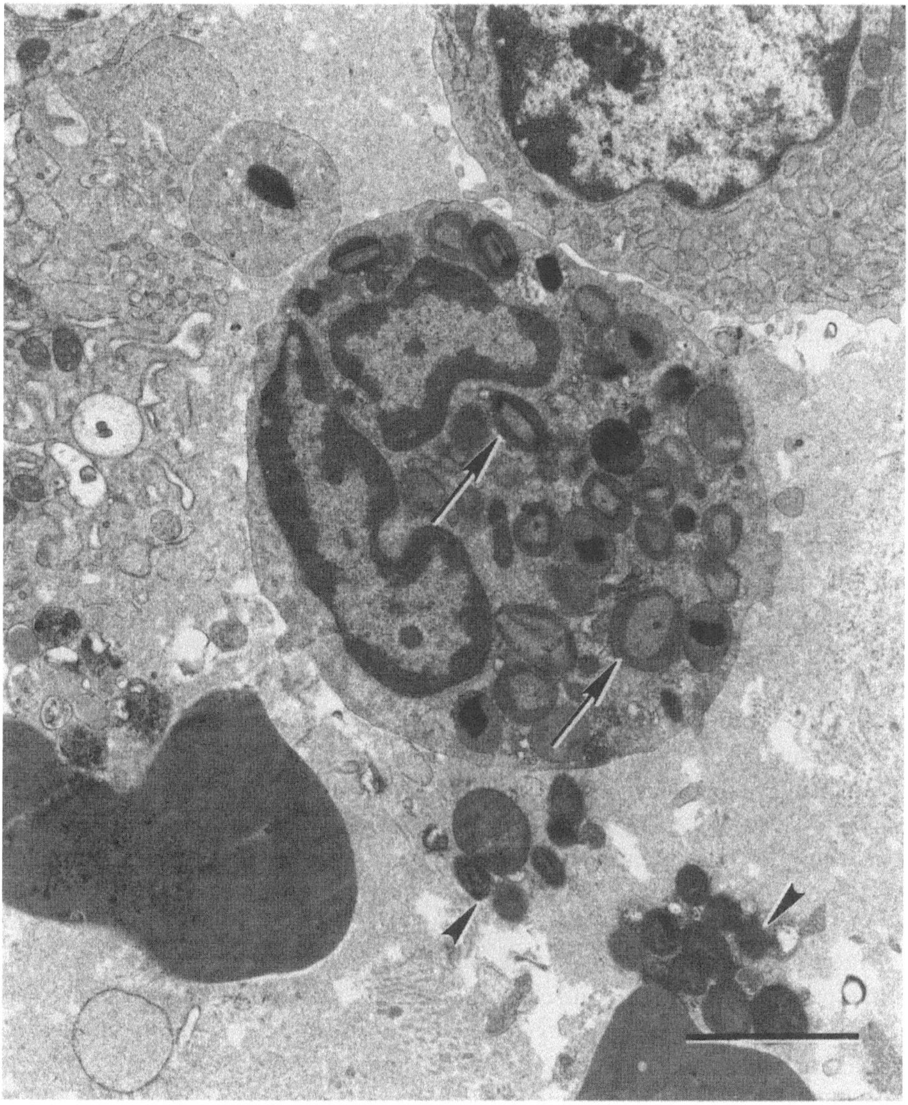

Figure 16
TEM of a bronchial biopsy in atopic asthma showing "piecemeal eosinophil degranulation". The granules within the cell have lost their major basic protein-rich and electron-dense core (arrows). This molecule is thought to damage airway tissues in asthma. Clusters of free eosinophil granules (C fegs) are also seen (arrowheads) as the result of eosinophil "cytolysis" (see Fig. 10). Scale bar = 2.5 μm.

Bronchitis

Acute bronchitis (or tracheobronchitis) and bronchiolitis

Acute inflammation of the conducting airways of the lower respiratory tract is common, (especially in young children and the elderly) varying much from year to year dependent upon the interactions of cold weather, atmospheric pollutants and the prevalence of infections such as influenza and measles. Gases including ammonia, sulphur dioxide, ozone, particularly those which are highly water soluble, induce inflammation in the larger conducting airways whereas those which are less soluble, such as oxides of nitrogen, high concentrations of oxygen and metal fumes affect the small airways and alveoli. Hydrocarbon combustion products and self-pollution by tobacco smoke also induce inflammation but these are usually associated with more chronic inflammation and its sequelae.

Viruses, including the influenza virus, parainfluenza viruses, respiratory syncytial virus (RSV), adenoviruses and herpes may induce acute airway inflammation at characteristic sites in the airway tree: e.g., RSV and adenovirus are especially prone to cause bronchiolitis in young children (see Fig. 5). The consequent pathology is to some extent dependent upon the type of virus involved but in general they either have a cytopathic effect on, usually, epithelial cells or induce their mitotic proliferation. In necrotizing bronchiolitis the bronchiolar epithelium is destroyed whereas in viral pneumonia it is the alveolar epithelium with consequent formation of hyaline membranes. During viral invasion, there is swelling and vascuolation of cell cytoplasm and nuclear degeneration and much or most of the surface epithelium is destroyed. There is oedema and hyperaemia of deeper tissues and moderate to marked infiltration by lymphocytes. Neutrophils are usually less common unless there is (as is often) the complication of secondary bacterial infection when neutrophils become the dominant inflammatory cell.

Acute *bacterial* infections of the lungs are still one of the commonest causes of death, especially in the young and elderly. Like viruses, bacteria may also be site specific as in, e.g., diphtheria which is generally limited to the pharynx. In complicating viral infections *Streptococcus pneumoniae* and *Staphylococcus aureus* are commonly involved whereas in chronic bronchitis it is commonly *Streptococcus pneumoniae* or *Haemophilus influenzae*. These bacteria and adhesive molecules on their cell walls have a great avidity for the mucus in the airway lumen and thrive on it (Fig. 17a). Providing the mucus is wafted by the cilia to the throat and swallowed or expectorated as sputum, the mucocilary system ensures the surface of the epithelium remains relatively free of bacteria. But if ciliary beating is compromised by viruses, bacterial exotoxins or atmospheric pollutants then the mucus stagnates, bacteria multiply and the exotoxins (e.g. pyocyanin) produced by them may induce sloughing of surface epithelial cells to which bacteria may then attach in large numbers (Fig. 17b) In lobar pneumonia there is congestion (lasting less than 24 h), dilation of alveolar capillaries and flooding of alveolar lumena (i.e., alveolar oedema) with fibronogen-rich fluid (and or erythrocytes) which clots to form interlacing strands of fibrin (referred to as red hepatisation). After 2–3 days, large numbers of neutrophils and then macrophages are recruited into the fibrinous matrix and there is reduction of capillary congestion (referred to as grey hepatisation). After the 8th or 9th day of illness, there then follows a spontaneous phase of resolution, lasting several weeks, which can be accelerated with treatment, during which there is liquefaction of the previously solid fibrinous constituent by enzymes thought to be released from neutrophils.

In bronchopneumonia there are patchy areas of inflammation which begin as widely dispersed bronchitis or bronchiolitis and are thus focused initially on the centres of the respiratory acinus. However, as the lesions spread, the bacteria induce an acute alveolar inflammation characterized by a copious exudation of fluid and neutrophil recruitment to alveolar walls and spaces. In these cases, healing by fibrosis, bronchiolar obliteration or emphysema rather than resolution is common. Similar inflammatory changes can be induced experimentally by the intratracheal instillation of lipopolysaccharide [89, 90].

Chronic (smokers) bronchitis

Chronic bronchitis (mucous hypersecretion) is defined by the presence of chronic cough and recurrent increases in bronchial secretions sufficient to cause expectoration. The secretions are present on most days for a minimum of 3 months a year, for at least two successive years, and cannot be attributed to other pulmonary or cardiac causes [91–93]. Chronic airways hypersecretion can occur in the absence of airflow limitation. Analysis of sputum in smokers chronic bronchitis shows a pattern of inflammation in which macrophages predominate and eosinophils and metachromatic (mast) cells are scarce [94]. Electron microscopic and immunohistochemical techniques are only just beginning to be applied to examine the nature of the inflammatory infiltrate in chronic bronchitis. There is evidence of inflammation in bronchial biopsies of subjects with stable disease and in exacerbations of bronchitis (Fig. 18) [95–99]. Bronchial mononuclear cells appear to form a predominant cell type with few neutrophils and in contrast to asthma there are relatively few eosinophils (in the absence of an exacerbation of infection). The mononuclear component comprises lymphocytes, plasma cells and macrophages [97, 100]. Significant increases are reported in the numbers of CD45 (total leucocytes), CD3 (T lymphocytes), CD25 activated and VLA-1 (late activation) positive cells and of macrophages [97]. There is a moderate increase in the number of tissue eosinophils compared to that found in normal healthy controls and it has been suggested that, in contrast to asthma, the tissue eosinophils found in chronic bronchitis do not degranulate [95]. However, Saetta and co-workers find that the numbers of tissue eosinophils are only increased when there are exacerbations of bronchitis [99, 101].

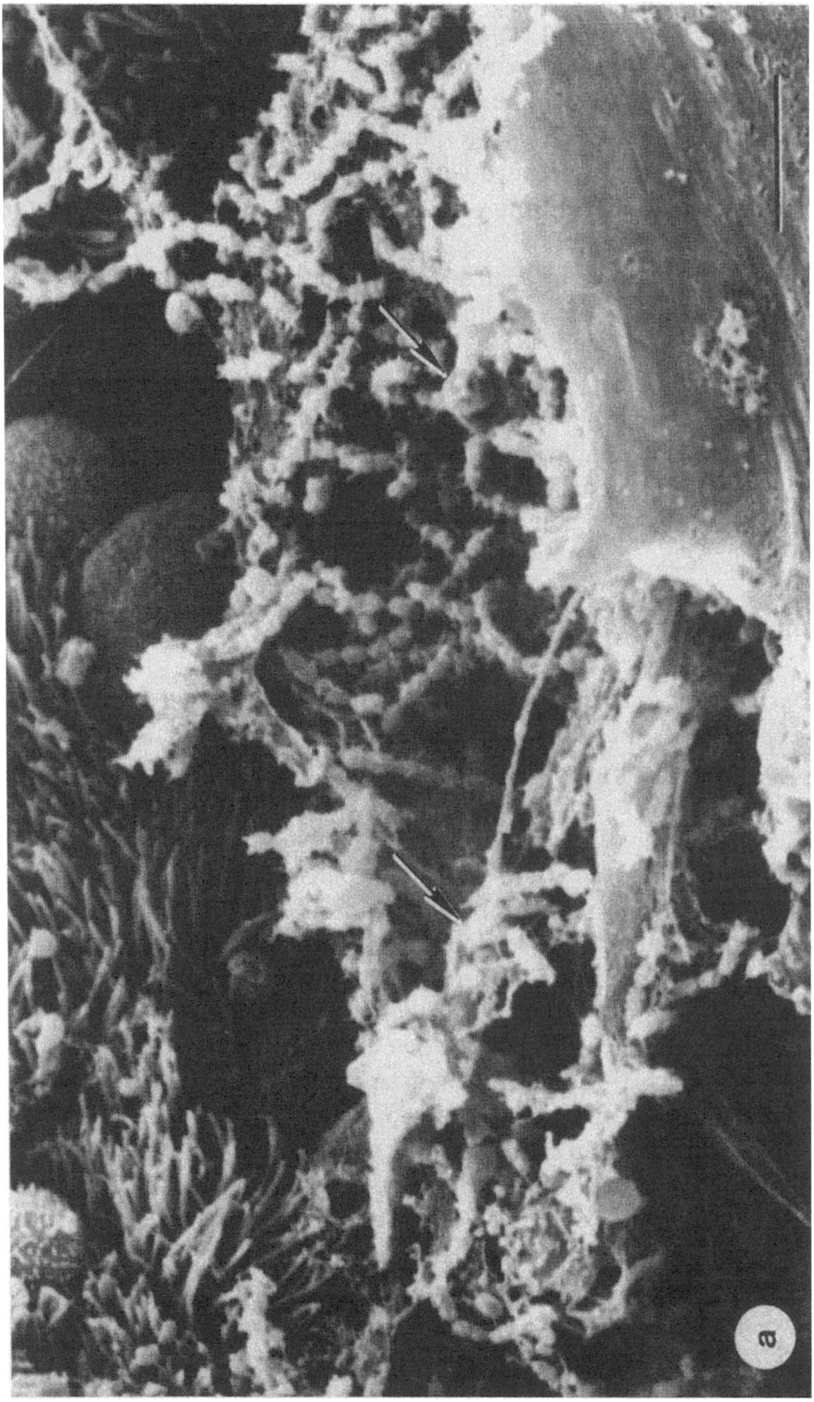

Figure 17a
SEM of human airway epithelial surface. There is colonisation of the overlying mucus but not the underlying epithelial cells by bacteria (Pneumococcus sp) (arrows). Scale bar = 5 µm.

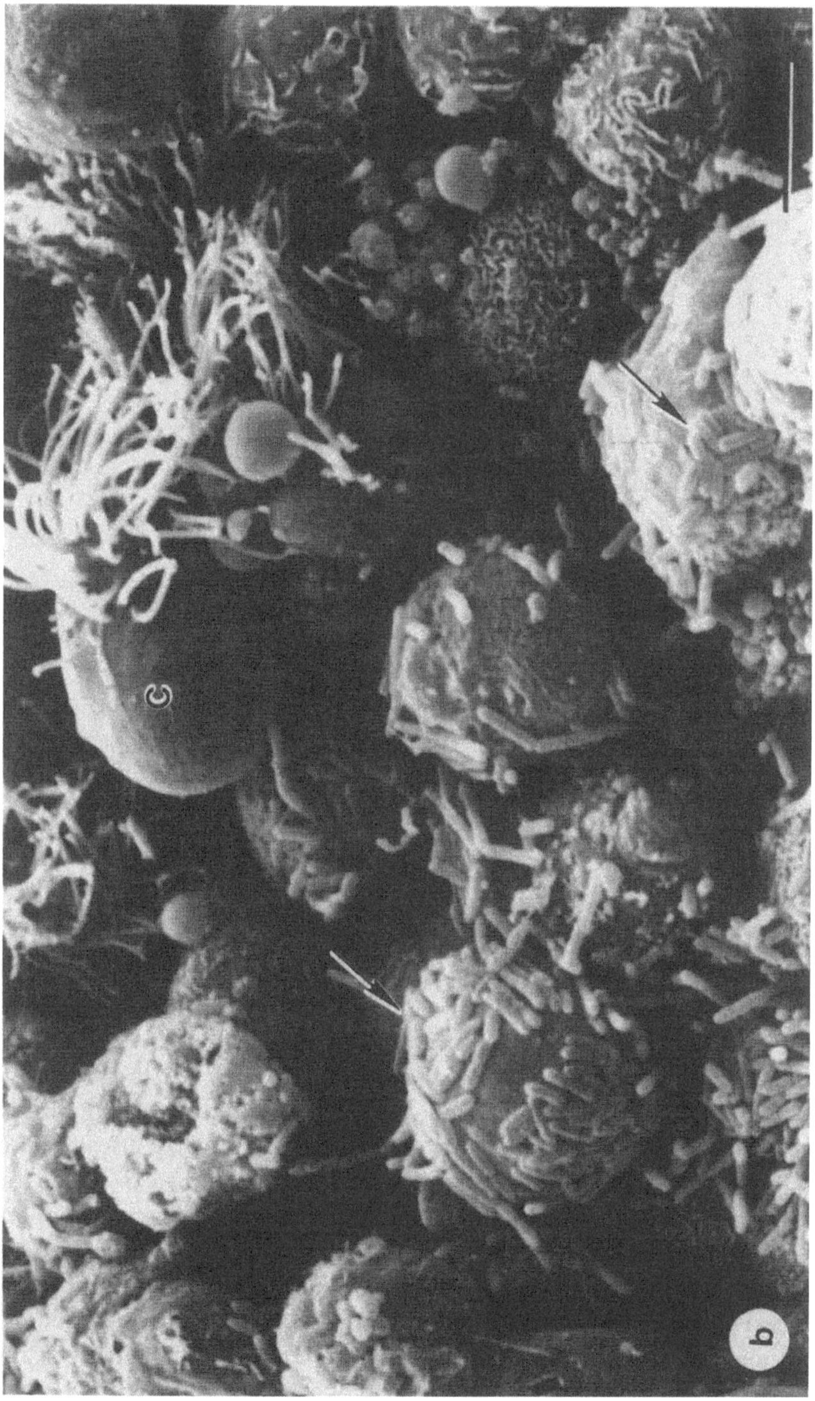

Figure 17b
SEM of sloughing airway epithelial cells illustrating the effects of bacterial toxins (Haemophilus sp)*. The ciliated (C) and non-ciliated cells are damaged and bacteria now attach avidly to their surfaces (arrows). Scale bar = 5 μm.*

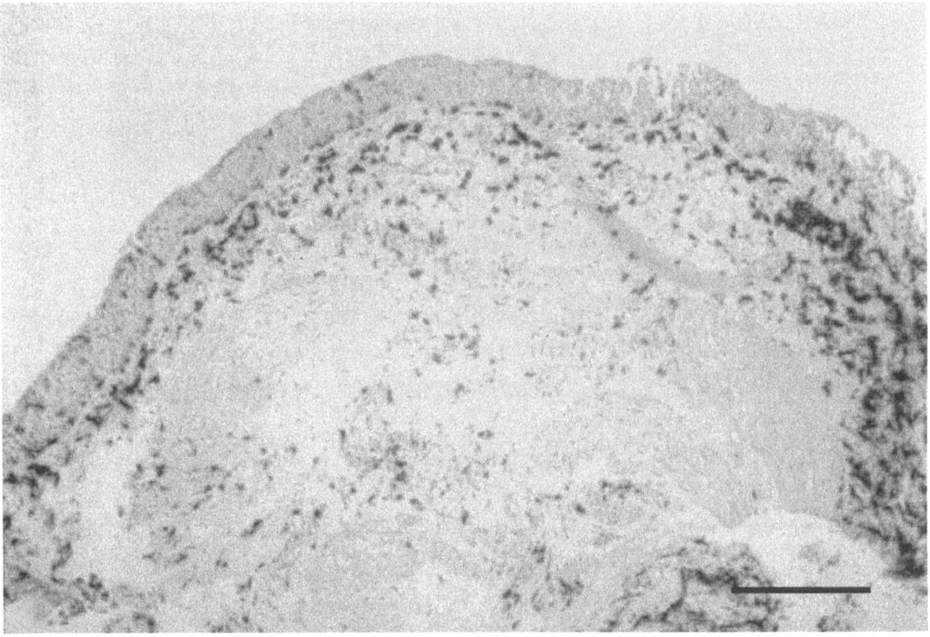

Figure 18
Histological section of a mucosal biopsy obtained from a patient with smokers bronchitis during an exacerbation. There are large numbers of CD8 positive cells infiltrating the mucosa. Scale bar = 150 μm.
(Immunostained by Dr. D. Li using the APAAP technique to stain $CD8^+$ cells red; biopsy specimen kindly obtained by Dr. M. Saetta, Padua)

The same group of workers together with another report increases in the cell surface adhesion molecules associated with such inflammation [98, 99].

The increase in sputum production may be initiated by the inflammatory process [102]. Cough and sputum production are the symptoms most frequently experienced by the 15–20% of smokers who succumb to respiratory disease: both mechanisms are effective in clearing large proximal airways (down to about the sixth generation of branching), acting to protect the more distal respiratory portion of the lung from damage. Sputum and respiratory tract secretions are a mixture of constituents including glycoproteins, glycosaminoglycans, lipids and transudate. Normally, respiratory tract secretions probably amount to less than 10 ml/day [103] and has been suggested to consist primarily of glycosaminoglycans [104, 105]. Chronic irritation by pollutants including cigarette smoke causes alterations in the number and activity of secretory cells in the mucosa, i.e. an enlargement of submucosal glands (by an increase in both the number and size of their cells) and an increase in the number of secretory cells in the surface epithelium. Mucous gland enlargement and hyperplasia of secretory cells are the histological hallmarks of chronic bronchitis and the tissue correlate of sputum production [106]. Epithelial changes may include atrophy [107], focal squamous metaplasia108 and decreases of both ciliated cell number and mean ciliary length [109–111]. Ultrastructural changes in cilia such as the development of compound cilia have been attributed directly to the effects of cigarette smoke [112] but in the author's opinion these changes are non-specific or more likely consequences of complicating exacerbations of infection and due to the bacterial exotoxins known to be ciliotoxic [113]. The presence of a gel-like mucus is essential to mucocilary clearance – normally the mucus is present as discrete flakes but in bronchitis it is thought to be present as a continuous sheet or blanket. Whilst bronchial goblet cell hyperplasia and submucosal gland enlargement are reported in chronic bronchitis [54], in emphysema (see above), gland enlargement is very much less marked and shows extensive overlap with the normal range [28]. Disproportionate reduction of serous acini of the submucosal glands which contain lysozyme, lactoferrin antibacterial agents and a small molecular weight anti-protease, tends to favour bacterial colonisation and also proteolytic damage to airways. Whilst bronchial goblet cell hyperplasia may be a feature of both asthma and bronchitis, the appearance of goblet cells in bronchioli where goblet cells are normally absent or sparse (referred to as mucous metaplasia) and their increase in number, and consequent hypersecretion of mucus in airways of less than 2 mm diameter is a key alteration contributing to small airways disease and the airflow obstruction which is the feature of COPD [114, 115].

Chronic obstructive pulmonary disease (COPD)

Chronic obstructive pulmonary disease (COPD) is a major cause of morbidity and mortality. In Europe, COPD and asthma, together with pneumonia, are the third most common cause of death. In North America, COPD is the fourth leading cause of death, and mortality rates and prevalence are increasing. The incidence and morbidity from COPD are rising. The main risk factors are cigarette smoking and occupational exposure.

The definition of COPD is much debated and the clinical definitions are still imprecise (see ERS guidelines [116]). The difficulties of definition are compounded by the recognition that both COPD and asthma are not disease entities but rather each is a complex of conditions which contribute to airflow limitation (obstruction). Unlike asthma, in COPD the limitation, particularly to expiratory airflow, is usually, but not always, persistent and typically shows a more rapid progressive deterioration with age than is normal. Accordingly the most recent and generally accepted definition in Europe is: "Chronic obstructive pulmonary disease (COPD) is a disorder characterized by reduced maximum expiratory flow and slow forced emptying of the lungs; features which do not change markedly over several months" [116]. Three conditions may contribute to airflow limitation to varying degree in each patient: (i) chronic bronchitis defined clinically (see above), (ii) adult chronic bronchiolitis (small or peripheral airways disease) which is difficult to define clinically but which may be recognized by sophisticated tests of small airway function (i.e. airways of 2 mm diameter or less), and (iii) emphysema which is defined anatomically by permanent, destructive enlargement of airspaces distal to the terminal bronchioli without obvious fibrosis [117]. Those changes which contribute most to the progressive and accelerated decline in lung function are chronic bronchiolitis and emphysema.

Inflammation associated with airflow limitation (large airways)

Biopsy studies of 2–3 order bronchi demonstrate few neutrophils and eosinophils in bronchial biopsies of stable bronchitic smokers with or without chronic bronchitis pulmonary disease (COPD). However as airflow limitation progressively worsens (measured by assessment of the forced expiratory volume in one second), T lymphocytes and neutrophils increase in the surface epithelium as do T lymphocytes and macrophages in the subepithelium. We have reported that it is the $CD8^{+}$ve lymphocyte subset which increases in number and proportion in COPD and have shown that the increase of $CD8^{+}$ cells is significantly associated with decline in lung function [100]. Importantly this contrasts with the predominance and activation of the $CD4^{+}$ T cell subset which is characteristicly increased in mild atopic asthma. Increasing pigmentation of sputum-derived macrophages and increased numbers of neutrophils are also associated with poor lung function [118]. Broncho-alveolar lavage fluid (BALF) from subjects with chronic bronchitis also demonstrates high numbers of neutrophils [95, 119]. The total number of inflammatory cells recovered by lavage is lower in COPD than in chronic bronchitis without airflow obstruction, however increased glutathione (GSH), myeloperoxidase (MPO, a marker of neutrophils) and eosinophil cationic protein (ECP) are associated with reduced FEV_1 [120]. Increased GSH may represent an airway epithelial response to persistent oxidant attack by both cigarette smoke and the highly toxic oxygen species released by inflammatory cells recruited from the vasculature, which migrate through tissues to the airway lumen. Interestingly the high numbers of neutrophils and MPO found in lavage fluid from subjects with COPD is not reflected in their numbers in the bronchial mucosa, at least in the subepithelial zone (often referred to as the lamina propria) of biopsies obtained from the same subjects [95, 100, 121]. This may represent the inability of bronchoscopy to sample distal portions of the lung to which neutrophils may be preferentially recruited in COPD or it might be due to the relatively rapid migration of neutrophils across the airway wall of the more proximal airways, sampled by bronchoscopy. Alternatively, the location of the histological section in which the inflammatory cells are counted may not be that in which neutrophils accumulate. It is our (unpublished) experience that whilst neutrophil counts in the subepithelium may be low, they preferentially accumulate within the surface epithelium during their presumed passage to the airway lumen: this is a biopsy site often not included in counts of inflammatory cells [122].

Adult chronic bronchiolitis (small airways disease)

Airflow limitation, as determined by FEV_1, usually occurs late in the course of cigarette smoke-related events, whereas inflammation in small airways (i.e. bronchioli < 2–3 mm diameter) occurs relatively early and may be detected physiologically well before the age of 30 years [123, 124]. The small airway defect is characterised by persistent airflow limitation which may show progressive deterioration in the absence of emphysema. Whilst the site of the lesion and diagnosis is, as yet, difficult to pinpoint by lung function, experimental physiologists (*inter alia* [125, 126]) have indicated that the dominant site lies in bronchioli of less than 3 mm diameter. Histologically one of the most consistently observed early effects of cigarette smoke is a marked increase in the number of macrophages and neutrophils, both in man and experimentally in animal studies. The increase is seen within both the lung interstitium and alveolar air space and can be detected in bronchoalveolar lavage fluid (BAL) [127]. Early smoking-related inflammatory changes occurring in small airways have been described in studies comparing lungs of young smokers and controls of similar age from a group who had experienced sudden non-hospital deaths [114, 128, 129]. It is suggested that the primary lesion is progressive inflammation leading to peribronchiolar fibrosis. Evidence of destructive emphysema and right ventricular hypertrophy is common in COPD; in contrast, both are uncommon findings in asthma. The resultant narrowing of small bronchioli has been well demonstrated in bronchiolar casts of patients with COPD by Bignon and colleagues [130]. The peribronchiolar inflammation consisting of lymphocytes and fibrosis may also predispose to the development of centrilobular emphysema and may be responsible for the subtle abnormalities detected by lung function (Fig. 19). The T cell functional phenotype and cytokine profile of bronchiolar inflammation in smokers is yet to be characterized. Associated loss of alveolar attachments to the airway perimeter contribute to loss of elastic recoil and favour increased tortuosity and early closure of bronchioli (which lack cartilagenous support) during expiration [131–133]. Cosio and colleagues [114] have described lesions in smokers dying suddenly: inflammation in bronchioles and a respiratory bronchiolitis consisting of pigmented macrophages associated with mucous metaplasia, smooth muscle hypertrophy, mural oedema, peribronchiolar fibrosis and an excess of air-

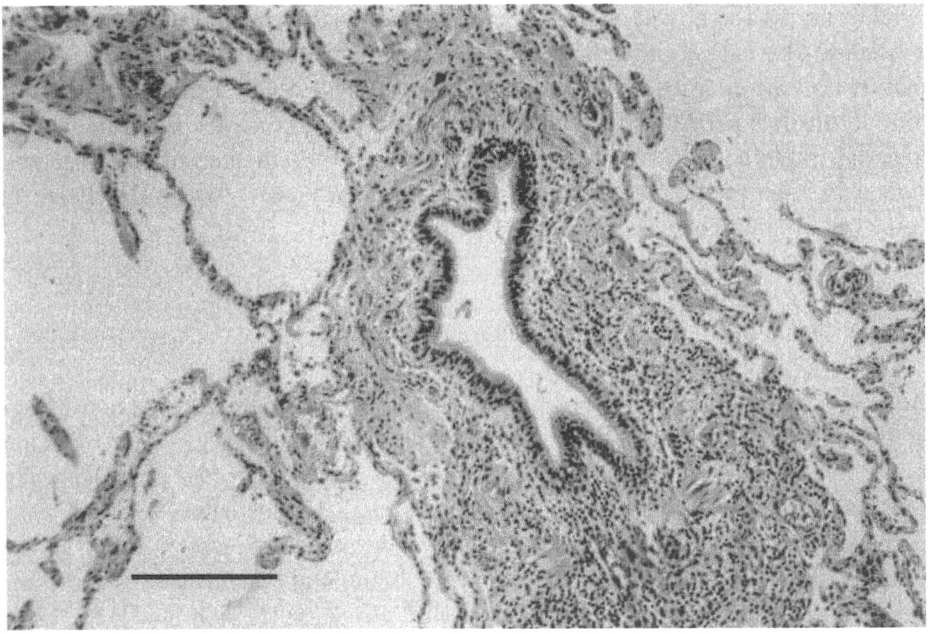

Figure 19a
H&E stained section of the centriacinar region of a case of COPD in which there is a small airway with marked peribronchiolitis surrounded by abnormally large alveolar spaces. Scale bar = 1000 μm.

ways < 400 μm diameter were the main lesions in these smokers [114, 128, 134]. Associated stenotic narrowing of bronchioli have been demonstrated and inflammatory changes to small airways appear to be related to clinical airflow obstruction in COPD.

In bronchioli, secretory and ciliated cells are the main cell types [135, 136] and, of them, the Clara cell is the major secretory and progenitor cell. It has been suggested that the Clara cell normally produces both a hypophase component of bronchiolar surfactant [137] and a low molecular weight protease inhibitor (syn. antileukoprotease or bronchial mucosal protease inhibitor [138]). The latter is the main anti-elastase screen in sputum and normally prevents autolysis of airway tissues [139]. In smokers, Clara cells are replaced by mucous cells [115] and mucus appears in peripheral airways and its secretion is abnormally increased therein [140]. The increase in mucus at this distal site is difficult to clear by cough and dramatically increases surface tension favouring early closure of airways during expiration [141].

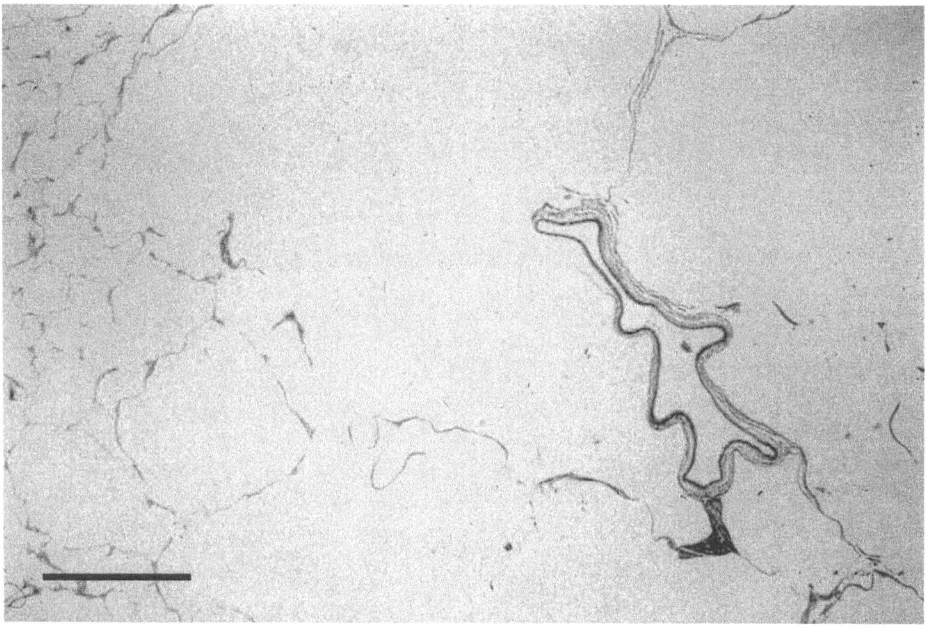

Figure 19b
H&E stained section through emphysematous lung in which there is destruction of alveolar attachments to the bronchiolar wall, resulting in a tortuous appearance and probably early collapse during expiration. Scale bar = 2000 μm.

Emphysema

Laennec gave us the first clear anatomic descriptions of emphysema in 1826. He also recognized that cough, expectoration of mucus, air-flow obstruction, and shortness of breath on effort were the clinical correlates in life of the finding of emphysema at autopsy.

The early changes leading to emphysema have been thought to include subtle disruption to elastic fibres with accompanying loss of elastic recoil, bronchiolar and alveolar distortion and the appearance of fenestrae which enlarge [142] eventually leading to loss of interalveolar septa. In smokers with emphysema there is loss of alveolar wall tissue even in regions removed from those with obvious macroscopic lesions: recent data have shown that this is accompanied by a net increase in the mass of collagen. This suggests that, contrary to the current internationally accepted definition (see above) that there is active alveolar wall fibrosis in the tissues which remain in otherwise emphysematous lungs [143].

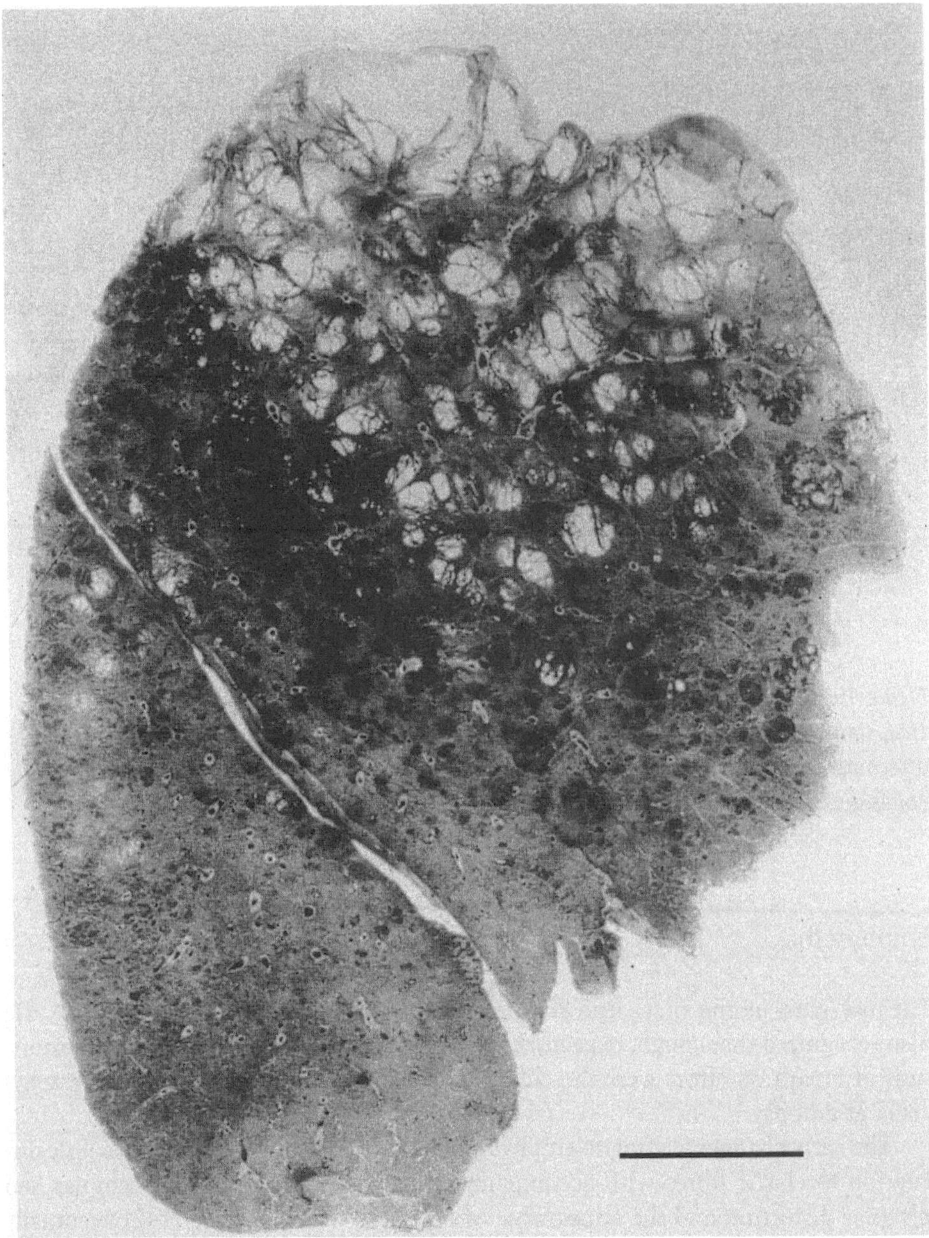

Figure 20
Gross appearance of the cut surface of a lung resected from a smoker showing severe centri-acinar emphysema with destruction predominantly present in the upper aspects of each lobe. Scale bar = 5 cm. (Courtesy of Prof. B. Heard)

Two main forms of emphysema are described. They are distinguished by the part of the acinus affected. *Centriacinar* emphysema is characterised by focal destruction restricted to respiratory bronchioli and the central portions of the acinus, each focus surrounded by areas of grossly normal lung parenchyma. This form of emphysema is usually more severe in the upper lobes of the lung (Fig. 20). *Panacinar* emphysema involves some degree of destruction of the walls in a fairly uniform manner of all the air spaces beyond the terminal bronchiolus. This form of emphysema is characteristic of patients who develop smoking-related emphysema relatively early in life and, in contrast to the centriacinar form, has a tendency to involve the lower lobes more than the upper. In the familial form of panacinar emphysema it is usually associated with α_1-antitrypsin deficiency [144].

Epidemiological studies have demonstrated a significant relationship between cigarette smoking and severity of emphysema [145] but the mechanism(s) by which cigarette smoke causes such damage is still the subject of much research. One current working hypothesis is that emphysema is the result of an imbalance between proteolytic enzymes and protease inhibitors in the lung, favouring an excess of enzyme and in particular elastases. In addition, the imbalance between oxidants and antioxidants contributes also by allowing an excessive oxidant burden to degrade the normal protease inhibitor screen [146, 147]. The proposed mechanism involves interactions between cigarette smoke, alveolar macrophages, chemoattractants, neutrophils, elastases, endogenous and exogenous oxidants, protease inhibitors, antioxidants and lung connective tissue, primarily elastin, which undergoes repeated destruction, synthesis and degradation [148]. The *in vitro* effects of cigarette smoke on pulmonary connective tissue are consistent with the protease/antiprotease and oxidant/antioxidant hypotheses. In spite of this, experimental animal models of cigarette smoke-induced emphysema have proved difficult to develop. The destruction of the respiratory zone in emphysema is also considered to be the result of an inflammatory reaction, much of this centred on respiratory bronchioli and largely initiated by products of inhaled tobacco smoke [147, 149]. As with the more proximal airways T lymphocytes (recently suggested to be of the CD8 phenotype) and macrophages appear to play a role in the lung parenchyma also [150, 151]. Factors chemotactic for neutrophils, and which will induce their emigration from the microcirculation are released by smokers' alveolar macrophages [152] and the alveolar neutrophil population may increase from 1% to 5% of inflammatory cells. Cigarette smoke may, itself, contains substances chemoattractant for neutrophils [153], a possibility that is supported by the associated peripheral blood leukocytosis which is widely reported [154]. Cigarette smoke or factors released from cigarette smoke-exposed macrophages induce the release elastases from neutrophils which degrade lung elastin even in the presence of antiprotease [155–157]. The approximation of neutrophils with interstitial connective tissue is a close one even when they are retained in the pulmonary circulation (Fig. 21). The average diameter of circulating neutrophils is 7.0 µm which necessitates their deformation as they squeeze through

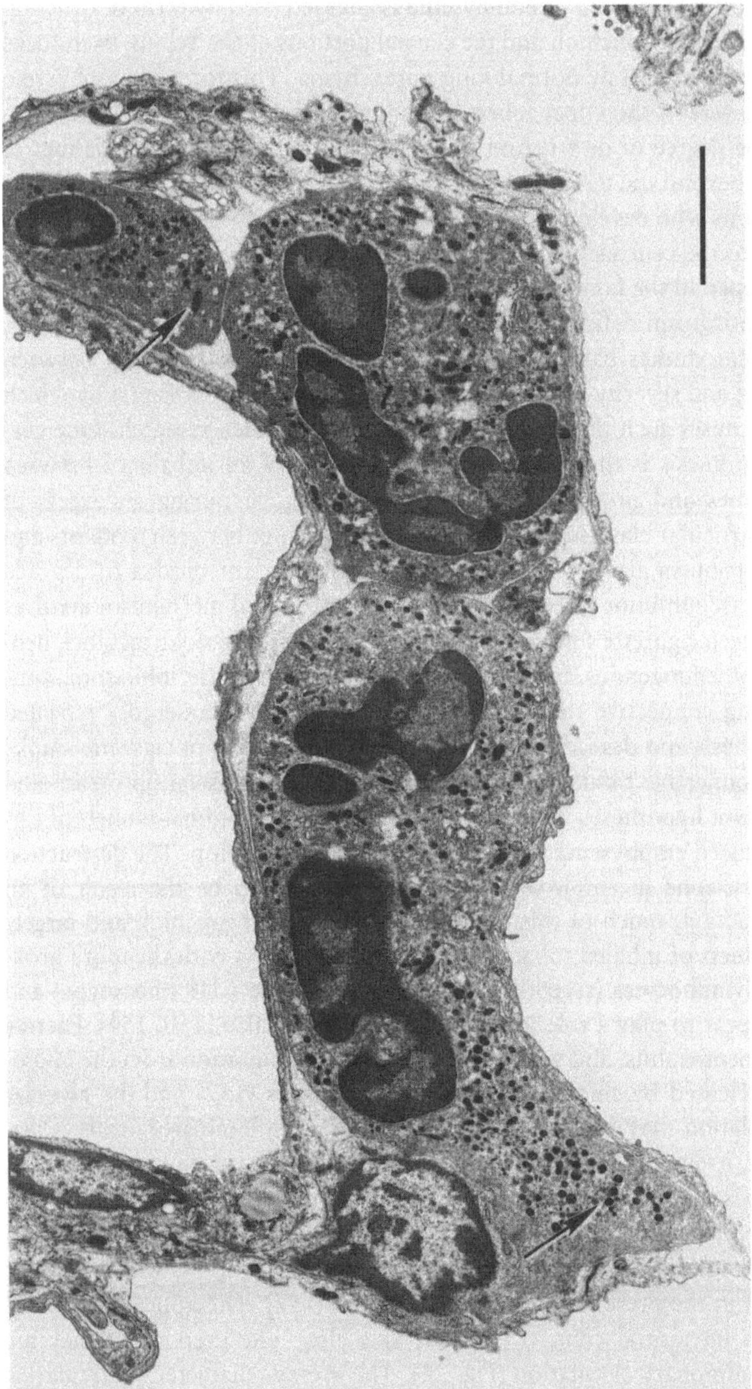

Figure 21
TEM appearance of capillaries in the alveolar wall in which neutrophils have been retained in response to experimentally-induced acute lung injury. The capacity of neutrophils to deform their shape is essential if they are to pass through the capillary network. Their stasis and activation likely leads to release of electron-dense lysosomal granules (arrows) causing elastolysis and breakdown of the alveolar wall and enlargement of alveolar spaces. Scale bar = 2.5 μm.

capillary segments of 5 μm diameter. Neutrophil traffic through the capillaries of the lung is normally slower (i.e. there is a higher transit time) than that of red blood cells as they are 700 times less deformable than RBCs [158]. Recent studies with radioactively labelled neutrophils have demonstrated that the normal delay in neutrophil transit is further exaggerated, transiently, even in healthy subjects during smoking [159]. Exposure of neutrophils to cigarette smoke *in vitro* and *in vivo* results in decreased deformability associated with polymerisation of actin microfilaments [158, 160]. This is the likely mechanism of the observed cigarette smoke-induced increase in transit time.

Elastin fragments created by the elastase activity of both neutrophil and macrophages attract monocytes from the circulating pool of blood leukocytes from which alveolar macrophages mature [161]. When activated, alveolar macrophages release a variety of oxidants which damage tissues [154, 162]. Cigarette smoke itself also contributes significantly to the exogenous oxidant burden and may reduce antiprotease activity of the lungs anti-elastase screen. It is estimated that each puff contains 10^{14} free radicals in each of the soluble and particulate phases and that many of these are relatively long-lived [163]. Cigarette smoke-derived oxidants may damage directly host tissue or act by inhibiting α_1-antitrypsin.

Whilst the major pathological changes are thought to occur in the small airways and parenchyma, in patients with more advanced COPD, changes also occur to the pulmonary circulation, the right heart, and respiratory muscles. With alveolar hypoxia, the medial vascular smooth muscle of pulmonary arterioles extends distally to vessels that normally lack muscle and there is intimal thickening. In addition, loss of the vascular bed occurs as a consequence of emphysema. Right ventricular enlargement due to dilatation and/or hypertrophy is not uncommon and atrophy of the diaphragm occurs in some cases. In contrast, these changes are not features of asthma.

Lastly, but importantly, many life-long smokers do not succumb to the development of emphysema and constitutional factors are likely to predispose individuals and make them especially susceptible to the effects of tobacco smoke. Genetic deficiency of α_1-antitrypsin is a well documented extreme example and smoking in this group clearly advances the onset of emphysema and accelerates its subsequent progression. Other genetic factors such as variation in cellular response to cytotoxicity, phagocytosis and enzyme release may also be important determinants of an individual's susceptibility to cigarette smoke [164]. O'Shaughnessy and colleagues [100] suggest that susceptibility to the effects of cigarette smoke will be greater in those individuals who already have a genetically determined low CD4/$CD8^+$ cell ratio in their peripheral blood [165]. This is a novel explanation as to why only a relatively small proportion of smokers succumb to its deleterious effects: the hypothesis requires, however, testing and epidemiological proof. Long-term studies (soon to be reported) of inhaled corticosteroids in COPD are currently in progress to test the hypothesis that airways inflammation bears a relationship with rate of decline in

FEV_1: if the relationship is a direct one then there should be a slowing of the rate of decline following attenuation of the inflammatory reaction.

Table 1 summarizes the main distinctions between COPD and asthma. There is evidence of inflammation in both but there are marked differences in terms of the predominant inflammatory cell phenotype and the site and functional consequence of such inflammation. The distinctions are however not absolute and the two conditions may co-exist in any one patient.

Fibrosing alveolitis

Finally fibrosing alveolitis (FA) represents scar formation of the lung and fibrous thickening of the alveolar walls. The fibrosis may be intra-luminal or interstitial. In the former case it may represent organization of eosinophilic or bacterial pneumonia or its aetiology may be unknown (i.e., cryptogenic). In its interstitial form it may include (i) the organization of exudates, hyaline membranes or of a chronic interstitial oedema (such as that which may follow diffuse alveolar damage caused by toxic fumes, irradiation, virus or regurgitated gastric acid or (ii) the granulomatous conditions (including sarcoidosis, extrinsic allergic alveolitis and eosinophilic granuloma). Cryptogenic fibrosing alveolitis (CFA; also referred to as idiopathic pulmonary fibrosis) and that associated with the collagen-vascular disease, systemic sclerosis (FASSc), are also inflammatory conditions of the lung which result in collagenous thickening of the alveolar wall rather than its emphysematous destruction. An understanding of the reasons for the very different outcomes of the inflammatory processes of emphysema and FA is required. We know that activated T lymphocytes (i.e. CD25 and CD45Ro positive cells) are also present in increased numbers in FA. Gene expression for IL-4 and IL-5, whilst characteristic, is not unique to asthma and this Th2 pattern occurs in CFA also [166]. By contrast the inflammation of FASSc is associated with gene expression for IL-4, -5 and interferon γ (IFNγ) (i.e. a mixed Th2/Th1 phenotype). Interestingly both fibrotic conditions are associated with increases of IL-8 gene expression [167].

Conclusion

In conclusion the severity and nature of the inflammation and its consequences (be they obstructive or restrictive) depend much on the type, dose and persistence of the insult and the predominant site in the lung at which it occurs. By comparing and understanding the subtleties of the inflammatory and molecular processes of these pathologically distinct conditions and the contributions made by different inflammatory, and also structural cells, we will be able to understand better their interaction with the genetic factors which predispose an individual to the development of

Table 1 - Simplified comparison of COPD and asthma

	COPD	Asthma
Airflow obstruction	Progressive deterioration of lung function (± reversible component)	Variable (± irreversible component)
Post-mortem	Excessive mucus (mucoid/purulent) Small airway disease, emphysema	Hyperinflation airway plugs (exudate + mucus) No or little emphysema
Sputum	Macrophage Neutrophil (infective exacerbation)	Eosinophilia Metachromatic cells Creola bodies
Surface epithelium	Fragility undetermined	Fragility/loss
Bronchiolar mucous cells	Metaplasia/hyperplasia	Mucous metaplasia is debated
Reticular basement membrane	Variable or normal	Homogeneously thickened and hyaline
Congestion/oedema	Variable/fibrotic	Present
Bronchial smooth muscle	Enlarged mass (small airways)	Enlarged mass (large ainNays) Enlarged mass
Bronchial glands	Enlarged mass (increased acidic glycoprotein)	(no change in mucin histochemistry)
Cellular infiltrate	Predominantly CD3, CD8, CD68, CD25 VLA-1 and HLA-DR +ve Mild eosinophilia (? not degranulated) Mast cell increase	Predominantly CD3, CD4, CD25 (IL-2R) +ve Marked eosinophilia (EG2 +ve) (degranulated) Mast cell increase (decrease in severe/fatal)
Cytokines (ISH)	GM-CSF protein, IL-4 & IL-5 gene expression	IL-4 & IL-5 but not IFN gene expression (TH_2 profile)

these inflammatory conditions of the airways and lung and know better how to design more effective and incisive treatment.

Acknowledgements
I thank many colleagues who have worked with me and with whom I have shared interesting discussion. I am particularly grateful to Miss Leone Oscar for her help in typing the manuscript and for her careful attention to detail and Mr Andrew Rogers for his care in preparing the illustrations.

References

1 Horsfield K (1974) The relation between structure and function in the airways of the lung. *Br J Dis Chest* 68: 145–160
2 Lumsden AB, McLean A, Lamb D (1984) Goblet and Clara cells of human distal airways: evidence for smoking-induced changes in numbers. *Thorax* 39: 844–853
3 Jeffery PK (1983) Morphology of airway surface epithelial cells and glands. *Am Rev Respir Dis* 128: S14–S20
4 Jeffery PK (1995) Structural, immunologic, and neural elements of the normal human airway wall. In: WW Busse, ST Holgate (eds): *Asthma and rhinitis.* Blackwell Scientific Publications, Oxford, 80–106
5 Staunton D, Merluzzi V, Rothlein R, Barton R, Marlin S, Springer T (1989) A cell adhesion molecule, ICAM-1, is the makor surface receptor for rhinoviruses. *Cell* 56: 849–53
6 Papi A, Wilson S, Johnston S (1996) Rhinoviruses increase production of cell adhesion molecules (CAM) and NF-alpha B. *Am J Resp Crit Care Med* 153: A866 (abstract)
7 Devalia JL, Davies RJ (1993) Airway epithelial cells and mediators of inflammation. *Resp Med* 87: 405–408
8 Jeffery PK (1994) Innervation of the airway mucosa: Structure, function and changes in airway disease. In: RG Goldie (ed): Immunopharmacology of epithelial barriers. Academic Press, London, 85–118
9 Barnes PJ (1986) State of art: neural control of human airways in health and disease. *Am Rev Respir Dis* 134: 1289–1314
10 Bousquet J, Jeffery PK (1998) Methods for assessment of airways inflammation. *Eur Respir J* 11 (suppl 26): 1s–58s
11 Chakir J, Laviolette M, Boutet M, Laliberte R, Dube J, Boulet LP (1996) Lower airways remodeling in nonasthmatic subjects with allergic rhinitis. *Lab Invest* 75: 735–744
12 Mygind N, Winther B (1979) Light- and scanning electron-microscopy of the nasal mucosa. *Acta Otorhinolaryngol (Belg)* 33 (4): 591–602
13 Smith IM (1983) Epidemiology and natural history of asthma, allergic rhinitis and allergic dermatitis (eczema). In: E Middleton, CE Reed, EF Ellis (eds): *Allergy: Principles and Practice,* 2nd ed. CV Mosby Company, St. Louis, 771–804

14 Varney VA, Jacobson MR, Sudderick RM et al (1992) Immuno-histology of the nasal mucosa following allergen-induced rhinitis: identification of activated T lymphocytes, eosinophils and neutrophils. *Am Rev Respir Dis* 146: 170

15 Bentley AM, Jacobson MR, Cumberworth V et al (1992) Immunohistology of the nasal mucosa in seasonal allergic rhinitis: increases in activated eosinophils and epithelial mast cells. *J Allergy Clin Immunol* 89: 821–829

16 Bradding P, Feather IH, Wilson S et al (1993) Immunolocalization of cytokines in the nasal mucosa of normal and perennial rhinitic subjects. *J Immunol* 151: 3853–3865

17 Gomez E, Clague JE, Gatland D, Davies RJ (1988) Effect of topical corticosteroids on seasonally induced increases in nasal mast cells. *BMJ* 296: 1572–1573

18 Durham SR (1997) Mechanisms and treatment of allergic rhinitis. In: IS Mackay, TR Bull (eds): *Rhinology*, 6th ed. Butterworth-Heinemann, Oxford, 4/6/1–4/6/16

19 Howarth PH (1995) The cellular basis for allergic rhinitis. *Allergy* 50: 6–10

20 Ayars GH, Altman LC, McManus MM et al (1989) Injurious effect of the eosinophil peroxide-hydrogen peroxide-halide system and major basic protein on human nasal epithelium *in vitro*. *Am Rev Respir Dis* 140 (1): 125–131

21 Minshall EM, Cameron L, Lavigne F et al (1997) Eotaxin mRNA and protein expression in chronic sinusitis and allergen-induced nasal responses in seasonal allergic rhinitis. *Am J Respir Cell Mol Biol* 17: 683–690

22 Holgate ST, Bodey KS, Janezic A, Frew AJ, Kaplan AP, Teran LM (1997) Release of RANTES, MIP-1 alpha, and MCP-1 into asthmatic airways following endobronchial allergen challenge. *Am J Respir Crit Care Med* 156: 1377–1383

23 Sim TC, Reece LM, Hilsmeier KA, Grant JA, Alam R (1995) Secretion of chemokines and other cytokines in allergen-induced nasal responses: inhibition by topical steroid treatment. *Am J Respir Crit Care Med* 152: 927–933

24 Kuna P, Lazarovich M, Kaplan AP (1996) Chemokines in seasonal allergic rhinitis. *J Allergy Clin Immunol* 97: 104–112

25 Sur S, Hirohito K, Gleich GJ, Chenier TC, Hunt LW (1990) Eosinophil recruitment is associated with IL-5, but not with RANTES, twenty-four hours after allergen challenge. *J Allergy Clin Immunol* 97: 1272–1278

26 Meggs WJ, Elsheik T, Metzger WJ, Albernaz M, Bloch RM (1996) Nasal pathology and ultrastructure in patients with chronic airway inflammation (RADS and RUDS) following an irritant exposure. *J Toxicol Clin Toxicol* 34 (4): 383–396

27 Dunnill MS (1960) The pathology of asthma, with special reference to changes in the bronchial mucosa. *J Clin Pathol* 13: 27–33

28 Dunnill MS, Massarella GR, Anderson JA (1969) A comparison of the quantitative anatomy of the bronchi in normal subjects, in status asthmaticus, in chronic bronchitis, and in emphysema. *Thorax* 24: 176–179

29 List SJ, Findlay BP, Forstner GG, Forstner JF (1978) Enhancement of the viscosity of mucin by serum albumin. *Biochem J* 175: 565–571

30 Gleich GJ, Motojima S, Frigas E, Kephart GM, Fujisawa T, Kravis LP (1980) The

eosinophilic leucocyte and the pathology of fatal bronchial asthma: evidence for pathologic heterogeneity. *J Allergy Clin Immunol* 80: 412–415
31 Azzawi M, Johnston PW, Majumdar S, Kay AB, Jeffery PK (1992) T-lymphocytes and activated eosinophils in asthma and cystic fibrosis. *Am Rev Respir Dis* 145: 1477–1482
32 Sur S, Crotty TB, Kephart GM et al (1993) Sudden onset fatal asthma: a distinct entity with few eosinophils and relatively more neutrophils in the airway submucosa? *Am Rev Respir Dis* 148: 713–719
33 Jeffery PK, Wardlaw A, Nelson FC, Collins JV, Kay AB (1989) Bronchial biopsies in asthma: an ultrastructural quantification study and correlation with hyperreactivity. *Am Rev Respir Dis* 140: 1745–1753
34 Beasley R, Roche W, Roberts JA, Holgate ST (1989) *Cell*ular events in the bronchi in mild asthma and after bronchial provocation. *Am Rev Respir Dis* 139: 806–817
35 Laitinen LA, Heino M, Laitinen A, Kava T, Haahtela T (1985) Damage of the airway epithelium and bronchial reactivity in patients with asthma. *Am Rev Respir Dis* 131: 599–606
36 Ayers M, Jeffery PK (1988) Proliferation and differentiation in adult mammalian airway epithelium: a review. *Eur Respir J* 1: 58–80
37 Erjefalt JS, Erjefalt I, Sundler F, Persson CGA (1994) Airway microcirculation-derived factors in epithelial repair. *Microvasc Res* 48: 161–178
38 Shoji S, Ertl RF, Linder J, Romberger DJ, Rennard SI (1990) Bronchial epithelial cells produce chemotactic activity for bronchial epithelial cells: Possible role for fibronectin in airway repair. *Am Rev Respir Dis* 141: 218–225
39 Soderberg M, Hellstrom S, Sandstrom T, Lungren R, Bergh A (1990) Structural characterization of bronchial mucosal biopsies from healthy volunteers: a light and electron microscopical study. *Eur Respir J* 3: 261–266
40 Naylor B (1962) The shedding of the mucosa of the bronchial tree in asthma. *Thorax* 17: 69–72
41 Elia C, Bucca C, Rolla G, Scappaticci E, Cantino D (1988) A freeze-fracture study of tight junctions in human bronchial epithelium in normal, bronchitic and asthmatic subjects. *J Submic Cytol Pathol* 20: 509–517
42 Godfrey RWA, Severs NJ, Jeffery PK (1992) Freeze-fracture morphology and quantification of human bronchial epithelial tight junctions. *Am J Respir Cell Molec Biol* 6: 453–458
43 Jeffery PK (1994) Innervation of the airway mucosa: Structure, function and changes in airway disease. In: R Goldie et al (eds): *Immunopharmacology of epithelial barriers. Handbook of immunopharmacology,* vol. 8 (series ed. C Page). Academic Press, London, 85–118
44 Sparrow MP, Mitchell HW (1991) The epithelium acts as a barrier modulating the extent of bronchial narrowing produced by substances perfused through the lumen. *Br J Pharmacol* 103: 1160–1164
45 Hogg JC, Eggleston PA (1984) Is asthma an epithelial disease? *Am Rev Respir Dis* 129: 207–208

46 VanHoutte PM (1989) Eithelium-derived relaxing factor(s) and bronchial reactivity. *J Allergy Clin Immunol* 83: 855–861

47 Callerame MD, Condemi MD, Bohrod MD, Vaughan JH (1971) Immunologic reactions of bronchial tissues in asthma. *N Engl J Med* 284: 459–464

48 Roche WR, Beasley R, Williams JH, Holgate ST (1989) Subepithelial fibrosis in the bronchi of asthmatics. *Lancet* i: 520–523

49 Nowak J (1969) Anatomopathologic changes in the bronchial walls in chronic inflammation, with special reference to the basement membrane, in the course of bronchial asthma. *Acta Med Polona* 2: 151–172

50 Sobonya RE (1984) Quantitative structural alterations in long-standing allergic asthma. *Am Rev Respir Dis* 130: 289–292

51 Crepea SB, Harman JW (1955) The pathology of bronchial asthma. I. The significance of membrane changes in asthmatic and non-allergic pulmonary disease. *J Allergy* 26: 453–460

52 Brewster CEP, Howarth PH, Djukanovic R, Wilson J, Holgate ST, Roche WR (1990) Myofibroblasts and subepithelial fibrosis in bronchial asthma. *Am J Respir Cell Mol Biol* 3: 507–511

53 Gizycki MJ, Adelroth E, Rogers AV, O'Byrne PM, Jeffery PK (1997) Myofibroblast involvement in the allergen-induced late response in mild atopic asthma. *Am J Respir Cell Mol Biol* 16: 664–673

54 Reid L (1954) Pathology of chronic bronchitis. *Lancet* i: 275–279

55 Wanner A (1988) Airway mucus and the mucociliary system. In: E Middleton, CE Reed, EF Ellis, NF Adkinson, JW Uunginer (eds): *Allergy: Principles and practice.* C.V. Mosby, St. Louis, Washington DC, Toronto, 541–548

56 Cluroe A, Holloway L, Thomson K, Purdie G, Beasley R (1989) Bronchial gland duct ectasia in fatal bronchial asthma : association with interstitial emphysema. *J Clin Pathol* 42: 1026–1031

57 Carroll N, Elliot A, Morton A, James A (1993) The structure of large and small airways in nonfatal and fatal asthma. *Am Rev Respir Dis* 147: 405–410

58 James AL, Pare PD, Hogg JC (1989) The mechanics of airway narrowing in asthma. *Am Rev Respir Dis* 139: 242–246

59 Moreno RH, Hogg JC, Pare PD (1986) Mechanisms of airway narrowing. *Am Rev Respir Dis* 133: 1171–1180

60 Wiggs BR, Moreno R, Hogg JC, Hilliam C, Pare PD (1990) A model of the mechanics of airway narrowing. *J Appl Physiol* 69: 849–860

61 Wiggs BR, Bosken C, Pare PD, James A, Hogg JC (1992) A model of airway narrowing in asthma and in chronic obstructive pulmonary disease. *Am Rev Respir Dis* 145: 1215–1218

62 Heard BE, Hossain S (1983) Hyperplasia of bronchial muscle in asthma. *J Pathol* 110: 319–331

63 Bousquet J, Chanez P, Lacoste JY et al (1992) Asthma: a disease remodeling the airways (review). *Allergy* 47 (1): 3–11

64 Jeffery PK (1994) Structural changes in asthma. In: C Page, J Black (eds): *Airways and vascular remodelling in asthma and cardiovascular disease*. Academic Press, London, 3–19
65 Stewart AG, Tomlinson PR, Wilson J (1993) Airway wall remodelling in asthma: a novel target for the development of anti-asthmatic drugs. *TiPS* 14: 275–279
66 Widdicombe J (1993) New perspectives on basic mechanisms in lung disease: Why are the airways so vascular? *Thorax* 48: 290–295
67 Saetta M, Di Stefano A, Rosina C, Thiene G, Fabbri LM (1991) Quantitative structural analysis of peripheral airways and arteries in sudden fatal asthma. *Am Rev Respir Dis* 143: 138–143
68 Synek M, Beasley R, Frew AJ et al (1996) Cellular infiltration of the airways in asthma of varying severity. *Am J Resp Crit Care Med* 154: 224–230
69 Carroll N, Carello S, Cooke C, James A (1996) Airway structure and inflammatory cells in fatal attacks of asthma. *Eur Respir J* 9: 709–715
70 Azzawi M, Bradley B, Jeffery PK et al (1990) Identification of activated T-lymphocytes and eosinophils in bronchial biopsies in stable atopic asthma. *Am Rev Respir Dis* 142: 1407–1413
71 Li D, Wang D, Griffiths-Johnson DA et al (1997) Eotaxin protein gene expression in guinea-pigs: constitutive expression and upregulation after allergen challenge. *Eur Respir J* 10: 1946–1954
72 Persson CGA, Erjefalt JS (1997) Eosinophil lysis and free granules: an *in vivo* paradigm for cell activation and drug development. *TiPS* 18: 117–123
73 Erjefalt JS, Sundler F, Persson CGA (1996) Eosinophils, neutrophils and venular gaps in the airway mucosa at epithelial removal-resitution. *Am J Respir Crit Care Med* 153: 1666–1674
74 Laitinen LA, Laitinen A, Haahtela T (1993) Airway mucosal inflammation even in patients with newly diagnosed asthma. *Am Rev Respir Dis* 147: 697–704
75 Jeffery PK, Godfrey RWA, Adelroth E, Nelson F, Rogers A, Johansson S-A (1992) Effects of treatment on airway inflammation and thickening of reticular collagen in asthma: a quantitative light and electron microscopic study. *Am Rev Respir Dis* 145: 890–899
76 Bentley AM, Maestrelli P, Saetta M et al (1992) Activated T-lymphocytes and eosinophils in the bronchial mucosa in isocyanate-induced asthma. *J Allergy Clin Immunol* 89: 821–829
77 Bentley AM, Menz G, Storz Chr et al (1992) Identification of T-lymphocytes, macrophages and activated eosinophils in the bronchial mucosa in intrinsic asthma: Relationship to symptoms and bronchial responsiveness. *Am Rev Respir Dis* 146: 500–506
78 Filley WV, Holley KE, Kephart GM, Gleich GJ (1982) Identification by immunofluorescence of eosinophil granule major basic protein in lung tissue of patients with bronchial asthma. *Lancet* 1: 11–16
79 Gerblich AA, Campbell AE, Schuyler MR (1984) Changes in T-lymphocyte subpopula-

tions after antigenic bronchial provocation in asthmatics. *N Engl J Med* 310: 1349–1352
80 Wardlaw AJ, Dunnett S, Gleich GJ, Collins JV, Kay AB (1988) Eosinophils and mast cells in bronchoalveolar lavage in mild asthma: relationship to bronchial hyperreactivity. *Am Rev Respir Dis* 137: 62–69
81 Adelroth E, Rosenhall L, Johansson S-A, Linden M, Venge P (1990) Inflammatory cells and eosinophilic activity in asthmatics investigated by bronchoalveolar lavage: the effects of anti-asthmatic treatment with budesonide or terbutaline. *Am Rev Respir Dis* 142: 91–99
82 Bradding P, Feather IH, Howarth PH et al (1992) Interleukin 4 is localized to and released by human mast cells. *J Exp Med* 176: 1381–1386
83 Denburg JA, Telizyn S, Belda A, Dolovich J, Bienenstock J (1985) Increased numbers of circulating basophil progenitors in atopic patients. *J Allergy Clin Immunol* 76: 466–472
84 Ollerenshaw SL, Woolcock AJ (1993) Quantification and location of vasoactive intestinal peptide immunoreactive nerves in bronchial biopsies from subjects with mild asthma. *Am Rev Respir Dis* 147: A285
85 Ollerenshaw SL, Jarvis D, Sullivan CE, Woolcock AJ (1991) Substance P immunoreactive nerves in airways from asthmatics and non-asthmatics. *Eur Respir J* 4: 673–682
86 Howarth PH, Springall DR, Redington AE, Djukanovic R, Holgate ST, Polak JM (1995) Neuropeptide-containing nerves in endobronchial biopsies from asthmatic and non-asthmatic subjects. *Am J Respir Cell Mol Biol* 13: 288–296
87 Sharma R, Jeffery PK (1990) Airway B-adrenoceptor number in cystic fibrosis and asthma. *Clin Sci* 78: 409–417
88 Sharma RK, Jeffery PK (1990) Airway V.I.P. receptor number is reduced in cystic fibrosis but not asthma. *Am Rev Respir Dis* 141: A726
89 Li D, Jeffery PK (1996) Experimental induction of goblet cell hyperplasia *in vivo*. In: DF Rogers (ed): *Airway mucus: basic mechanisms and clinical perspectives*. Birkhäuser Verlag, Basel
90 Harkema JR, Hotchkiss J (1992) *In vivo* effects of endotoxin on intraepithelial mucosubstances in rat pulmonary airways. *Am J Pathol* 141: 307–317
91 Medical Research Council (1965) Definition and classification of chronic bronchitis for clinical and epidemiological purposes. A report to the Medical Research Council by their Committee on the etiology of chronic bronchitis. *Lancet* i: 775–780
92 Thurlbeck WM (1977) Aspects of chronic airflow obstruction. *Chest* 72: 341–349
93 Fletcher CM, Pride MB (1984) Definition of emphysema, chronic bronchitis, asthma and airflow obstruction: twenty-five years on from the CIBRA symposium. *Thorax* 39: 81–85
94 Gibson PG, Girgis-Gabardo A, Morris MM et al (1989) Cellular characteristics of sputum from patients with asthma and chronic bronchitis. *Thorax* 44: 693–699
95 Lacoste JY, Bousquet J, Chanez P et al (1993) Eosinophilic and neutrophilic inflammation in asthma, chronic bronchitis, and chronic obstructive pulmonary disease. *J Allerg Clin Immunol* 92: 537–548

96 Ollerenshaw SL, Woolcock AJ (1992) Characteristics of the inflammation in biopsies from large airways of subjects with asthma and subjects with chronic airflow limitation. *Am Rev Respir Dis* 145: 922–927

97 Saetta M, Di Stefano A, Maestrelli P et al (1993) Activated T-lymphocytes and macrophages in bronchial mucosa of subjects with chronic bronchitis. *Am Rev Respir Dis* 147: 301–306

98 Vignola AM, Campbell AM, Chanez P et al (1993) HLA-DR and ICAM-1 expression on bronchial epithelial cells in asthma and chronic bronchitis. *Am Rev Respir Dis* 148: 689–694

99 Di Stefano A, Maestrelli P, Roggeri A et al (1994) Upregulation of adhesion molecules in the bronchial mucosa of subjects with chronic obstructive bronchitis. *Am J Respir Crit Care Med* 149: 803–810

100 O'Shaughnessy TC, Ansari TW, Barnes NC, Jeffery PK (1997) Inflammation in bronchial biopsies of subjects with chronic bronchitis: inverse relationship of $CD8^+$ T-lymphocytes with FEV1. *Am J Respir Crit Care Med* 155: 852–857

101 Saetta M, Di Stefano A, Maestrelli P et al (1994) Airway eosinophilia in chronic bronchitis during exacerbations. *Am J Respir Crit Care Med* 150: 1646–1652

102 Mullen JBM, Wright JL, Wiggs BR, Pare PD, Hogg JC (1987) Structure of central airways in current smokers and ex-smokers with and without mucus hypersecretion. *Thorax* 42: 843–846

103 Toremalm NH (1960) The daily amount of tracheobronchial secretions in man: a method for continuous tracheal aspiration in largyngectomized and tracheostimized patients. *Acta Otolarynology* 158: 43–53

104 Lopez-Vidriero MT, Reid L (1985) Bronchial mucus in asthma. In: EB Weiss, MS Segal, M Stein (eds): *Bronchial asthma: Mechanisms and therapeutics*. Little, Brown & Company, Boston, 218–235

105 Coles SJ, Bhaskar KR, O'Sullivan BD, Neill KH, Reid LM (1984) Airway mucus: composition and regulation of its secretion by neuropeptides *in vitro*. In: J Nugent, M O'Connor (eds): *Mucus and mucosa*. Ciba Foundation Symposium 109. Pitman Medical, London, 40–60

106 Reid L (1954) Pathology of chronic bronchitis. *Lancet* 1: 275–279

107 Wright RR, Stuart CM (1965) Chronic bronchitis with emphysema: a pathological study of the bronchi. *Medicina Thoracalis* 22: 210

108 Klienerman J, Boren HG (1974) Morphologic basis of chronic obstructive lung disease. In: GL Baum (ed): *Textbook of pulmonary disease*. Little Brown Company, Boston, 571

109 Chang SC (1957) Microscopic properties of whole mounts and sections of human bronchial epithelium of smokers and non-smokers. *Cancer (Phila)* 10: 1246–1262

110 Wanner A (1977) Clinical aspects of muco-ciliary transport. *Am Rev Respir Dis* 116: 73–125

111 Misokovitch G, Appel J, Szule J (1974) Ultrastructural changes of ciliated columnar epithelium and goblet cells in chronic bronchitis biopsy material. *Acta Morphol Acad Sci Hung* 22: 91–103

112 Ailsby RL, Ghadially FN (1973) Atypical cilia in human bronchial mucosa. *J Pathol* 109: 75–77

113 Wilson R, Pitt T, Taylor G et al (1987) Pyocyanin and 1-hydroxyphenazine produced by *Pseudomonas aeruginosa* inhibit the beating of human respiratory cilia *in vitro*. *J Clin Invest* 79: 221–229

114 Cosio MG, Hale KA, Niewoehner DE (1980) Morphologic and morphometric effects of prolonged cigarette smoking on the small airways. *Am Rev Respir Dis* 122: 265–271

115 Ebert RV, Terracio MJ (1975) The bronchiolar epithelium in cigarette smokers: observations with the scanning electron microscope. *Am Rev Respir Dis* 111: 4–11

116 Siafakas NM, Vermeire P, Pride NB et al (1995) Optimal assessment and management of chronic obstructive pulmonary disease (COPD). *Eur Respir J* 8: 1398–1420

117 Snider GL, Kleinerman J, Thurlbeck WM (1985) The definition of emphysema. Report of a National Heart and Blood Institute, division of lung diseases, Workshop. *Am Rev Respir Dis* 132: 182–185

118 Swan GE, Roby TJ, Hodgkin JE, Mittman C, Peters JA, Jacobo N (1994) Relationship of cytomorphology to spirometric findings in cigarette smokers. *Acta Cytologica* 38: 547–553

119 Thompson AB, Daughton D, Robbins RA, Ghafouri MA, Oehlerking M, Rennard SI (1989) Intraluminal airway inflammation in chronic bronchitis. Characterization and correlation with clinical parameters. *Am Rev Respir Dis* 140: 1527–1537

120 Linden M, Rasmussen JB, Piitulainen E et al (1993) Airway inflammation in smokers with nonobstructive and obstructive chronic bronchitis. *Am Rev Respir Dis* 148: 1226–1232

121 Lacoste J-Y, Bousquet J, Chanez P et al (1993) Eosinophilic and neutrophilic inflammation in asthma, chronic bronchitis, and chronic obstructive pulmonary disease. *J Allergy Clin Immunol* 92: 537–548

122 O'Shaughnessy TC, Ansari TW, Barnes NC, Jeffery PK (1996) Inflammatory cells in the airway surface epithelium of smokers with and without bronchitic airflow obstruction. *Eur Respir J* 9 (suppl 23): 14s

123 Buist S, Ghezzo H, Anthonisen NR et al (1979) Relationship between the single breath N2 test and age, sex and smoking habits in three North American cities. *Am Rev Respir Dis* 120: 305–318

124 Nemery B, Moavero NE, Brasseur L, Stanescu DC (1981) Significance of small airways test in middle-aged smokers. *Am Rev Respir Dis* 124: 232–238

125 Hogg JC, Macklem PT, Thurlbeck WM (1968) Site and nature of airway obstruction in chronic obstructive lung disease. *N Engl J Med* 278: 1355–1360

126 Verbeken EK, Cauberghs M, Mertens I, Lauweryns JM, van de Woestijne KP (1992) Tissue and airway impedance of excised normal, senile, and emphysematous lungs. *Am Phys Soc* 2343–2353

127 Reynolds HY (1987) Bronchoalveolar lavage. *Am Rev Respir Dis* 135: 250–263

128 Niewoehner DE, Klienerman J, Rice D (1974) Pathologic changes in the peripheral airways of young cigarette smokers. *N Engl J Med* 291: 755–758

129 Mitchell RS, Stanford RE, Johnson JM, Silvers GW, Dart G, George MS (1976) The morphologic features of the bronchi, bronchioles and alveoli in chronic airway obstruction: a clinicopathologic study. *Am Rev Respir Dis* 114: 137–145
130 Bignon J, Khoury F, Evan P, Andre J, Brouet G (1969) Morphometric study in chronic obstructive broncho-pulmonary disease. *Am Rev Respir Dis* 99: 669–695
131 Saetta M, Ghezzo H, Wong Dong Kim et al (1985) Loss of alveolar attachments in smokers. A morphometric correlate of lung function impairment. *Am Rev Respir Dis* 132: 894–900
132 Linhartova A, Anderson AE Jr, Foraker AG (1977) Further observations on lumenal deformity and stenosis of non respiratory bronchioles in pulmonary emphysema. *Thorax* 32: 50–53
133 Anderson AE, Foraker AG (1962) Relative dimensions of bronchioles and parenchymal spaces in lungs from normal subjects and emphysematous patients. *Am J Med* 32: 218–226
134 Wright JL, Hobson JE, Wiggs B, Pare PD, Hogg JC (1988) Airway inflammation and peribronchiolar attachments in the lungs of nonsmokers, current and ex-smokers. *Lung* 166: 277–286
135 Jeffery PK, Reid L (1975) New observations of rat airway epithelium: a quantitative electron microscopic study. *J Anat* 120: 295–320
136 Jeffery PK, Corrin B (1984) Structural analysis of the respiratory tract. In: J Bienenstock (ed): *Immunology of the lung*. McGraw-Hill, New York, 1–27
137 Gil J, Weibel E (1971) Extracellular lining of bronchioles after perfusion-fixation of rat lungs for electron microscopy. *Anat Rec* 169: 185–200
138 Mooren HWD, Kramps JA, Franken C, Meijer CJLM, Dijkman JA (1983) Localisation of a low-molecular weight bronchial protease inhibitor in the peripheral human lung. *Thorax* 38: 180–183
139 Kramps JA, Franken C, Dijkman JH (1984) ELISA for quantitative measurement of low-molecular-weight bronchial protease inhibitor in human sputum. *Am Rev Respir Dis* 129: 959–963
140 Ebert RV, Hanks PB (1981) Mucus secretion by the epithelium of the bronchioles of cigarette smokers. *Br J Dis Chest* 75: 277–282
141 Macklem PT, Proctor DF, Hogg JC (1970) The stability of peripheral airways. *Resp Physiol* 8: 191–203
142 Gillooly M, Lamb D (1993) Microscopic emphysema in relation to age and smoking habit. *Thorax* 48: 491–495
143 Lang MR, Fiaux GW, Gilooly M, Stewart JA, Hulmes DJS, Lamb D (1994) Collagen content of alveolar wall tissue in emphysematous and non-emphysematous lungs. *Thorax* 49: 319–326
144 Eriksson S (1964) Pulmonary emphysema and alpha 1-antitrypsin deficiency. *Acta Med Scand* 175: 197–205
145 Auerbach O, Hammond EC, Garfinkel L, Benante C (1972) Relation of smoking and age to emphysema. *N Engl J Med* 286: 853–858

146 Gadek JE, Fells GA, Crystal RG (1979) Cigarette smoking induces functional antiprotease deficiency in the lower respiratory tract of humans. *Science* 206: 1315–1316

147 Cantin A, Crystal RG (1985) Oxidants, antioxidants and the pathogenesis of emphysema. *Eur J Respir Dis* 66 (suppl 139): 7–17

148 Kimbel P (1985) Proteolytic damage and emphysema pathogenesis. In: TL Petty (ed): *Chronic obstructive pulmonary disease*, vol 28. Dekker, New York, 105–128

149 Jeffery PK (1990) Tobacco smoke-induced lung disease. In: RD Cohen, B Lewis, KGMM Alberti, AM Denman (eds): The metabolic and molecular basis of acquired disease. Balliere Tindall, London, 466–495

150 Finkelstein R, Fraser RS, Ghezzo H, Cosio MG (1995) Alveolar inflammation and its relation to emphysema in smokers. *Am J Respir Crit Care Med* 152: 1666–1672

151 Majo J, Ghezzo H, Hogg J, Cosio MG (1996) Alveolar wall inflammation in lungs of smokers. *Am J Respir Crit Care Med* 153 (4): A821

152 Hunninghake GW, Crystal RG (1983) Cigarette smoking and lung destruction: accumulation of neutrophils in the lungs of cigarette smokers. *Am Rev Respir Dis* 128: 833–838

153 Kilburn KH, McKenzie W (1975) Leucocyte recruitment to airways by cigarette smoke and particle phase in contrast to cytotoxicity of vapour. *Science* 189: 634–636

154 Ludwig WP, Hoidal JR (1982) Alterations in leucocyte oxidative metabolism in cigarette smokers. *Am Rev Respir Dis* 126: 977–980

155 Eliraz A, Kimbell P, Weinbaum G (1977) Canine alveolar macrophage and neutrophil exposure to cigarette smoke: regulation of elastase secretion. *Chest* 72: 239

156 Cohen AB, James HL (1982) Reduction of the elastase inhibitory capacity of alpha 1-antitrypsin by peroxides in cigarette smoke: an analysis of brands and filters. *Am Rev Respir Dis* 126: 25–30

157 Sandhaus RA (1983) Migration-induced elastolysis: directed migration of human neutrophils causes connective tissue proteolysis in the absence of alpha 1-protease inhibitor. *Am Rev Respir Dis* 127: 2815

158 MacNee W, Selby C (1993) New perspectives on basic mechanisms in lung disease: 2. Neutrophil traffic in the lungs: role of haemodynamics, cell adhesion and deformability. *Thorax* 48: 79–88

159 MacNee W, Wiggs B, Belzberg AS, Hogg JC (1989) The effect of cigarette smoking on neutrophil kinetics in human lungs. *N Engl J Med* 321: 924–928

160 Drost EM, Selby C, Lannan S, Lowe GDO, MacNee W (1992) Changes in neutrophil deformability following *in vitro* smoke exposure: mechanisms and protection. *Am J Resp Cell Mol Biol* 6: 287–295

161 Senior RM, Griffin GL, Mecham RP (1980) Chemotactic activity of elastin derived peptides. *J Clin Invest* 66: 859–863

162 Ward PA (1982) The chemotaxis system. In: RS Cohan, N Kaufmann (eds): *Current topics in inflammation and infection.* Williams & Wilkins, Baltimore, 54–61

163 Pryor WA (1977) The role of free radical reactions in biological systems. In: WA Pryor (ed): *Free radicals in biology*, vol 1. Academic Press, New York, 1–22

164 Hopkin JM, Tomlinson CS, Jenkins RM (1981) Variations in response to cytotoxicity of cigarette smoke. *Br Med J* 283: 1209–1211
165 Amadori A, Zamarchi R, De Silvestro G et al (1995) Genetic control of the CD4/CD8 T-cell ratio in humans. *Nature Med* 1: 1279–1283
166 Jeffery PK, Hamid Q, Majumdar S et al (1993) Antigen-primed T cells and expression of cytokine mRNA for IL4, IL5 and INF-gamma in fibrosing alveolitis associated with systemic sclerosis. *J Pathol* 170: 380A (abstract)
167 Southcott AM, Jones KP, Li D et al (1995) Interleukin-8 differential expression in lone fibrosing alveolitis and systemic sclerosis. *Am J Respir Crit Care Med* 151: 1604–1612

Role of basophils in airways inflammation

Gianni Marone, Massimo Triggiani, Giuseppe Spadaro, Anna Maria Onorati and Arturo Genovese

Division of Clinical Immunology and Allergy, University of Naples Federico II, Via S. Pansini 5, 80131 Napoli, Italy

Introduction

Human basophils were first identified by Paul Ehrlich (1878) thanks to the metachromatic staining properties of their cytoplasmic granules [1, 2]. In all mammalian species analysed so far, basophils and mast cells are the only cells that synthesize histamine and express plasma membrane receptors that bind with high affinity the Fcε portion of IgE (FcεRI) [3]. Human basophils derive from precursors that originate in the bone marrow and in foetal liver and that circulate in peripheral blood. Under normal conditions, basophils are never found in human healthy tissues. Basophils differentiate and mature in the bone marrow and circulate in the blood with a prevalence of ≅ 0.5% of total leukocytes [4]. Under certain circumstances, basophils can be recruited into the inflamed tissue during specific IgE-dependent reactions and in association with a variety of pathologic conditions [5–8]. Increasing evidence suggests that basophils and their mediators are involved in delayed-type hypersensitivity reactions in the human skin and in the lung [5, 6, 8, 9].

Identification of basophils in the airways of asthmatics

Basophils have been identified in human bronchoalveolar lavage fluid in late phase responses [8]. Basophils have also been found *post mortem* in the airway's lumen, in the bronchial epithelium and in the submucosa of fatal asthma patients [7]. Interestingly, basophils in sputum of asthmatics increase just before an asthmatic attack and after allergen-induced asthmatic responses [5]. Finally, annual changes in basophils in peripheral blood have been correlated to airways responsiveness [9]. These anatomical observations suggest that basophils and their mediators play a role in various aspects of allergic inflammation. It is important to note that degranulated basophil leukocytes can no longer be recognized by routine light microscopy.

Cellular Mechanisms in Airways Inflammation, edited by Clive P. Page, Katharine H. Banner and Domenico Spina

Table 1 - Effects of IL-3 on human basophils

Growth factor
Increases survival
Increases basophil releasability
Activates basophils to release histamine
Potentiates the release of histamine and LTC_4
Potentiates the immunologic release of IL-4
Induces chemotaxis
Stimulates adherence to vascular endothelium

Growth factor for human basophils

The principal growth and differentiation factor for human basophils appears to be IL-3 [10, 11]. IL-3 exerts multiple effects on human basophils (Tab. 1). IL-3 increases the survival of basophils *in vitro*, and is also a chemotactic and activating factor for human basophils [10–13]. In addition, preincubation of human basophils with IL-3 significantly potentiates the release of histamine, cysteinyl leukotriene C_4 (LTC_4) and IL-4 from human basophils immunologically challenged with anti-IgE or anti-FcεRI [12, 13] (Fig. 1).

Basophil adhesion molecules

Although the human basophil is predominantly a circulating cell, they have also been identified in skin at sites of contact hypersensitivity, erythema multiforme, bullous pemphigoid, and cutaneous basophil hypersensitivity reactions and in the airways of subjects with allergic rhinitis and asthma [5–8]. In addition, an influx of basophils accompanies the allergic late phase response that occurs after antigen challenge of the skin and airways [5, 6]. Thus, basophils, like other granulocytes, can migrate from the intravascular compartment into specific tissues. The observation that basophils accumulate at certain inflammatory sites suggests that they are activated and recruited to these locations. This process implies that basophils interact with endothelial cells and extracellular matrix proteins as they undergo margination and transendothelial migration, and enter the tissue space. This process involves the interaction of basophil cell surface adhesion molecules with specific adhesion molecule counter-receptors [14]. Two publications provide excellent overviews of basophil adhesion molecule biology [4, 15].

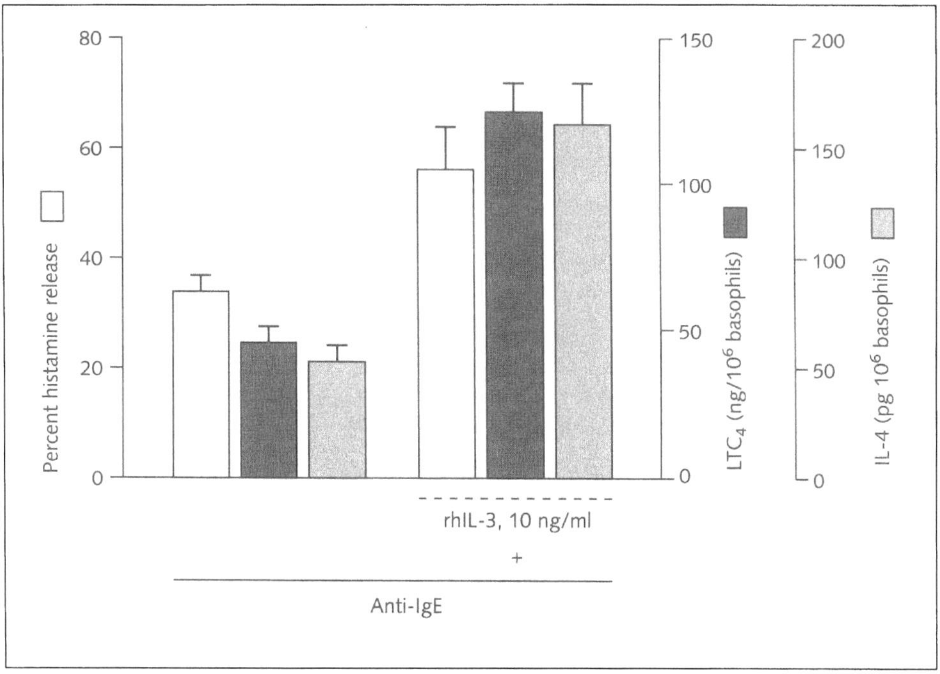

Figure 1
Effects of priming of basophils with rhIL-3 on anti-IgE-induced release of histamine, LTC_4 and IL-4. Basophils were treated or not with IL-3 (10 ng/ml for 2 h at 37° C) before the addition of anti-IgE (0.3 µg/ml). After 4 h, the cell-free supernatants were harvested for histamine, LTC_4 and IL-4 measurements. The results are presented as the mean ± SEM of four preparations of basophils.

With respect to the expression of cell adhesion molecules, basophils have on their surface several molecules belonging to the integrin, selectin, and immunoglobulin gene superfamilies, as well as carbohydrate molecules that are ligands for selectins (Tab. 2). These molecules are primarily constitutively expressed and their expression is not usually altered by cell activation. However, a major exception to this is the finding that activation by certain secretagogues, cytokines, or chemoattractans results in a rapid increase in the cell surface expression of β2 integrins (e.g., CD11b but not CD11a) and CD35 (CR1). Associated with these changes is a more gradual decline in surface expression of L-selectin [16, 17]. Identical phenotypic changes in the expression of CD11b and L-selectin appear to have occurred in basophils that have been recruited into the lower airways after segmental allergen challenge *in vivo* [18].

Human basophils express sialyl Lewis^x, a counter-receptor for selectins that mediates rolling of leukocytes on vascular cell surfaces before adhesion and trans-

*Table 2 - Expression of adhesion molecules on human basophils**

Type (Integrins)	Name (CD designation)	Ligands	Expressed on basophils
β1 (VLA) family	VLA-1, α1β1 (CD49a/CD29)	Collagen, laminin	No
	VLA-2, α2β1 (CD49b/CD29)	Collagen, laminin	No
	VLA-3, α3β1 (CD49c/CD29)	Collagen, laminin, others	No
	VLA-4, α4β1 (CD49d/CD29)	VCAM-1, fibronectin	Yes
	VLA-5, α5β1 (CD49e/CD29)	Fibronectin	Yes
	VLA-6, α6β1 (CD49f/CD29)	Laminin	No
β2 family	LFA-1, αLβ2 (CD11a/CD18)	ICAM-1, ICAM-2, ICAM-3	Yes
	Mac-1, αMβ2 (CD11b/CD18)	C3bi, ICAM-1, others	Yes
	p150,95, αXβ2 (CD11c/CD18)	C3bi, fibrinogen, others	Yes
	αdβ2	ICAM-3	Yes
β3 family	αIIbβ3 (CD41/CD61)	Fibrinogen, fibronectin, others	No
	αvβ3 (CD51/CD61)	Vitronectin, others	No
Others	α6β4 (CD49f/CD104)	Laminin	No
	Act-1, α4β7	MAdCAM-1, VCAM-1, fibronectin	Yes
	HML-1, αEβ7 (CD 103)	E-Cadherin	No
Selectins	L-selectin (CD62L)	GlyCAM-1, CD34, MAdCAM-1	Yes
	E-selectin (CD62E)	Sialyl-Lewis^{x}, others	No
	P-selectin (CD62P)	Sialyl-Lewis^{x}, others	No
Immunoglobulin gene superfamily	PECAM-1 (CD31)	CD31, others	Yes
	ICAM-1 (CD54)	LFA-1	Yes
	ICAM-2 (CD102)	LFA-1	Yes
	ICAM-3 (CD50)	LFA-1, αdβ2	Yes
Carbohydrates	Lewis^{x} (CD15)	P-selectin	No
	Sialyl-Lewis^{x} (CD15s)	E- and P-selectin	Yes
	Sialyl-dimeric Lewis^{x}	E-selectin	Yes
	PSGL-1	P-selectin	Yes

**Modified from S.S. Saini, K. Matsumoto and B.S. Bochner (Ref. [15])*

migration. Endothelial cell receptors expressed on human basophils include the β1 integrin very late activation antigen-4 (VLA-4) and the β2 integrin leukocyte function antigen-1 (LFA-1) [4, 15]. These integrins are composed of an α and β chain. Human basophils express the common β chain of β1 integrins (CD29) and β2 integrins (CD18), as well as VLA-4α (CD49d) and LFA-1α chain (CD11a). VLA-4 is a receptor for vascular cell adhesion molecule-1 (VCAM-1) expressed on activated endothelial cells and LFA-1 is a receptor for intercellular adhesion molecule-1 (ICAM-1). Binding of basophils to activated endothelium is primarily mediated *via* VCAM-1, E-selectin and ICAM-1 interactions [4]. Basophils also express the laminin receptor VLA-5, but lack CD49f, CD51/CD61 (VNR), and the β4 integrin. Human mast cells express VLA-4, VLA-5, and the vitronectin receptor α and β chain, but lack LFA-1 (CD11a/18) and CD104 [19].

Another adhesion receptor on basophils is the Pgp-1 homing receptor (CD44). The ICAM-1 antigen (CD54) is expressed on basophils. Basophils and mast cells also express ICAM-2 (CD102), ICAM-3 (CD50), and the LFA-3 antigen (CD58) on their surface, but not LFA-2 (CD2) [4]. In addition, basophils bear PECAM-1 (CD31) and L-selectin (CD62L). The x-hapten Lewis X, (CD15) is located on the basophil surface but is masked by sialic acid. Thus, basophils express CD15 when exposed to neuraminidase or to sialidase-producing viruses. Table 2 provides a summary of many of the adhesion receptors expressed on human basophils.

Immunologic and non-immunologic stimuli activating human basophils

Human basophils purified from peripheral blood can be activated by a large number of immunologic stimuli. Antigen challenge of human FcεRI$^+$ cells results in the release of preformed mediators stored in the cytoplasmic granules (e.g., histamine) and in the *de novo* synthesis and release of lipid mediators such as LTC_4 and platelet-activating factor (PAF). Antibodies raised against human Fcε (anti-IgE) or against an epitope of the α subunit of FcεRI also induce a secretory process in human basophils called "reverse anaphylaxis", similar but not identical to direct anaphylaxis [20–22].

The latter process might be important *in vivo* because there is increasing evidence that autoantibodies anti-IgE and anti-FcεRI are present in some patients with chronic urticaria and atopic syndromes [23–27]. IgG anti-IgE purified by affinity chromatography from serum of some atopic patients can induce mediator release from human basophils and mast cells [25].

Activation of basophils can also be induced by a growing list of immunological stimuli including anaphylatoxins (C3a and C5a), cytokines (IL-3, etc.), chemokines and naturally occurring (pepstatin A) or synthetic peptides (f-Met-Leu-Phe: FMLP), all of which interact with specific membrane receptors independent of the IgE receptor [28–33] (Tab. 3). Interestingly, most of the immunologic stimuli that activate

Table 3 - Immunological activators of human basophils and mast cells isolated from lung parenchyma (HLMC) and bronchoalveolar lavage (BAL-MC)

Activators	Basophils	HLMC	BAL-MC
Antigen	+	+	+
Anti-IgE	+	+	+
Anti-FcεRI	+	+	+
C3a, C5a	+	–	–
rhSCF	–	+	+
MCP-1, MCP-2	+	–	–
MCP-3, MCP-4	+	–	–
RANTES	+	–	–
Eotaxin	+	–	–
MCAF	+	–	–
Concanavalin A	+	–	–
rhIL-3	+	–	–
rhIL-8	±	–	–
Protein L from *P. magnus*	+	+	+
Protein A from *S. aureus*	+	–	–
Protein Fv	+	+	+
PAF	+	–	–

human basophils do not induce mediator release from mast cells isolated from lung parenchyma (HLMC) and bronchoalveolar lavage (BAL-MC).

Several cytokines activate human FcεRI+ cells by interacting with specific membrane receptors. Human basophils, but not mast cells, from 30% of normal and atopic donors can be activated by IL-3 [34–36]. IL-3 not only induces basophil degranulation *per se* but enhances mediator release in response to immunological and non-immunological stimuli [37–39]. In addition, IL-3 primes basophils to synthesize LTC_4 in response to stimuli such as C5a, which by themselves are unable to trigger the release of *de novo* synthesized mediators [38]. Interestingly, human basophils primed by IL-3 produce IL-4 in response to IgE receptor stimulation [40].

Chemotactic cytokines of the CC subfamily (CC chemokines) are major mediators of allergic inflammation. Several chemokines activate human basophils by interacting with at least three specific CCR receptors [41]. Basophils can be activated by the monocyte chemotactic protein (MCP) 1, MCP-2, MCP-3, MCP-4, RANTES and eotaxins to release histamine [41–47]. In particular, CCR3 receptors appear important for basophils chemotaxis, and CCR2 for mediator release from basophils [41]. Basophils can also be activated by such lipid mediators as PAF [48].

Table 4 - Basophil and mast cell mediator-releasing cytokines

	Human basophils		Human lung mast cells	
Cytokine	Trigger	Modulator	Trigger	Modulator
rhIL-1α	–	+	–	–
rhIL-1β	–	+	–	–
rhIL-2	–	–	–	–
rhIL-3	+	++	–	–
rhIL-4	–	–	–	–
rhIL-5	–	+	–	–
rhIL-6	–	–	–	–
rhIL-7	–	–	–	–
rhIL-8	±	–	–	–
rhIL-9	–	–	–	–
rhIL-10	–	–	–	–
rhGM-CSF	–	+	–	–
rhSCF	–	+	+	+
NGF	–	+	–	–
TNFα	–	–	–	–
IFNγ	–	–	–	–

The fact that a wide range of stimuli other than antigens and anti-IgE can induce mast cell and basophil activation suggests that these cells might be critical effectors not only in IgE-dependent immediate hypersensitivity disorders (allergic rhinitis, bronchial asthma and atopic dermatitis), but in a variety of diseases not involving IgE.

Besides IL-3, other cytokines, such as IL-1α and IL-1β, GM-CSF, IL-5 and NGF modulate the release of mediators from basophils [34, 37, 49] (Tab. 4). Interestingly, these cytokines do to induce or modulate mediator release from HLMC and BAL-MC. Stem cell factor (SCF) or *c-kit* receptor ligand (KL), a potent stimulator of human bone marrow progenitor cell proliferation, particularly in synergy with other growth factors (IL-6) [50], is the only cytokine so far identified that induces mediator release fron human skin, lung, heart and synovial mast cells and enhances histamine secretion induced by anti-IgE [32, 51, 52].

The results listed in Tables 3, 4 and 5 indicate that many of the activators of human basophils do not activate mast cells isolated from human tissues. For example, basophils can be activated by naturally occurring (pepstatin A) or synthetic peptides (FMLP), phorbol esters and bryostatins [53], and anaphylatoxins C3a and C5a

Table 5 - Non-immunologic activators of human basophils and mast cells isolated from lung parenchyma (HLMC) and bronchoalveolar lavage (BAL-MC)

Activators	Basophils	HLMC	BAL-MC
Ca^{2+} ionophores (A23187 and ionomycin)	+	+	+
Mitotoxin	+	+	+
Compound 48/80	–	–	–
Deuterium oxide	+	–	–
Eosinophil major basic protein	+	–	–
FMLP and Pepstatin A	+	–	–
General anesthetics*	–	+	+
Hyperosmolality	+	±	+
Morphine	–	–	–
Muscle relaxants**	–	+	N.D.
PAF	+	–	–
Phorbol esters and bryostatins	+	–	–
Substance P	–	–	N.D.

*N.D., not demonstrated; *, ketamine and propofol; **, atracurium and vecuronium*

[28] or by bioactive lipids such as PAF [48], which do not induce the release of mediators from lung mast cells. Conversely, anaesthetic drugs selectively induce histamine release from lung and skin mast cells, but not from basophils [54–56]. These results highlight some of the biochemical and immunological differences between human basophils and mast cells.

Preformed mediators of human basophils

Histamine is the only biogenic amine detected so far in human mast cells and basophils. Each basophil contains, on average, 1 pg of histamine, whereas human mast cells contain approximately 3 pg of histamine/cell [21, 22] (Tab. 6). Mast cells recovered from BAL from normal donors and asthmatics contain less histamine than parenchymal lung mast cells [21]. Mast cell granules contain high concentrations of proteases such as tryptase and chymase [22, 57, 58]. Negligible amounts of tryptase are found in human basophils, making this enzyme a specific mast cell marker.

Staining of $Fc\varepsilon RI^+$ cells with basic dyes and the expression of metachromasia are due to the highly sulphated proteoglycans contained in the secretory granules. Two classes of proteoglycans, heparin and chondroitin sulphate, have been described.

Table 6 - Chemical mediators synthesized by human basophils and mast cells isolated from lung parenchyma (HLMC)

Mediators	Basophils	HLMC
Preformed		
Histamine (pg/cell)	~ 1	~ 3
Tryptase (pg/cell)	< 0.04	~ 10
Chymase (pg/cell)	< 0.04	±
Heparin	–	+
Chondroitin sulphate A	+	–
Chondroitin sulphate E	–	+
De novo synthesized		
LTC_4 (ng/10^6 cells)*	~ 60	~ 60
PGD_2 (ng/10^6 cells)*	< 0.006	~ 60
TxA_2 (ng/10^6 cells)*	≈ 0.005	~ 5
PAF (ng/10^6 cells)*	~ 0.2**	~ 1
AAGPC (ng/10^6 cells)*	~ 0.3**	~ 3

*N.D., not demonstrated; *, amount released upon IgE-mediated challenge; **, as measured by the incorporation of radiolabelled acetate.*

Heparin is the major proteoglycan in human lung and skin mast cell granules, whereas different chondroitin sulphates are prevalent in the granules of basophils and of intestinal mast cells [59–61].

Lipid metabolism in human basophils

Large quantities of arachidonic acid are stored in membrane glycerolipids of human basophils. Upon cell activation, arachidonic acid is mobilized from the storage pools by various phospholipases and is converted to leukotrienes by 5-LO and to prostanoids by cyclooxygenases (COX) [62]. The profile of eicosanoids generated by activated human basophils and mast cells has been extensively studied [62–64].

Lung and skin mast cells synthesize approximately 60 ng of $PGD_2/10^6$ cells when challenged with IgE-mediated stimuli [55, 65]. In contrast, basophils do not produce PGD_2 or any other known cyclo-oxygenase metabolite. Arachidonic acid can also be metabolized by 5-lipoxygenase (5-LO) to the unstable metabolite leukotriene A_4 (LTA_4) [64]. The enzyme, normally located in the cytosol, is translocated to the membrane upon cell activation to form a stable complex with other components of the leukotriene synthetic pathway and with a membrane protein named "5-lipoxygenase activating protein" (FLAP). Formation of the FLAP-5-LO complex is essential to regulate the interaction of 5-LO with its substrate, arachidonic acid. Once formed, LTA_4 can be converted either to leukotriene B_4, a potent chemotactic factor for polymorphonuclear leukocytes, by LTA_4 hydrolase [66], or to LTC_4 by conjugation with reduced glutathione, catalyzed by the specific enzyme LTC_4 synthase [67]. Once secreted, LTC_4 is metabolized sequentially to the two metabolites leukotrienes D_4 (LTD_4), by removal of glutamine, and E_4 (LTE_4), by removal of glycine. Cysteinyl-leukotrienes C_4, D_4, and E_4 make up the biological mixture that used to be referred to as the "slow-reacting substance of anaphylaxis" (SRS-A) [68].

Immunologically activated human basophils and lung mast cells generate approximately 60 ng of $LTC_4/10^6$ cells on average [69], whereas skin mast cells challenged with IgE- and non-IgE-mediated stimuli generate little or none [70].

Cysteinyl-leukotrienes C_4, D_4 and E_4 have been implicated in the pathogenesis of allergic rhinitis and bronchial asthma. Upon inhalation, they reduce airway conductance in asthmatics [71]. Levels of cysteinyl-leukotrienes are elevated in biological fluids from asthmatics. Moreover, LTD_4 receptor antagonists [72, 73] or inibitors of 5-LO activity [74, 75] have an appreciable effect on bronchial and nasal antigen challenge.

The biochemical basis of the different profiles of eicosanoids released by basophils and mast cells isolated from different anatomical sites is not known. However, our knowledge of the mechanisms of eicosanoid synthesis in basophils and mast cells took a step forward with the identification of novel enzymes and regulatory molecules involved in arachidonic acid metabolism [65, 76]. At least two major phospholipases A_2 (PLA_2) are involved in arachidonate mobilization in mast cells: a high molecular weight cytosolic PLA_2 ($cPLA_2$) and a low molecular weight secretory PLA_2 ($sPLA_2$) [77, 78]. $cPLA_2$ is an arachidonate-selective PLA_2 activated by micromolar Ca^{2+} concentrations [79]. Upon translocation to the nuclear membrane, $cPLA_2$ generates free arachidonate that is mostly converted to leukotrienes. There are two mechanisms of upregulation of $cPLA_2$ in mast cells activated by IgE-dependent stimuli: a rapid mechanism occurring within minutes after cell activation based on phosphorylation mediated by MAP kinase, and a delayed mechanism based on transcription and expression of new enzyme molecules [80]. The latter mechanism requires several hours to be effective and is strongly modulated by cytokines [81].

$sPLA_2$ is stored within cytoplasmic granules of quiescent mast cells [82] and is rapidly released when the cells are activated by immunological stimuli or by such cytokines as SCF. $sPLA_2$ is a non arachidonate-selective enzyme and requires for its activation millimolar concentrations of Ca^{2+}, such as those found in the extracellular milieu. $sPLA_2$ can be considered for many aspects a mediator of inflammation because: (1) it is released in discrete amounts in the extracellular environment after immunological activation of mast cells [82]; (2) it can be measured *in vivo* in such inflammatory fluids as the bronchoalveolar lavage of asthmatic patients [83] and the synovial fluid of patients with rheumatoid arthritis [84] and (3) its administration reproduces signs and symptoms of inflammation [85]. Once released, $sPLA_2$ can hydrolyze phospholipids on the outer layer of the cytoplasmic membrane of mast cells thereby generating arachidonate that is mostly converted to prostanoids such as PGD_2. In addition, recent evidence suggests the presence of a specific membrane receptor for $sPLA_2$ on murine mast cells [86]. Activation of this receptor, which is blocked by heparin, induces the release of both preformed (histamine and proteases) and *de novo* synthesized mediators (eicosanoids). The existence of an $sPLA_2$ receptor on human mast cells has not yet been demonstrated.

PAF, originally discovered as a factor synthesized by immunologically activated rabbit basophils [87], an ether-linked phospholipid (1-alkyl-2-acetyl-*sn*-glycero-3-phosphocholine: AGEPC) [88], can be synthesized by human lung mast cells challenged with anti-IgE (~ 1 ng/10^6 cells) [89]. Human basophils produce much smaller amounts of PAF than do mast cells [90]. Besides PAF, the 1-acyl analog of PAF (1-acyl-2-acetyl-*sn*-glycero-3-phosphocoline: AAGPC) is synthesized by human lung mast cells, and basophils in amounts two to four times greater than PAF [90]. These results introduced the concept of "2-acetylated phospholipids", i.e., molecules having the common feature of an acetyl group at the *sn*-2 position of the glycerol backbone.

Cytokine and chemokine expression in human basophils

Several groups of investigators have demonstrated the generation and secretion of IL-4 by human basophils after IgE-dependent activation. Brunner et al. presented the first evidence for the release of IL-4 from normal basophils purified by combining countercurrent elutriation and negative selection techniques [40]. IL-4 protein levels increased substantially, as did leukotriene C_4 (LTC_4) generation, if basophil cultures were pretreated with IL-3 for 18 h before stimulation. Arock et al. using human leukemic and bone marrow-derived basophils, found that IL-3 was essential for the development of cells expressing IL-4 message and secreting protein [91]. Sustained pretreatment with IL-3 before stimulation with anti-IgE antibody was not an absolute requirement for the secretion of IL-4 from pure (88% to 99%) basophils [92]. However, preincubation with IL-3 markedly potentiated the immunologic release of IL-4 from purified basophils.

The kinetics of IL-4 secretion from basophils suggest that this cytokine is generated de novo on immunologic activation and is not stored and released on degranulation, as has been suggested for some mast cell-derived cytokines. Unlike the release of histamine that occurs within minutes after IgE cross linking, approximately 2 h are needed before IL-4 protein is first detected in basophil cultures, with levels peaking at 4 to 5 h. The ability of cycloheximide to ablate the secretion of IL-4 indicates that protein synthesis is necessary for the generation of this cytokine in basophils. However, the kinetics of IL-4 release from basophils is considerably less than the 12 to 16 h required for IL-4 production by antigen-stimulated T lymphocytes. Resting basophils constitutively express IL-4 mRNA, as shown by Northern blot and reverse transcriptase polymerase chain reaction analysis. In addition, IL-4 mRNA accumulates in response to stimulation. Experiments investigating the dose-response relationship of anti-IgE stimulation showed that IL-4 secretion is optimal at lower concentrations than those necessary for optimal histamine release. Interestingly, highly purified preparations of basophil suspensions generated less IL-4 in response to IgE-mediated stimulation. These observations suggest that basophils subjected to the stress occurring during purification produce less IL-4 protein in response to IgE-dependent stimulation than do those in freshly isolated enriched cultures, and that IL-3 pretreatment may function to restore cytokine releasability after purification.

There is compelling evidence that immunologically activated human basophils also release IL-13 [93, 94]. Expression of IL-4 and other cytokines typically associated with a Th2 phenotype (IL-3, IL-5, IL-13, and GM-CSF) has been so far documented in mast cells from different human tissues [95–99]. Immunohistochemical data indicate that human mast cells contain IL-4, IL-5, IL-6 and TNFα [95, 96]. We have recently demonstrated by immunogold staining the presence of SCF, the principal growth differentiating, chemotactic and activating factor of human mast cells, in secretory granules of human mast cells [100, 101].

Basophils purified from peripheral blood express immunoreactive MIP-1α upon stimulation with anti-IgE [102]. Preincubation with IL-3 (15 min to 18 h) augmented anti-IgE-induced MIP-1α production from basophils. MIP-1α has potent proinflammatory and histamine-releasing activities and, therefore, its production by basophils suggests the existence of a positive feedback for allergic inflammation.

Several studies have focused on IL-4 gene transcription in transformed mouse mast cell lines. However, few studies have been conducted to date to analyze the mechanisms of gene expression in basophils. Human basophils express mRNA for nuclear proteins GATA-2 and GATA-3, suggesting a role of these proteins in gene regulation in these cells [103]. The role of nuclear factor of activated T cells (NFAT)-1 and related proteins has been investigated in cytokine expression in FcεRI$^+$ cells. NFAT-1 has been involved in the transcription of most cytokine genes expressed in mast cells and basophils, among which IL-3, IL-4 IL-5, GM-CSF, TNFα, and, perhaps, IL-13 [103, 104]. An NFAT-1-immunoreactive protein has been recently detected by immunofluorescence staining of human basophils (V. Casolaro, personal communication). Like NFAT-1, this protein is constitutively expressed in the cytoplasm, while IgE- or Ca^{2+}-mediated stimulation induces its translocation to the nucleus. This phenomenon occurs rapidly (within 5 min) and is typically blocked by cyclosporin A or FK-506. Taken together, these findings raise the possibility that unique transcription factors contribute to basophil- or mast cell-restricted cytokine gene expression.

The observation that several cytokines can be synthesized by human basophils and mast cells indicates that these cells play a complex role in chronic inflammation of the upper and lower airways in man.

Basophils and mast cells as effector cells of allergic inflammation

Histological, biochemical, and pharmacological findings supports the involvement of basophils and mast cells and their mediators in the pathogenesis of allergic disorders of the upper and lower respiratory tract. Airway inflammation has long been recognized as a prominent feature of fatal asthma attacks [7, 105, 106]. Recently, inflammatory findings have been reported in bronchial biopsies of even mild asthmatics [107]. There is now evidence that inflammation of the airways is a critical feature presumably leading to bronchial hyper-responsiveness [108], which is a typical feature of asthma. These changes are very likely produced by the proinflammatory mediators, cytokines and chemokines released from inflammatory cells residing in the airways.

Kimura et al. reported an increase in the number of basophils in the sputum from asthmatic patients before the onset of an asthmatic attack, and the number of basophils was related to the severity of the relapse [109]. Basophils have been observed in nasal secretions of allergic patients challenged with antigens, and their presence has been closely related to mediator release and clinical symptoms [110, 111]. A higher percentage of mast cells is recovered from the BAL of asthmatics than controls [112] and the histamine and PGD_2 concentrations in the BAL are also higher in these patients [21].

The release of chemical mediators from $Fc\varepsilon RI^+$ cells is influenced both by surface density of IgE molecules, and by a biochemical process, defined "releasability" [113–115]. Basophil and mast cell releasability are independently controlled [21] and the former appears to be under genetic control [114, 116]. An increase in IgE- and non-IgE-mediated basophil releasability has been detected in patients with allergic rhinitis and bronchial asthma [21]. Interestingly, basophil reactivity to anti-IgE was significantly higher in asthmatics than in patients with allergic rhinitis [21]. The IgE-mediated releasability of BAL mast cells from mild asthmatics is also greater than in normal age-matched donors [21]. Thus, basophil and mast cell releasability in response to IgE-mediated stimuli is increased in respiratory allergy, and more so in bronchial asthma. Infiltrating basophils contribute with eosinophils and other cells to the chronic inflammatory events of allergic disease. The growing evidence that IgE cross-linking initiates synthesis and secretion of several cytokines and chemokines by human basophils [91–94, 102] and mast cells [95–99, 101] supports the hypothesis that these cells play not only a proinflammatory but an immunomodulatory role in allergic disorders.

The role of mast cells and basophils in the pathogenesis of allergic disorders is indirectly supported by pharmacological evidence. Drugs active in the prevention or treatment of these disorders such as methylxanthines [117], corticosteroids [118], β-adrenergic agents [29, 30], cyclosporin A [119–121], and FK-506 [122–124] inhibit the release of histamine and other mediators from FcεRI$^+$ cells *in vivo* and *in vitro*.

Role of basophils in bacterial and viral infections

There is compelling evidence that viral respiratory tract infections are a major cause of wheezing in infants and adults with asthma. Viruses can exacerbate bronchial inflammation and provoke asthma through different immunologic mechanisms [125]. There is also the possibility that bacterial infections play a role in some allergic disorders [126, 127].

Although human basophils possess surface receptor for formyl-containing bacterial peptides [128], no evidence existed as to the *in vivo* significance of these cells in bacterial infections. Several reports have demonstrated that mast cells, which are selectively located at the portals of bacterial entry, are important for host defence [129, 130]. Mast cell-deficient mice (W/W^v) are significantly less efficient than normal +/+ littermates in clearing enterobacteria and this phenomenon is, at least in part, due to decreased TNFα production [129, 130]. Moreover, leukotriene-deficient mice manifest enhanced lethality from *Klebsiella pneumoniae* [131]. These results revealed a previously unrecognised role of mast cells in bacterial infections.

It is important to note that such bacterial factors as pepstatin A [128, 132], type 1 fimbriae of *Escherichia coli* [133], protein A of *Staphylococcus aureus* [29], and protein L of *Peptostreptococcus magnus* [32] can activate human basophils and/or mast cells through different immunologic mechanisms. Interestingly, such viral products as gp120 of HIV-1 and protein Fv, *in vivo* induced during viral hepatitis, can also activate human basophils and mast cells to release proinflammatory mediators and immunoregulatory cytokines [33, 33a]. In collaboration with Jean-Pierre Bouvet, we have found that protein Fv, which is an endogenous superantigen released *in vivo* in patients suffering from viral hepatitis [134], stimulated not only the release of histamine from purified peripheral blood basophils, but also the *de novo* synthesis of IL-4 [100, 100a]. Taken together, these observations suggest that basophils can play a role during viral and bacterial infections.

Immunopharmacology of human basophils and mast cells

Numerous studies have focused on the *in vitro* and *in vivo* effects of drugs that modulate the release of preformed and *de novo* synthesized mediators from human basophils and mast cells isolated from different tissues [29, 117–124]. Significant differences have been documented: (a) between mast cells and basophils as regards the pharmacological agents and the mediators they produce; (b) between mast cells isolated from different anatomical sites; and (c) between compounds of the same pharmacologic class. In addition, this approach has significantly contributed to clarifying the biochemical mechanisms by which these cells release mediators in response to immunologic and non-immunologic stimuli [29, 117–124].

Closing remarks

Basophils, which are absent from healthy human tissues, are found at sites of allergen challenge in the nose, and in the upper and lower airways [5, 7–9]. In particular, the density of basophils at sites of allergen-induced inflammation is relatively large compared with their limited numbers in the circulation. Activated basophils have been detected in the airways of post-mortem cases of fatal asthma [7].

These *in vivo* observations suggest that basophils, like other granulocytes, can emigrate from the intravascular compartment into specific tissues. Tremendous effort has been put into trying to understand the molecular mechanisms mediating the adhesion of basophils to endothelial cells and their recruitment to allergic and other inflammatory lesions [15]. The availability of large panels of monoclonal antibodies has prompted extensive phenotypic analyses of human basophils [4, 15–18].

Basophils express a unique of pattern of cell surface adhesion molecules and the expression of some of these molecules, such as β2 integrins and L-selectin, is altered during cell activation [17]. Interestingly, similar phenotypic changes occur in basophils recruited into the upper and lower airways after allergen challenge *in vivo* [18]. Parallel studies have identified two types of stimuli that are responsible for the preferential recruitment of basophils at sites of allergic inflammation. Several chemotactic factors (C5a, FMLP and PAF), cytokines (IL-3) and IgE-dependent stimuli (allergen and anti-IgE) can stimulate basophil adhesion to endothelial cells *in vitro*. In addition, several C-C chemokines (RANTES, MIP-1α, MCP-1, MCP-2, MCP-3 and MCP-4) can promote basophil chemotaxis and/or activation [41–43]. Taken together, these findings account, at least in part, for the selective basophil recruitment and activation during late-phase allergic reactions of the upper and lower respiratory tract [5, 8, 18].

Another interesting feature of human basophils, distinct from mast cells, is their susceptibility to activation and priming by several cytokines. Besides IL-3, which is the most effective cytokine in terms of basophil activation and priming, other such cytokines as IL-1α and IL-1β, GM-CSF, IL-5 and NGF can modulate the release of pro-inflammatory mediators (histamine and cysteinyl leukotriene C_4) and indeed cytokines themselves, i.e., IL-4 [34, 37–40, 49]. These observations imply that once basophils are recruited at sites of allergic inflammation and exposed to high levels of local cytokines, they become hyper-responsive to a variety of immunologic stimuli.

The clinical relevance of the basophils/cytokine inter-relationship clearly emerges from the demonstration that immunologically activated basophils synthetise and release cytokines, i.e., IL-4 and IL-13 [40, 92, 93] and the MIP-1α chemokine [102].

Finally, it is now evident that human basophils play a major and dual role in the immediate and late phases of allergic inflammation of the upper and lower airways. First through the release of pro-inflammatory and fibrogenetic mediators (histamine, leukotrienes etc.), and second through the production of immunoregulatory cytokines and chemokines. These observations provide the rationale for the concept that basophils and their mediators represent critical targets for an immunopharmacological approach to allergic disorders of the airways.

Acknowledgments

This work was supported by grants from the C.N.R. (Targeted Project Biotechnology No. 99.00216.PF31 and 99.00401.PF49), the M.U.R.S.T. and Ministero della Sanità-Istituto Superiore Sanità (AIDS Project 40B.64 and 40.B1) (Rome, Italy).

References

1 Ehrlich P (1878) *Beiträge zur Theorie und Praxis der histologischen Färbung*. Leipzig, Thesis

2 Ehrlich P (1879) Beiträge zur Kenntniss der granulirten Bindegewebszellen und der eosinophilen Leukocythen. *Arch Anat Physiol* 166–169

3 Scharenberg AM, Kinet J-P (1995) Early events in mast cell signal transduction. In: Marone G (ed): *Human basophils and mast cells: biological aspects*. Karger, Basel, 72–87

4 Valent P (1995) Immunophenotypic characterization of human basophils and mast cells. In: Marone G (ed): *Human basophils and mast cells: biological aspects*. Karger, Basel, 34–48

5 Liu MC, Hubbard WC, Proud D, Stealey BA, Galli SJ, Kagey-Sobotka A, Bleecker ER, Lichtenstein LM (1991) Immediate and late inflammatory responses to ragweed antigen challenge of the peripheral airways in allergic asthmatics. Cellular, mediator, and permeability changes. *Am Rev Respir Dis* 144: 51–58

6 Charlesworth EN, Kagey-Sobotka A, Schleimer RP, Norman PS, Lichtenstein LM (1991) Prednisone inhibits the appearance of inflammatory mediators and the influx of eosinophils and basophils associated with the cutaneous late-phase response to allergen. *J Immunol* 146: 671–676

7 Koshino T, Teshima S, Fukushima N, Takaishi T, Hirai K, Miyamoto Y, Arai Y, Sano Y,

Ito K, Morita Y (1993) Ientification of basophils by immunohistochemistry in the airways of post-mortem cases of fatal asthma. *Clin Exp Allergy* 23: 919–925
8 Guo C-B, Liu MC, Galli SJ, Bochner BS, Kagey-Sobotka A, Lichtenstein LM (1994) Identification of IgE-bearing cells in the late-phase response to antigen in the lung as basophils. *Am J Respir Cell Mol Biol* 10: 384–390
9 Sparrow D, O'Connor GT, Rosner B, Weiss ST (1994) Predictors of longitudinal change in methacholine airway responsiveness among middle-aged and older men: the normative aging study. *Am J Respir Crit Care Med* 149: 376–381
10 Valent P, Schmidt G, Besemer J, Mayer P, Zenke G, Liehl E, Hinterberger W, Lechner K, Maurer D, Bettelheim P (1989) Interleukin-3 is a differentiation factor for human basophils. *Blood* 73: 1763–1769
11 Kirshenbaum AS, Goff JP, Kessler SW, Mican JM, Zsebo KM, Metcalfe DD (1992) Effect of IL-3 and stem cell factor on the appearance of human basophils and mast cells from $CD34^+$ pluripotent progenitor cells. *J Immunol* 148: 772–777
12 de Paulis A, Ciccarelli A, Cirillo R, de Crescenzo G, Columbo M, Marone G (1992) Cytokine-induced modulation of human $Fc\varepsilon RI^+$ inflammatory cells. In: S Romagnani, TR Mosmann, AK Abbas (eds): *New advances on cytokines*. Raven Press, New York, 367–383
13 Brunner T, Heusser CH, Dahinden CA (1993) Human peripheral blood basophils primed by interleukin 3 (IL-3) produce IL-4 in response to immunoglobulin E receptor stimulation. *J Exp Med* 177: 605–611
14 Bochner BS, Sterbinsky SA, Briskin M, Saini SS, MacGlashan DW Jr (1996) Counter-receptors on human basophils for endothelial cell adhesion molecules. *J Immunol* 157: 844–850
15 Saini SS, Matsumoto K, Bochner BS (1997) Phenotypic and functional characteristics of adhesion molecules on human basophils. In: BS Bochner (ed): *Adhesion molecules in allergic disease*. Marcel Dekker, New York, 129–138
16 Bochner BS, McKelvey AA, Sterbinsky SA, Hildreth JEK, Derse CP, Klunk DA, Lichtenstein LM, Schleimer RP (1990) IL-3 augments adhesiveness for endothelium and CD11b expression in human basophils but not neutrophils. *J Immunol* 145: 1832–1837
17 Bochner BS, Sterbinsky SA (1991) Altered surface expression of CD11 and Leu 8 during human basophil degranulation. *J Immunol* 146: 2367–2373
18 Georas SN, Liu MC, Newman W, Beall WD, Stealey BA, Bochner BS (1992) Altered adhesion molecule expression and endothelial activation accompanies the recruitment of human granulocytes to the lung following segmental antigen challenge. *Am J Respir Cell Mol Biol* 7: 261–269
19 Columbo M, Bochner BS, Marone G (1995) Human skin mast cells express functional b1 integrins that mediate adhesion to extracellular matrix proteins. *J Immunol* 154: 6058–6064
20 Marone G, Kagey-Sobotka A, Lichtenstein LM (1981) IgE-mediated histamine release from human basophils: differences between antigen E- and Anti-IgE-induced secretion. *Int Archs Allergy Appl Immunol* 65: 339–348

21 Casolaro V, Spadaro G, Marone G (1990) Human basophil releasability. VI. Changes in basophil releasability in patients with allegic rhinitis or bronchial asthma. *Am Rev Respir Dis* 142: 1108–1111
22 Patella V, Marinò I, Lampärter B, Arbustini E, Adt M, Marone G (1995) Human heart mast cells. Isolation, purification, ultrastructure, and immunologic characterization. *J Immunol* 154: 2855–2865
23 Quinti I, Brozek C, Wood N, Geha RS, Leung DYM (1986) Circulating IgG autoantibodies to IgE in atopic syndromes. *J Allergy Clin Immunol* 77: 586–594
24 Marone G, Casolaro V, Quinti I, Paganelli R, Spadaro G, Stellato C (1989) Mast cell and basophil activation by human anti-IgE autoantibodies. In: JP Werner, MS Beda, C Dahinden, AR Pécoud, PC Frei, C Schneider, AL de Weck (eds): *Progress in allergy and clinical immunology.* Hogrefe & Huber Publishers, Toronto, 125–128
25 Marone G, Casolaro V, Paganelli R, Quinti I (1989) IgG anti-IgE from atopic dermatitis induces mediator release from basophils and mast cells. *J Invest Dermatol* 93: 246–252
26 Hide M, Francis DM, Grattan CEH, Hakimi J, Kochan JP, Greaves MW (1993) Autoantibodies against the high-affinity IgE receptor as a cause of histamine release in chronic urticaria. N Engl J Med 328: 1599–1604
27 Tong LJ, Balakrishnan G, Kochan JP, Kinét J-P, Kaplan AP (1997) Assessment of autoimmunity in patients with chronic urticaria. *J Allergy Clin Immunol* 99: 461–465
28 Glovsky MM, Hugli TE, Ishizaka T, Lichtenstein LM, Erickson BW (1979) Anaphylatoxin-induced histamine release with human leukocytes. *J Clin Invest* 64: 804–811
29 Marone G, Poto S, Petracca R, Triggiani M, De Lutio di Castelguidone E, Condorelli M (1982) Activation of human basophils by staphylococcal protein A. I. The role of cyclic AMP, arachidonic acid metabolites, microtubules and microfilaments. *Clin Exp Immunol* 50: 661–668
30 Marone G, Columbo M, Soppelsa L, Condorelli M (1984) The mechanism of basophil histamine release induced by pepstatin A. *J Immunol* 133: 1542–1546
31 MacGlashan DW Jr, Hubbard WC (1993) IL-3 alters free arachidonic acid generation in C5a-stimulated human basophils. *J Immunol* 151: 6358–6369
32 Patella V, Casolaro V, Björck L, Marone G (1990) Protein L. A bacterial Ig-binding protein that activates human basophils and mast cells. *J Immunol* 145: 3054–3061
33 Patella V, Bouvet J-P, Marone G (1993) Protein Fv produced during viral hepatitis is a novel activator of human basophils and mast cells. *J Immunol* 151: 5685–5698
33a Patella V, Florio G, Petraroli A, Marone G (2000) HIV-1 gp120 induces IL-4 and IL-13 release from human FcεRI$^+$ cells through interaction with the V_H3 region of IgE. *J Immunol* 164: 589–595
34 Haak-Frendscho M, Arai N, Arai K-i, Baeza ML, Finn A, Kaplan AP (1988) Human recombinant granulocyte-macrophage colony-stimulating factor and interleukin 3 cause basophil histamine release. *J Clin Invest* 82: 17–20
35 MacDonald SM, Schleimer RP, Kagey-Sobotka A, Gillis S, Lichtenstein LM (1989)

Recombinant IL-3 induces histamine release from human basophils. *J Immunol* 142: 3527–3532
36 de Paulis A, Valentini G, Spadaro G, Lupoli S, Tirri G, Marone G (1991) Human basophil releasability. VIII. Increased basophil releasability in patients with scleroderma. *Arthritis Rheum* 34: 1289–1296
37 Bischoff SC, de Weck AL, Dahinden CA (1990) Interleukin 3 and granulocyte/macrophage-colony-stimulating factor render human basophils responsive to low concentrations of complement component C3a. *Proc Natl Acad Sci USA* 87: 6813–6817
38 Kurimoto Y, de Weck AL, Dahinden CA (1991) The effect of interleukin 3 upon IgE-dependent and IgE-independent basophil degranulation and leukotriene generation. *Eur J Immunol* 21: 361–368
39 de Paulis A, Cirillo R, Ciccarelli A, Condorelli M, Marone G (1991) FK-506, a potent novel inhibitor of the release of proinflammatory mediators from human FcεRI⁺ cells. *J Immunol* 146: 2374–2381
40 Brunner T, Heusser CH, Dahinden CA (1993) Human peripheral blood basophils primed by interleukin 3 (IL-3) produce IL-4 in response to immunoglobulin E receptor stimulation. *J Exp Med* 177: 605–611
41 Uguccioni M, Mackay CR, Ochensberger B, Loetscher P, Rhis S, LaRosa GJ, Rao P, Ponath PD, Baggiolini M, Dahinden CA (1997) High expression of the chemokine receptor CCR3 in human blood basophils. Role in activation by eotaxin, MCP-4, and other chemokines. *J Clin Invest* 100: 1137–1143
42 Weber M, Uguccioni M, Ochensberger B, Baggiolini M, Clerk-Lewis I, Dahinden CA (1995) Monocyte chemotactic protein MCP-2 activates human basophil and eosinophil leukocytes similar to MCP-3. *J Immunol* 154: 4166–4172
43 Uguccioni M, Loetscher P, Forssmann U, Dewald B, Li H, Lima SH, Li Y, Kreider B, Garotta G, Thelen M et al (1996) Monocyte chemotactic protein 4 (MCP-4), a novel structural and functional analogue of MCP-3 and eotaxin. *J Exp Med* 183: 2379–2384
44 Pasmans SGMA, Aalbers M, Daha MR, Knol EF, Jansen HM, Aalberse RC (1996) Histamine-releasing activity in supernatants of mononuclear cells: contribution of monocyte chemotactic protein-1 activity compared with IgE-dependent activity. *J Allergy Clin Immunol* 98: 962–968
45 MacDonald SM, Rafnar T, Langdon J, Lichtenstein LM (1995) Molecular identification of an IgE-dependent histamine-releasing factor. *Science* 269: 688–690
46 Kuna P, Reddigari SR, Rucinski D, Oppenheim JJ, Kaplan AP (1992) Monocyte chemotactic and activting factor is a potent histamine-releasing factor for human basophils. *J Exp Med* 175: 489–493
47 Alam R, Lett-Brown MA, Forsythe PA, Anderson-Walters DJ, Kenamore C, Kormos C, Grant JA (1992) Monocyte chemotactic and activating factor is a potent histamine-releasing factor for basophils. *J Clin Invest* 89: 723–728
48 Columbo M, Casolaro V, Warner JA, MacGlashan DW Jr, Kagey-Sobotka A, Lichtenstein LM (1990) The mechanism of mediator release from human basophils induced by platelet-activating factor *J Immunol* 145: 3855–3861

49 Bürgi B, Otten UH, Ochensberger B, Rihs S, Heese K, Ehrhard PB, Ibanez CF, Dahinden CA (1996) Basophil priming by neurotrophic factors. Activation through the trk receptor. *J Immunol* 157: 5582–5588

50 Saito H, Ebisawa M, Tachimoto H, Shichijo M, Fukagawa K, Matsumoto K, Likura Y, Awaji T, Tsujimoto G, Yanagida M et al (1996) Selective growth of human cells induced by steel factor, IL-6, and prostaglandin E_2 from cord blood mononuclear cells. *J Immunol* 157: 343–350

51 Columbo M, Horowitz EM, Botana LM, MacGlashan DW Jr, Bochner BS, Gillis S, Zsebo KM, Galli SJ, Lichtenstein LM (1992) The human recombinant c-kit receptor ligand, rhSCF, induces mediator release from human cutaneous mast cells and enhances IgE-dependent mediator release from both skin mast cells and peripheral blood basophils. *J Immunol* 149: 599–608

52 de Paulis A, Ciccarelli A, Cirillo R, de Crescenzo G, Columbo M, Marone G (1992) Modulation of human lung mast cell function by the c-kit receptor ligand. *Int Arch Allergy Immunol* 99: 326–329

53 Patella V, Casolaro V, Ciccarelli A, Pettit GR, Columbo M, Marone G (1995) The antineoplastic bryostatins affect human basophils and mast cells differently. *Blood* 85: 1272–1281

54 Stellato C, de Paulis A, Cirillo R, Mastronardi P, Mazzarella B, Marone G (1991) Heterogeneity of human mast cells and basophils in response to muscle relaxants. *Anesthesiology* 74: 1078–1086

55 Stellato C, Casolaro V, Ciccarelli A, Mastronardi P, Mazzarella B, Marone G (1991) General anaesthetics induce only histamine release selectively from human mast cells. *Br J Anaesthesia* 67: 751–758

56 Stellato C, Cirillo R, de Paulis A, Casolaro V, Patella V, Mastronardi P, Mazzarella B, Marone G (1992) Human basophil/mast cell releasability. IX. Heterogeneity of the effects of opioids on mediator release. *Anesthesiology* 77: 932–940

57 Patella V, de Crescenzo G, Marinò I, Genovese A, Adt M, Gleich GJ, Marone G (1996) Eosinophil granule proteins activate human heart mast cells. *J Immunol* 157: 1219–1225

58 de Paulis A, Marinò I, Ciccarelli A, de Crescenzo G, Concardi M, Verga L, Arbustini E, Marone G (1996) Human synovial mast cells. I. Ultrastructure *in situ* and *in vitro* immunologic characterization. *Arthritis Rheum* 39: 1222–1233

59 Metcalfe DD, Lewis RA, Silbert JE, Rosenberg RD, Wasserman SI, Austen KF (1979) Isolation and characterization of heparin from human lung. *J Clin Invest* 4: 1537–1543

60 Metcalfe DD, Bland CE, Wasserman SI (1984) Biochemical and functional characterization of proteoglycans isolated from basophils of patients with chronic myelogenous leukaemia. *J Immunol* 132: 1943–1950

61 Chieffi Baccari G, de Paulis A, Di Matteo L, Gentile M, Marone G, Minucci S (1998) *In situ* characterization of mast cells in the frog Rana esculenta. *Cell & Tissue Res* 292: 151–162

62 Triggiani M, Casolaro V, Genovese A, Spadaro G, Marone G (1993) Heterogeneity of human FcεRI-bearing cells. *Ann Allergy* 71: 133–138

63 Dahinden CA, Clancy RM, Gross M, Chiller JM, Hugli TE (1985) Leukotriene C_4 production by murine mast cells: evidence of a role for extracellular leukotriene A_4. *Proc Natl Acad Sci USA* 82: 6632–6636

64 Triggiani M, Oriente A, de Crescenzo G, Marone G (1995) Metabolism of lipid mediators in human basophils and mast cells. In: G Marone (ed): *Human basophils and mast cells: biological aspects*. Karger, Basel, 135–147

65 Triggiani M, Oriente A, Marone G (1994) Differential roles for triglyceride and phospholipid pools of arachidonic acid in human lung macrophages. *J Immunol* 152: 1394–1403

66 Orning L, Krivi G, Fitzpatrick FA (1991) Leukotriene A_4 hydrolase. Inhibition by bestatin and intrinsic aminopeptidase activity establish its functional resemblance to metallohydrolase enzymes. *J Biol Chem* 266: 1375–1378

67 Yoshimoto T, Soberman RJ, Spur B, Austen KF (1988) Properties of highly purified leukotriene C_4 synthase of guinea pig lung. *J Clin Invest* 81: 866–871

68 Lewis RA, Austen KF, Soberman RJ (1990) Leukotrienes and other products of the 5-lipoxygenase pathway. *N Engl J Med* 323: 645–655

69 Marone G, Columbo M, Triggiani M, Cirillo R, Genovese A, Formisano S (1987) Inhibition of IgE-mediated release of histamine and peptide leukotriene from human basophils amd mast cells by forskolin. *Biochem Pharmacol* 36: 13–20

70 Genovese A, Patella V, de Crescenzo G, de Paulis A, Spadaro G, Marone G (1997) Loratadine and desethoxylcarbonyl-loratadine inhibit the immunological release of mediators from human $Fc\varepsilon RI^+$ cells. *Clin Exp Allergy* 27: 559–567

71 Adelroth E, Morris MM, Hargreave FE, O'Byrne PM (1986) Airway responsiveness to leukotrienes C_4 and D_4 and to methacholine in patients with asthma and normal controls. *N Engl J Med* 315: 480–484

72 Israel E, Juniper EF, Callaghan JT, Mathur PN, Morris MM, Dowell AR, Enas GG, Hargreave FE, Drazen JM (1989) Effect of a leukotriene antagonist, LY171883, on cold air-induced bronchoconstriction in asthmatics. *Am Rev Respir Dis* 140: 1348–1353

73 Manning PJ, Watson RM, Margolskee DJ, Williams VC, Schwartz JI, O'Byrne PM (1990) Inhibition of exercise-induced bronchoconstriction by MK-571, a potent leukotriene D_4-receptor antagonist. *N Engl J Med* 323: 1736–1739

74 Israel E, Dermarkarian R, Rosenberg M, Sperling R, Taylor G, Rubin P, Drazen JM (1990) The effects of a 5-lipoxygenase inhibitor on asthma induced by cold, dry air. *N Engl J Med* 323: 1740–1744

75 Knapp HR (1990) Reduced allergen-induced nasal congestion and leukotriene synthesis with an orally active 5-lipoxygenase inhibitor. *N Engl J Med* 323: 1745–1748

76 Triggiani M, De Marino V, Sofia M, Faraone S, Ambrosio G, Carratù L, Marone G (1997) Characterization of platelet-activating factor acetylhydrolase in human bronchoalveolar lavage. *Am J Respir Crit Care Med* 156: 94–100

77 Fonteh AN, Bass DA, Marshall LA, Seeds M, Samet JM, Chilton FH (1994) Evidence

that secretory phospholipase A_2 plays a role in arachidonic acid release and eicosanoid biosynthesis by mast cells. *J Immunol* 152: 5438–5446
78 Fonteh AN, Samet JM, Chilton FH (1995) Regulation of arachidonic acid, eicosanoid, and phospholipase A_2 levels in murine mast cells by recombinant stem cell factor. *J Clin Invest* 96: 1432–1439
79 Clark JD, Lin LL, Kriz RW, Ramesha CS, Sultzman LA, Lin AY, Milona N, Knopt JL (1991) A novel arachidonic-selective cytosolic PLA_2 contains a Ca^{2+}-dependent translocation domain with homology to PKC and Gap. *Cell* 65: 1043–1051
80 Nakatani Y, Murakami M, Kudo I, Inoue K (1994) Dual regulation of cytosolic phospholipase A2 in mast cells after cross-linking of Fcε-receptor. *J Immunol* 153: 796–803
81 Murakami M, Matsumoto R, Urade Y, Austen KF, Arm JP (1995) c-Kit ligand mediates increased expression of cytosolic phospholipase A_2, prostaglandin endoperoxide synthase-1, and hematopoietic prostaglandin D_2 synthase and increased IgE-dependent prostaglandin D_2 generation in immature mouse mast cells. *J Biol Chem* 270: 3239–3246
82 Murakami M, Kudo I, Suwa Y, Inoue K (1992) Release of 14-kDa group II phospholipase A_2 from activated mast cells and its possible involvement in the regulation of the degranulation process. *Eur J Biochem* 209: 257–265
83 Chilton FH, Averill FJ, Hubbard WC, Fonteh AN, Triggiani M, Liu MC (1996) Antigen-induced generation of lyso-phospholipids in human airways. *J Exp Med* 183: 2235–2245
84 Hara S, Kudo I, Chang H-W, Matsuta K, Miyamoto T, Inoue K (1989) Purification and characterization of extracellular phospholipase A_2 from human synovial fluid in rheumatoid arthritis. *J Biochem (Tokyo)* 105: 395–399
85 Edelson JD, Vadas P, Villar J, Mullen JBM, Pruzanski W (1991) Acute lung injury induced by phospholipase A_2. Structural and functional changes. *Am Rev Respir Dis* 143: 1102–1109
86 Murakami M, Kudo I, Inoue K (1991) Eicosanoid generation from antigen-primed mast cells by extracellular 14-kDa group II phospholipase A_2. *FEBS Lett* 294: 247–251
87 Benveniste J, Henson PM, Cochrane CG (1972) Leukocyte-dependent histamine release from rabbit platelets. The role of IgE, basophils, and a platelet-activating factor. *J Exp Med* 136: 1356–1377
88 Demopoulos CA, Pinckard RN, Hanahan DJ (1979) Platelet-Activating Factor. Evidence for 1-O-alkyl-2-acetyl-*sn*-glyceryl-3-phosphorylcholine as the active component (a new class of lipid chemical mediators). *J Biol Chem* 254: 9355–9358
89 Triggiani M, Hubbard WC, Chilton FH (1990) Synthesis of 1-acyl-2-acetyl-*sn*-glycero-3-phosphocholine by an enriched preparation of the human lung mast cell. *J Immunol* 144: 4773–4780
90 Triggiani M, Schleimer RP, warner JA, Chilton FH (1991) Differential synthesis of 1-acyl-2-acetyl-sn-glycero-3-phosphocholine and platelet-activating factor by human inflammatory cells. *J Immunol* 147: 660–666
91 Arock M, Merle-Béral H, Dugas B, Ouaaz F, Le Goff L, Vouldoukis I, Mencia-Huerta

J-M, Schmitt C, Leblond-Missenard V, Debre P et al (1993) IL-4 release by human leukemic and activated normal basophils. *J Immunol* 151: 1441–1447
92 MacGlashan D Jr, White JM, Huang S-K, Ono SJ, Schroeder JT, Lichtenstein LM (1994) Secretion of IL-4 from human basophils. The relationship between IL-4 mRNA and protein in resting and stimulated basophils. *J Immunol* 152: 3006–3016
93 Ochensberger B, Daepp G-C, Rihs S, Dahinden CA (1996) Human blood basophils produce interleukin-13 in response to IgE-receptor-dependent and -independent activation. *Blood* 88: 3028–3037
94 Li H, Sim TC, Alam R (1996) IL-13 released by and localized in human basophils. *J Immunol* 156: 4833–4838
95 Ohkawara Y, Yamauchi K, Tanno Y, Tamura G, Ohtani H, Nagura H, Ohkuda K, Takishima T (1992) Human lung mast cells and pulmonary macrophages produce tumor necrosis factor-a in sensitized lung tissue after IgE receptor triggering. *Am J Respir Cell Mol Biol* 7: 385–392
96 Bradding P, Roberts JA, Britten KM, Montefort S, Djukanovic R, Mueller R, Heusser C H, Howarth PH, Holgate ST (1994) Interleukin-4, -5, and -6 and tumor necrosis factor-a in normal and asthmatic airways: evidence for the human mast cell as a source of these cytokines. *Am J Respir Cell Mol Biol* 10: 471–480
97 Bradding P, Okayama Y, Howarth PH, Church MK, Holgate ST (1995) Heterogeneity of human mast cells based on cytokine content. *J Immunol* 155: 297–307
98 Krüger-Krasagakes S, Möller A, Kolde G, Lippert U, Weber M, Henz BM (196) Production of interleukin-6 by human mast cells and basophilic cells. *J Invest Dermatol* 106: 75–79
99 Burd PR, Thompson WC, Max EE, Mills FC (1995) Activated mast cells produce interleukin 13. *J Exp Med* 181: 1373–1380
100 Marone G, Casolaro V, Patella V, Florio G, Triggiani M (1997) Molecular and cellular biology of mast cells and basophils. *Int Arch Allergy Immunol* 114: 207–217
100a Patella V, Giuliano A, Bouvet J-P, Marone G (1998) Endogenous superallergen protein Fv induces IL-4 secretion from human FcεRI$^+$ cells through interaction with the V_H3 region of IgE. *J Immunol* 161: 5647–5655
101 Patella V, Marinò I, Arbustini E, Lamparter-Schummert B, Verga L, Adt M, Marone G (1998) Stem cell factor in mast cells and increased mast cell density in idiopathic and ischemic cardiomyopathy. *Circulation* 97: 971–978
102 Li H, Sim TC, Grant JA, Alam R (1996) The production of macrophage inflammatory protein-1α by human basophils. *J Immunol* 157: 1207–1212
103 Zon LI, Yamaguchi Y, Yee K, Albee EA, Kimura A, Bennett JC, Orkin SH, Ackerman SJ (1993) Expression of mRNA for the GATA-binding proteins in human eosinophils and basophils: potential role in gene transcription. *Blood* 81: 3234–3243
104 Rao A (1994) NF-ATp: a transcription factor required for the co-ordinate induction of several cytokine genes. *Immunol Today* 15: 274–281
105 Dunnill MS (1960) The pathology of asthma with special reference to changes in the bronchial mucosa. *J Clin Path* 13: 27–33

106 Glynn AA, Michaels L (1960) Bronchial biopsy in chronic bronchitis and asthma. *Thorax* 15: 142–151.

107 Laitinen LA, Heino M, Laitinen A, Kava T, Haahtela T (1985) Damage of the airway epithelium and bronchial reactivity in patients with asthma. *Am Rev Respir Dis* 131: 599–606

108 Chung KF (1986) Role of inflammation in the hyperreactivity of the airways in asthma. *Thorax* 41: 657–662

109 Kimura I, Tanizaki Y, Saito K, Takahashi K, Ueda N, Sato S (1975) Appearance of basophils in the sputum of patients with bronchial asthma. *Clin Allergy* 5: 95–98

110 Hastie R, Heroy JH III, Levy DA (1979) Basophil leukocytes and mast cells in human nasal secretions and scrapings studied by light microscopy. *Lab Invest* 40: 554–561

111 Creticos PS, Peters SP, Adkinson NF Jr, Naclerio RM, Hayes EC, Norman PS, Lichtenstein LM (1984) Peptide leukotriene release after antigen challenge in patients sensitive to ragweed. *N Engl J Med* 310: 1626–1630

112 Tomioka M, Ida S, Shindoh Y, Ishihara T, Takishima T (1984) Mast cells in bronchoalveolar lumen of patients with bronchial asthma. *Am Rev Respir Dis* 129: 1000–1005

113 Marone G, Casolaro V, Ayala F, Melillo G, Condorelli M (1990) Releasability in allergic disorders. In: G Melillo, PS Norman, G Marone (eds): *Respiratory allergy. Clinical immunology*, vol 2. B.C. Decker, Toronto, 67–77

114 Casolaro V, Spadaro G, Marone G (1993) Genetic studies of basophil releasability. In: DG Marsh, A Lockhart, ST Holgate (eds): *The genetics of asthma.* Blackwell Scientific Publications Ltd, Oxford, 22: 291–308

115 Marone G, Spadaro G, Patella V, Genovese A (1994) The clinical relevance of basophil releasability. *J Allergy Clin Immunol* 94: 1293–1303

116 Marone G, Poto S, Celestino D, Bonini S (1986) Human basophil releasability. III. Genetic control of human basophil releasability. *J Immunol* 137: 3588–3592

117 Marone G., Spadaro G., Genovese A (1995) Pharmacological modulation of human mast cell and basophil secretion *in vitro* and *in vivo*. In: Y Kitamura, S Yamamoto, SJGalli, MW Greaves (eds): Biological and molecular aspects of mast cell and basophil differentiation and function. Raven Press, New York, 193–210

118 Marone G, Stellato C, Renda A, Genovese A (1993) Anti-inflammatory effects of glucocorticoids and cyclosporin A on human basophils. *Eur J Clin Pharmacol* 45 (Suppl 1): S17–S20

119 de Paulis A, Ciccarelli A, Marinò I, de Crescenzo G, Marinò D, Marone G (1997) Human synovial mast cells. II. Heterogeneity of the pharmacologic effects of anti-inflammatory and immunosuppressive drugs. *Arthritis Rheum* 40: 469–478

120 Casolaro V, Spadaro G, Patella V, Marone G (1993) *In vivo* characterization of the anti-inflammatory effect of cyclosporin A on human basophils. *J Immunol* 151: 5563–5573

121 Stellato C, de Paulis A, Ciccarelli A, Cirillo R, Patella V, Casolaro V, Marone G (1992) Anti-inflammatory effect of cyclosporin A on human skin mast cells. *J Invest Dermatol* 98: 800–804

122 de Paulis A, Cirillo R, Ciccarelli A, Condorelli M, Marone G (1991) FK-506, a potent novel inhibitor of the release of proinflammatory mediators from human FcεRI⁺ cells. *J Immunol* 146: 2374–2381

123 de Paulis A, Cirillo R, Ciccarelli A, de Crescenzo G, Oriente A, Marone G (1991) Characterization of the anti-inflammatory effect of FK-506 on human mast cells. *J Immunol* 147: 4278–4285

124 de Paulis A, Stellato C, Cirillo R, Ciccarelli A, Oriente A, Marone G (1992) Anti-inflammatory effect of FK-506 on human skin mast cells. *J Invest Dermatol* 99: 723–728

125 Busse WW, Gern JE (1997) Viruses in asthma. *J Allergy Clin Immunol* 100: 147–150

126 Salvaggio J, Aukrust L (1981) Mold-induced asthma. *J Allergy Clin Immunol* 68: 327–346

127 Licorish K, Novey HS, Kozak P, Fairshter RD, Wilson AF (1985) Role of *Alternaria* and *Penicillium* spores in the pathogenesis of asthma. *J Allergy Clin Immunol* 76: 819–825

128 Marone G, Columbo M, Soppelsa L, Condorelli M (1984) The mechanism of basophil histamine release induced by pepstatin A. *J Immunol* 133: 1542–15

129 Echtenacher B, Männel DN, Hültner L (1996) Critical protective role of mast cells in a model of acute septic peritonitis. *Nature* 381: 75–77

130 Malaviya R, Ikeda T, Ross E, Abraham SN (1996) Mast cell modulation of neutrophil influx and bacterial clearance at sites of infection through TNF-α. *Nature* 381: 77–80

131 Bailie MB, Standiford TJ, Laichalk LL, Caffey MJ, Strieter R, Peters-Golden M (1996) Leukotriene-deficient mice manifest enhanced lethality from *Klebsiella pneumonia* in association with decreased alveolar macrophage phagocytic and bactericidal activities. *J Immunol* 157: 5221–5224

132 de Paulis A, Ciccarelli A, de Crescenzo G, Cirillo R, Patella V, Marone G (1996) Cyclosporin H is a potent and selective competitive antagonist of human basophil activation by N-formyl-methionyl-leucyl-phenylalanine. *J Allergy Clin Immunol* 98: 158–164

133 Malaviya R, Ross E, Jakschik BA, Abraham SN (1994) Mast cell degranulation induced by type 1 fimbriated *Escherichia coli* in mice. *J Clin Invest* 93: 1645–1653

134 Bouvet JP, Pirès R, Lunel-Fabiani F, Crescenzo-Chaigne B, Maillard P, Valla D, Opolon P, Pillot J (1990) Protein F. A novel F(ab)-binding factor, present in normal liver, and largely released in the digestive tract during hepatitis. *J Immunol* 145: 1176–1180

Platelets

Paolo Gresele[1] *and Roberta Vezza*[2]

[1]Institute of Internal and Vascular Medicine, University of Perugia, Via Enrico Dal Pozzo, 06126 Perugia, Italy; [2]Center for Experimental Therapeutics, University of Pennsylvania, School of Medicine, Philadelphia, USA

Introduction

With the increasing knowledge of the role that platelets play in the pathogenesis of ischemic cardiovascular disorders [1, 2] a great deal of attention has been focussed on these blood elements. This large research effort has lead to a series of significant advances in the understanding of the physiology of platelets and on their participation not only to haemostasis and thrombosis but also to non-haemostatic processes.

Important new achievements have been gained from the application of new methodologies, such as cytofluorimetry, molecular biology and gene manipulation, to the study of platelets or their precursors and the picture emerging is more and more that of the platelet as a multifunctional blood element. The aim of this chapter is to summarize the state of the art on platelet structure, physiology and pathophysiology with special emphasis on those aspects that appear of particular relevance for the potential involvement of these blood elements in airways inflammation.

Cellular structure

In circulating blood, platelets have a discoid shape with a diameter of about 2–4 μm [3]. From a morphologic point of view, several zones can be identified in the cellular structure of platelets [4].

(1) Peripheral zone
The peripheral zone represents the surface of the platelet and consists of the plasma membrane and associated structures. The most external part of the peripheral zone is called glycocalix and it is particularly rich in glycoproteins (see later); the middle layer is a typical plasma membrane, rich in phospholipids and it is particularly important for the interaction with coagulation factors; the inner layer is formed by

Cellular Mechanisms in Airways Inflammation, edited by Clive P. Page, Katharine H. Banner and Domenico Spina

short actin filaments, making up the membrane cytoskeleton. Longer actin filaments form the cytoplasmic cytoskeleton [4].

(2) Sol-gel zone
The sol-gel zone represents the platelet cytoplasm and its detergent-resistant elements referred as cytoskeleton. Different systems of fibers are present in the platelet matrix and, in particular, submembrane filaments, microtubules and microfilaments. Microtubules are formed by polymerized tubulin and are involved in maintaining the platelet in a discoidal shape. Microtubules allow the normal platelet contraction, although they are not contractile elements. Microfilaments are formed by actin, which is the most abundant platelet protein. Although actin is polymerized to some extent even in resting platelets, its polymerization state increases upon platelet activation; the organization of actin filaments in parallel bundles is important for platelet spreading and pseudopod formation [4].

(3) Organelles zone
The organelles zone consists of alpha granules, delta (or dense) granules, peroxysomes, lysosomes and mitochondria, that are dispersed in the cytoplasm. Organelles are involved in metabolic processes and store non-metabolic adenine nucleotides, enzymes, serotonin, calcium, and a variety of proteins.

(4) Membrane system
The open canalicular system consists of invaginations of the plasma membrane and, thus, it is surface connected. Canaliculi of the open canalicular system greatly increase the total surface area of the platelet exposed to plasma and to the chemicals present in it. In addition, these canaliculi represent conduits for substances extruded by platelets during the release reaction. The dense tubular system originates from the endoplasmic reticulum of megakaryocytes. Together with the dense granules, the dense tubular system is a site for calcium storage in platelets. Another important feature of the dense tubular system is that the enzyme cyclooxygenase is located on the membrane of these tubules. Although two cyclooxygenase isozymes have been identified and cloned [5], platelets only possess cyclooxygenase 1, the constitutive isoform of the enzyme [6, 7]. In fact, since cyclooxygenase 2 is an inducible enzyme, i.e. its expression requires protein synthesis, it is not present in the anucleated platelet.

The glycocalix

The glycocalix is the most external layer of the platelet membrane. It is rich in glycoproteins (GP) which function as receptors for a wide variety of stimuli and can be classified into five families [8].

(1) Integrins are heterodimeric proteins that mediate interactions between different cells or between cells and adhesive molecules.
(2) Leucine-rich glycoproteins (LRG) form the GPIb/V/IX complex, important as a receptor for von Willebrand factor (vWf) and thrombin.
(3) Selectins mediate the interaction of platelets and endothelial cells with leucocytes.
(4) Immunoglobulins, among which PECAM-1, which are present on the surface of platelets and in the gaps between endothelial cells.
(5) Quadraspanins, proteins of unknown function that span the membrane four times. Members of this family are p24/CD9 and the α granule protein ME491.

Another platelet glycoprotein that can not be classified as a member of the above described families, due to the low structural homology, is GPIV (or CD36) that functions as a collagen receptor.

The majority of the platelet glycoproteins belong to the integrin family. Integrins bind adhesive proteins and they are expressed, besides platelets, on endothelial cells, smooth muscle cells, leucocytes and fibroblasts. The name integrins implies that they integrate the ligands on the outside of the cell with the cytoskeleton apparatus in the inside of the cell [9].

Integrins are heterodimers formed by an α and a β subunit linked by non covalent bonds. Several α and one β subunits have been identified; the different heterodimers that can be formed are grouped into families with a common β subunit (β1, β2, β3 families) [8, 9]. The β1 family consists of 6 members formed by β1 that dimerizes with α1, α2, α3, α4, α5 and α6. Not all the members of this family are expressed in platelets (Tab. 1). The three members of the β2 family (αMβ2 or Mac-1; αLβ2 or LFA-1 and α150β2 or p150/95) are not expressed in platelets, but in leucocytes and mediate the adhesion of the latter cells to other leucocytes and to endothelial cells. Members of the β3 family present in platelets are αIIbβ3 (GPIIb/IIIa) and αVβ3 (Tab. 1).

GPIIb/IIIa

The most abundant integrin in platelets is a member of the β3 family (αIIbβ3) also called GPIIb/IIIa: it is the receptor for fibrinogen and it is essential not only for platelet adhesion, but also for aggregation. Indeed, patients with Glanzmann's thrombasthenia, characterized by defective or abnormal GPIIb/IIIa, have a dramatically impaired platelet aggregation and haemorrhagic diathesis [8]. A minority of patients possesses nearly normal amounts of GPIIb/IIIa but still fail to bind fibrinogen: point mutations in the cDNA for this receptor give dysfunctional proteins [10].

GPIIb/IIIa is present at approximately 50,000–100,000 copies per platelet [8] and is expressed only in cells of megakaryocytic lineage. 80% of the platelet GPIIb/IIIa is randomly exposed on the surface; the remaining 20% is located on the

Table 1 - A summary of the integrin families on platelets and their counterligands

Integrin	Ligand
β1 family	
α2β1 (VLA-2, GPIa/IIa, ECMR-II)	Collagen, laminin
α5β1 (VLA-5, GPIc/IIa)	Fibronectin
α6β1 (VLA-6, GPIc/IIa region)	Laminin, fibronectin
β2 family	
None	
β3 family	
αIIbβ3 (GPIIb/IIIa)	Fibrinogen, vWf, fibronectin, vitronectin, thrombospondin
αVβ3	Vitronectin, thrombospondin, vWF, fibronectin, fibrinogen

surface of the open canalicular system and in the inner membrane of the α granules [11].

The αIIb subunit consists of a heavy (GPIIba; 125 kDa) and a light (GPIIbb; 25 kDa) chain linked by a disulphide bond. The αIIb and β3 chains interact through their N-terminal (extracellular) portions and bivalent cations are necessary for this interaction [12]. The αIIb and β3 subunits have long extracellular domains while only 26 aminoacids of the light chain of αIIb and 45 aminoacids of β3 form the intracellular domains. The intracellular tails interact with the actin cytoskeleton through a series of linking proteins, among which talin and vinculin [10].

The N-terminal portion of GPIIb/IIIa contains the ligand binding site for several adhesive molecules usually containing a RGD sequence, such as fibrinogen, von Willebrand factor (vWf), vitronectin, fibronectin and thrombospondin [12]. In resting platelets, however, GPIIb/IIIa is unable to bind plasma fibrinogen or matrix-bound vWf with high affinity, preventing adhesion or aggregation in circulating blood. In addition, GPIIb/IIIa binding to vWf requires initial interaction of vWf with another integrin receptor, GPIb/V/IX (see later). Platelet activation by a wide variety of agonists leads to a conformational change of GPIIb/IIIa and to its activation; activated GPIIb/IIIa can bind fibrinogen or vWf with high affinity. Although the specific pathways leading to GPIIb/IIIa activation following platelet stimulation (inside-out signaling) are still not completely unravelled, protein kinase C (PKC) seems to play a role and phosphorylation of the integrin correlates with its activation [13]. Also other kinases, such as the phosphoinositide 3-kinase (PI 3-kinase), and the small GTP binding protein rhoA seem to be involved in GPIIb/IIIa activation, although the mechanism is not clear. Several lines of evidence demonstrate that the portion of the GPIIb/IIIa molecule important for activation mediated by intracellular signaling is the cytoplasmic domain [11,12]. This region is also important in mediating other events that follow GPIIb/IIIa activation and that are indicated as outside-in signaling. Indeed, once activated, GPIIb/IIIa induces reorganization of the cytoskeleton, elevation of intracellular calcium and pH, phosphoinositide metabolism, activation of serine/threonine and tyrosine kinases. Among the tyrosine phosphorylated proteins, the tyrosine kinase $pp125^{FAK}$ (focal adhesion kinase) has been described [11].

GPIa/IIa

Another integrin of the platelet glycocalix is the GPIa/IIa or α2β1 that represents one collagen receptor and it is important in mediating platelet adhesion to the collagen fibers (but not collagen monomers) of the subendothelium. The α2 subunit has only one polypeptide chain with a short intracellular domain and a longer extracellular domain. The N-terminus of α2 presents a I domain that is important for collagen binding, however it is not known if α2β1 changes its conformation and becomes active when platelets react with collagen fibers or other agents, or if the activation of α2β1 is required for adhesion and aggregation of platelets to collagen [14].

Other collagen receptors on platelets are the glycoproteins GPVI and GPIV (or GPIIIb or CD36) [14]. While patients with abnormalities in GPIa have a marked bleeding tendency, abnormalities in GPVI cause only a mild bleeding disorder; GPIV defect is not responsible for any clinical disorder, indicating that GPIV is probably not an essential factor for the interaction of platelets with collagen, although it might have some stimulatory effect in this reaction. It is important to note that in experimental conditions of flow, closely resembling a physiological situation under which thrombus occurs, platelets interact with vWf molecules bound to collagen; after this initial step, adherent platelets react with collagen through their collagen receptors, resulting in activation and aggregation [14].

Although the activation pathways initiated by platelet binding to collagen have not been fully elucidated, activation of phospholipase C (PLC) has been reported [15]. More recently, it has been found that stimulation of platelets by collagen leads to the phosphorylation of several proteins [16]. In particular, the non-receptor tyrosine kinase Syk, and PLCγ2 are phosphorylated and activated following platelet stimulation with collagen. The phosphorylation of Syk and PLCγ2 is dependent of α2β1, although this integrin is not sufficient to induce these phosphorylation events, suggesting that α2β1 functions in a co-stimulatory way with other collagen receptors [17]. Phosphorylation of the Fc receptor FcγRII by collagen has also been described [17] (see later).

GPIb/V/IX complex

While receptors for fibrinogen, vitronectin, laminin and the GPIa/IIa for collagen belong to the integrin family, other glycoproteins of the glycocalix are classified as leucine-rich glycoproteins (LRG) because they contain one or more sequences of 24 aminoacids rich in leucine. LRG proteins form the GPIb/V/IX complex, or CD42 [18], which is one of the major adhesion receptors on the platelet surface.

GPIb is formed by two subunits, α and β, covalently linked by a disulphide bond; GPIX is non covalently bound to GPIb in a 1:1 ratio, while GPV is only weakly associated to GPIb/IX in a 1:2 ratio [18, 19]. GPIb is the most important component of the complex in terms of mass and functional sites: it contains binding sites for vWf and thrombin in the N-terminal region and for 14-3-3ζ protein in the cytoplasmic tail. The association of GPIbα with the 14-3-3ζ protein may serve to transduce platelet activation signals initiated by adhesion of the cells to vWf [20].

In resting platelets, GPIb does not bind plasma vWf, but binding can occur in conditions of high shear associated with constricted vessels in advanced atherosclerosis.

Soluble vWf can bind to collagen and other molecules of the subendothelium, thus being immobilized onto complex extracellular matrices. Immobilized vWf plays important roles in platelet adhesion under high shear rates. The first step of this process is mediated by the binding of vWf to GPIbα through the A1 domain present in the vWf molecule. The interaction of vWf with GPIbα is rapid but has a fast dissociation rate: since this interaction is not stable, it can not provide bonds supporting irreversible adhesion, although it can slow down platelet velocity. This phenomenon is called rolling and new bonds between GPIbα and immobilized vWf are formed as different regions of the membrane of rolling platelets come in closer contact with the subendothelium. The platelet rolling continues until GPIIb/IIIa becomes activated and binds to vWf through the Asp-Gly-Arg-Ser (RGDS) sequence in the C-terminal domain of the vWf molecule. The bonds between vWf and GPIIb/IIIa have a low dissociation rate and, thus, they mediate irreversible adhesion [21].

Although binding of vWf to GPIb was thought to be a passive phenomenon (called agglutination), there are evidences that the stress caused by this binding causes further activation of platelets and GPIIb/IIIa activation [18]. One of the early events associated with vWf binding to platelets is the tyrosine phosphorylation of several proteins, including tyrosine kinases themselves.

GPIb also binds thrombin and, in particular, it represents the high affinity binding site for thrombin, while the G protein coupled receptor binds thrombin with a moderate affinity (see later). Little is known about the signal transduction events linked to thrombin binding to GPIb [19].

P selectin

Another glycoprotein of the platelet glycocalix is a member of the selectin family and is called P selectin or granule membrane protein 140 (GMP-140) or PADGEM.

Other selectins (E selectin and L selectin) are expressed in endothelial cells and leucocytes, but not in platelets.

P selectin is stored in platelet α granules and becomes expressed on the surface following platelet activation with, for example, thrombin, histamine, complement fragments, oxygen-derived free radicals and cytokines. The ligand for P selectin has not been identified, and also its functions are not well understood [8]. It has been hypothesized that P selectin expression on the platelet surface could lead to the formation of platelet-neutrophils intravascular aggregates through the combination of P selectin domains on platelets with specific ligands on neutrophils. P selectin can also participate in the attachment of platelets to the endothelium [22] and thus possibly in the diapedesis of platelets through the junctions between endothelial cells, explaining the platelet infiltrates which characterize some inflammatory tissue responses [23].

The cytoskeleton

The platelet cytoskeleton is formed by a network of cytoplasmic actin, a peripheral microtubule coil and the membrane skeleton that coats the internal face of the plasma membrane. The membrane skeleton by lining the plasma membrane regulates its contours and contributes to its stabilization, preventing it from fragmentation. Membrane skeleton is attached to glycoproteins and it may regulate their lateral distribution; GPIb/IX, for example, is present over the entire surface of the membrane in resting platelets, but it clusters when the membrane skeleton is disrupted [24].

Mainly formed by actin, the cytoskeleton also contains other proteins, such as actin-binding protein (ABP), α-actinin, tropomyosin, talin, vinculin and cortactin. In resting platelets, 30–40% of the total actin is in a polymerized form; upon activation, this figure rises up to 70–80%. The new filaments of polymerized actin form in at least two locations: a network is localized at the periphery of the cell, and bundles of filaments form in developing filopodia. Several mechanisms are involved in preventing actin polymerization in resting cells and, in particular, thymosin β4 seems to play an important role in sequestering monomeric actin in resting platelets, thus avoiding its massive polymerization. The release of actin monomers from thymosin β4, in addition to other mechanisms, allows actin polymerization following activation. Also other proteins, such as profilin and gelsolin, keep actin in a depolymerized state [3].

When platelets are activated, a reorganization of the cytoskeleton occurs, both in an aggregation-independent manner and in aggregating platelets. Within seconds of stimulation the cytoskeleton undergoes a reorganization which is observed even in non stirred platelets that, lacking cell-cell contacts, do not aggregate. This aggregation-independent reorganization consists of a redistribution of the cytoskeletal proteins: tropomyosin, distributed diffusely in resting platelets, is concentrated in filopodia in activated cells; also actin-binding protein becomes concentrated in the filopodia while α-actinin becomes concentrated in filopodia and in a submembrane location. Polymerized actin in the cytoplasm (and not that in the filopodia) can bind to phosphorylated myosin; this leads to platelet contraction and organelles centralization.

During platelet aggregation, other changes in the platelet cytoskeleton occur, following fibrinogen binding to GPIIb/IIIa. GPIIb/IIIa molecules cluster and the membrane skeleton associates with the underlying actin filaments leading to a more complex cytoskeleton reorganization. In addition to GPIIb/IIIa other proteins can be recovered in the organized cytoskeleton of aggregated platelets and, among these, protein kinase C, phosphoinositide 3-kinase, $pp60^{c\text{-}src}$ (the major tyrosine kinase present in platelets), $pp62^{c\text{-}yes}$, $pp59^{fyn}$, $pp125^{FAK}$, $p21^{ras}$, the small GTP-binding protein rap1b, phospholipase C, diacylglycerol kinase, the glycoprotein PECAM-1 [11, 12, 24–26].

Main receptors

In addition to glycoproteins, that are principally receptors for adhesive proteins, other receptors for a wide variety of platelet agonists are present on platelets. These receptors are located in the plasma membrane and most of them belong to the family of the G protein-coupled receptors (GPCR), since they activate effector systems through an interaction with G proteins. GPCR are formed by a single polypeptide chain with an extracellular N-terminus, an intracellular C-terminus and seven hydrophobic transmembrane domains that are separated by three extracellular and three intracellular loops. Receptors for thromboxane A_2 (TxA_2) and other prostanoids (prostaglandin (PG) E_2, PGD_2, PGI_2), for thrombin, epinephrine, platelet activating factor (PAF), vasopressin, serotonin, all belong to the GPCR family. Less is known about the ADP receptors, although data exist that indicate that also one of the possible ADP receptors is a GPCR.

In this section, we will briefly review the characteristics of the main platelet receptors. It is noteworthy that some platelet stimuli, such as serotonin, TxA_2 and other prostanoids, in particular PGE_2, and thrombin, are also immunological/inflammatory stimuli.

TxA_2

TxA_2 is synthesized by activated platelets upon metabolism of the arachidonic acid liberated from the plasma membrane. Arachidonic acid is cleaved from phospholipids by phospholipase A_2 (PLA_2) and, in platelets, it is transformed by cyclooxygenase 1 in the prostaglandin endoperoxides PGG_2 and PGH_2. These reactions are accompanied by free radical generation that contributes to the participation of platelets to inflammatory reactions [27].

Different enzymes, among which thromboxane synthase, transform PGH_2 into different prostanoids (TxA_2, PGE_2, PGD_2 and, in endothelial cells, PGI_2) [28]. Once formed, TxA_2 can diffuse across the plasma membrane and, being a powerful aggregating agent, it amplifies the initial platelet response to stimulation [29]. TxA_2 is also a powerful vasoconstrictor and a bronchoconstrictor [29, 30].

Prostanoid receptors specific for TxA_2, PGE_2, PGD_2, PGI_2 and $PGF_{2\alpha}$ are named TP, EP, DP, IP and FP, respectively [31].

Two TxA_2 receptors have been cloned to date [32, 33] and called TPα the first cloned isoform, and TPβ the second. TPα and TPβ are splice variants of the same gene product and they differ at the level of the carboxy terminal tail: the 15 aminoacids sequence in the COOH terminus of TPα are replaced by a 79 aminoacids sequence in TPβ. TPα has been cloned from a placental library and also from megakaryocytic cell lines [32, 34] while TPβ has been cloned from an endothelial library [33].

Recently, using RT-PCR techniques, it has been demonstrated that platelets express both TPα and TPβ although it seems that they do not correspond to the two classes of TxA_2 binding sites described previously in platelets that have been extensively studied using ligand binding and biochemical approaches [35].

Although TPα and TPβ are differently coupled to adenylate cyclase, they both activate PLC in an overexpression system [35]. In platelets, stimulation with TxA_2 or its analogues causes activation of PLC (in particular the PLCβ isoform) with consequent diacylglycerol (DG) and inositol 1,4,5 triphosphate (IP_3) formation and calcium mobilization, activation of PKC, phosphorylation of pleckstrin and of myosin light chain, activation of GPIIb/IIIa. Platelets express at least PLCβ and PLCγ, although only PLCβ seems to be activated by G proteins. PLCβ1 and PLCβ3 respond predominantly to the α subunit of G proteins, while PLCβ2 may respond better to the βγ subunits. Thromboxane receptors are apparently coupled to PLCβ1 through Gα subunits [36]. In platelets, TxA_2 also activates PLA_2 [35].

Several G proteins have been demonstrated to couple to the TxA_2 receptor, in platelets or in overexpression systems. Among these, Gq [37, 38], G12 and G13 [39], G16 and its murine counterpart, G15 [40]; contrasting data exist about the coupling with Gi [37, 41, 42], while recent studies suggest a coupling of the thromboxane receptor with a newly described G protein called Gh [43].

Other prostanoids

PGH_2 can be substrate not only for thromboxane synthase, but also for other enzymes that, in platelets, form small amounts of PGE_2, PGD_2 and $PGF_{2\alpha}$. In endothelial cells PGI_2 (and in the microvasculature PGE_2) is the major product of arachidonic acid metabolism [28].

PGD_2 and PGI_2 act on platelets as antiaggregatory substances through DP and IP receptors, respectively, while PGE_2 exerts a proaggregatory effect when used in combination with other stimuli [44]. $PGF_{2\alpha}$ appears to be inactive in platelets, so the characteristics of its receptor will not be discussed in this chapter.

All the prostanoid receptors belong to the GPCR family and they have some conserved regions, in particular in the seventh transmembrane domain, second intracellular loop and third transmembrane domain. The overall homology is quite low (20–30%) but higher homology is observed when comparing receptors for the same ligand from different species, such as human and mouse [45]. While only one DP and only one IP receptor have been described, several EP receptors exist and they are called EP1, EP2, EP3 and EP4. The EP3 receptor exists in different splice variants. Six different splice variants of EP3 receptor have been cloned from human uterus and called EP3a, EP3b, EP3c, EP3d, EP3e, EP3f [46], while bovine EP3 receptors are called EP3A, EP3B, EP3C and EP3D. Alternative splicing has been demonstrated also in the mouse and rabbit EP3 receptor [45].

An EP3 receptor has been cloned from human erythroleukemia cells (HEL), a megakaryocytic cell line and, when expressed in COS-1 cells, found to be coupled to inhibition of adenylate cyclase [47]. It should be noted that in mock transfected cells, PGE_2 increased cAMP indicating that COS-1 cells have, *per se*, an EP receptor that stimulates adenylate cyclase [47]. This circumstance can confuse the picture; in addition, a sole inhibition of adenylate cyclase can not fully explain the proaggregatory activity of PGE_2 observed in platelets [44]. For these reasons, it is not yet clear which EP receptor subtype is present in platelets; it is possible that only one receptor, coupled to different signal transduction mechanisms, exists or that more than one EP receptor, still to be identified, is expressed in human platelets.

While several details on the signal transduction mechanism(s) linked to the activation of the EP receptor(s) in human platelets await clarification, it is well known that the IP receptor is linked to Gs and, thus, it causes an increase of intraplatelet cAMP. The physiologic role of PGI2 and its receptor in limiting platelet activation *in vivo* is highlighted by the recent report that mice lacking the prostacyclin receptor (IP receptor knock-out) present an enhanced susceptibility to arterial thrombosis [48]. Although less potent, also PGD_2 causes a cAMP increase through Gs [45], resulting in inhibition of platelet functions [49]. Consistent with the fact that $PGF_{2\alpha}$ does not play relevant roles in platelet functions, FP-deficient mice do not seem to have platelet abnormalities [50].

Thrombin

Thrombin is a serine/threonine protease generated by the sequential activation of the enzymes of the coagulation cascade. Since phospholipids of the activated platelets accelerate the blood clotting cascade, platelets promote thrombin generation. Thrombin, in turn, activates platelets. In addition to high affinity thrombin receptors represented by GPIb (see above), platelets have a GPCR with moderate affinity (roughly 1,800 copies/platelet) also referred as PAR-1 [51]. Another protease receptor has been described and cloned and called PAR-2, but this receptor is not present in human platelets [52].

PAR-1 in its N-terminus contains a site for cleavage by thrombin, located between Arg41 and Ser42. The region immediately C-terminal to the cleavage site is a tethered ligand able to activate the receptor, apparently interacting with sites located in the second extracellular loop and in the N-terminus near the first transmembrane domain [51, 53].

Not only thrombin, but also other proteases can cleave the thrombin receptor, although at sites different from that cleaved by thrombin. In particular, following tissue injury or inflammation, proteases such as cathepsin G, granzyme and tryptase can be secreted locally by leucocytes and mast cells. Cathepsin G and other proteases (chymotrypsin and plasmin) cleave the thrombin receptor at sites different from that of thrombin, thus disabling the receptor. Cathepsin G can cleave the thrombin receptor also at the same site where thrombin cleaves, thus explaining why cathepsin G can activate platelets. If the platelet activation induced by cathepsin G is due to a preferential cleavage at the Arg41-Ser42 site (instead of at Phe55-Trp56), or if it is due to the presence, in platelets, of additional receptors, remains to be determined [51].

Activation of platelets with thrombin causes activation of phospholipases such as PLC, PLA_2 (with consequent TxA_2 synthesis) and PLD, of kinases such as PKC and mitogen activated protein kinase (MAPK), calcium mobilization, protein phosphorylation and decrease of cAMP. Thrombin is thought to activate PLCβ, in particular the isoform PLCβ2, through the $\beta\gamma$ subunits released by activated Gi, while the α subunit of this G protein inhibits adenylate cyclase. Thrombin can also activate PLCβ isoforms through the α subunit of Gq, although in platelets the Gi route seems to be predominant; indeed, thrombin-induced phosphoinositide hydrolysis in platelets can be inhibited by pertussis toxin, that inhibits Gi [36, 51]. Also the thrombin receptor, as the thromboxane receptor, can couple with G16 and its murine counterpart G15 [40] and G12 and G13 [39, 54]. Using membranes of infected Sf9 cells, it has been recently demonstrated that thrombin also activates Gz, a G protein only expressed in platelets and in some neural tissues. Similar experiments did not show, as expected, coupling of the thrombin receptor with Gs [54].

ADP

ADP is an aggregating agent released by damaged endothelial or red blood cells. Platelets store ADP in their dense granules, and release it upon stimulation with other agonists, thus reinforcing aggregation. Platelet stimulation with ADP causes shape change, calcium influx, activation of GPIIb/IIIa and reversible aggregation if physiological concentrations of calcium are present in the medium (see below). Irreversible aggregation occurs following synthesis of TxA_2 from the activated platelets. ADP is, at most, only a weak activator of platelet PLC; ADP inhibits stimulated adenylate cyclase although this effect can not explain ADP-induced aggregation.

The nature of the platelet ADP receptor is still not yet completely elucidated, although recent studies have contributed to our understanding on this issue. The platelet ADP receptor has been initially called P2T purinoreceptor [56] but recent studies indicate that platelets have at least two ADP receptors thus the P2T receptor must be considered a pharmacological concept more than a molecular entity.

Inhibition of adenylate cyclase probably occurs after binding of ADP to a GPCR, possibly coupled to Gi2 [55]. Although cloning of the platelet ADP receptor has been to date unsuccessful, it has been demonstrated that platelets, as well as megakaryocytic cell lines, have the mRNA for the $P2Y_1$ receptor; this finding suggests that the $P2Y_1$ receptor is the platelet ADP receptor coupled to G protein(s) and responsible for aggregation and inhibition of adenylate cyclase.

ADP also induces a rapid influx of calcium from the extracellular medium and this effect seems to be mediated by a $P2X_1$ receptor. This receptor may be linked to a calcium channel and this early calcium influx could be responsible for ADP-induced shape change. The involvement of $P2X_1$ ionotropic receptors in shape change needs, however, to be confirmed: indeed, an ATP derivative able to induce calcium influx does not cause shape change [55].

Epinephrine

Epinephrine is a circulating hormone synthesized by adrenal medulla; it is also stored by platelets in the dense granules and it can be released during the release reaction [57]. Epinephrine is a peculiar platelet agonist: it induces aggregation and fibrinogen binding to GPIIb/IIIa without causing shape change. Recent investigations suggest that epinephrine is not a platelet agonist *per se* and that it only potentiates aggregation induced by other inducers, such as ADP, collagen, arachidonic acid, thrombin, serotonin, vasopressin, PAF [57, 58]. Epinephrine does not induce PLC activation per se: the PLC activation induced by epinephrine is due to TxA_2 synthesis by activated platelets. Epinephrine activates the H^+/Na^+ antiporter, causing alkalinization of the cytoplasm, and it inhibits adenylate cyclase [36, 57].

Platelet adrenergic receptors belong to the α2A subtype, coupled to inhibition of adenylate cyclase through Gi2 [59]. Although much less abundant, platelets also have β2 adrenoreceptors that, contrary to α2A receptors, induce increase of cyclic AMP. Some authors hypothesize that the epinephrine effects in platelets are the result of activation of both α2A and β2 receptors, but since α2A receptors are in abundance, the overall effect is a stimulation of platelet aggregation [57].

Platelet activating factor (PAF)

PAF is a phospholipid-like substance derived from phosphatidylcholine; it is released from neutrophils and from platelets following activation by thrombin or collagen and is itself a potent aggregating stimulus. PAF is an extremely potent inflammatory agent and it has been implicated as a mediator of inflammation and asthma [30]. The platelet PAF receptor belongs to the family of the GPCR and it is linked, through an unknown G protein, to PLC [60].

Serotonin

Serotonin, or 5-hydroxytryptamine (5HT), is stored in platelet dense granules and it is released upon activation by a variety of stimuli. 5HT is both a platelet agonist and a vasoconstrictor. Platelets have a very efficient uptake system for 5HT, so that the plasma concentrations of this amine are usually very low: concentrations of 5HT capable of activating platelets are reached only after platelets have undergone the release reaction [61].

Serotonin is a weak platelet agonist and it only induces shape change and small reversible aggregation with human platelets. Irreversible aggregation can occur when serotonin is used in combination with subthreshold doses of other agonists, such as ADP or TxA_2 analogues [62]. The platelet serotonin receptor is a GPCR member of the 5HT2 family. Platelets possess another binding site for 5HT that is used for the uptake process but this can not be considered a receptor in a functional way [61, 63]. Serotonin is also an inflammatory substance: besides inducing vasoconstriction it increases vascular permeability.

Vasopressin

Vasopressin is stored, together with adenine nucleotides, calcium ions and serotonin, in the platelet dense granules [57]. V1 receptors for vasopressin are present on platelets, but the concentration of the ligand required to activate platelets is several orders of magnitude higher than that normally achieved in the circulation [61] and the mechanism for vasopressin-induced platelet aggregation is not well elucidated. It has been shown that vasopressin inhibits adenylate cyclase, but only in isolated platelet membranes and not in whole cells [64].

Adenosine

Adenosine is an antiaggregatory and vasodilatory agent. Platelet adenosine receptors are represented by the GPCR A_{2A}. A_{2A} receptors are coupled to adenylate cyclase through Gs, thus causing cyclic AMP increase and inhibition of platelet activation [65, 66]. The physiologic role of adenosine in reducing platelet reactivity *in vivo* is highlighted by the recent description of mice with disrupted gene encoding for the A2aR (A2aR-knockout). Platelets from these animals are hyperresponsive to ADP [67]. It is worth noting that adenosine may play a role in bronchoconstriction [30].

Immunoglobulins (Ig)

Platelets also possess receptors for immunoglobulins, in particular of the IgE and IgG class. Receptors for IgE belong to the FcεRII type and have a lower affinity and are present in a lower number of copies as compared to those present in mast cells and basophils [27]. The cross-linking of an antigen with platelet-bound IgE causes release of inflammatory mediators. IgE receptors have also been implicated in cytotoxic response against parasites: activation of the IgE receptor by exposure of sensitized platelets to an appropriate antigen results in the production of oxygen radicals in concentrations sufficient to kill parasites [30]. The presence of IgE receptors suggests a potential role of platelets in allergic reactions.

Receptors for IgG belong to the family of the FcγRII receptor and are activated by aggregated IgG and IgG immune complex while monomeric IgG (that are normally present in large quantities in blood) do not activate this receptor. The physiological role of the FcγRII receptor is not well known, while it is more clear that this receptor can play a role in certain disease, such as auto-immune thrombocytopenia, thrombocytopenia associated with HIV infection and with sepsis. Some antiplatelet antibodies can activate platelets through the clustering of the FcγRII receptor; this causes platelet aggregation and, thus, an accelerated clearance of platelets and thrombocytopenia [68].

Interestingly, FCγRII can be phosphorylated following platelet stimulation with collagen through a α2β1-independent pathway suggesting that this phosphorylation is mediated by binding of collagen to a receptor different from α2β1, such as GPIV [17]. The exact role of FcγRII in collagen signaling remains, to date, unclear. As for collagen, stimulation of platelets through FcγRII causes PLCγ2 phosphorylation [69].

Platelet organelles

Several types of organelles can be detected in the platelet cytoplasm [4].

(1) Mitochondria are similar to those found in other cells and have a characteristic plication of their internal membrane; they provide ATP for the cytoplasmic metabolic pool.
(2) Peroxysomes are granules that resemble the peroxysomes found in other cells. Peroxysomes contain catalase [4] and synthesize superoxide anion, a cytotoxic mediator of inflammation.

(3) Lysosomes (or λ granules) contain acid hydrolases such as β-hexosaminidase, β-glucoronidase, β-galactosidase and small concentrations of other glycosidases. The secretion of the lysosomal enzymes requires higher levels of intracellular calcium than the secretion of α and dense granules and it is not complete: only 30–60% of the hydrolases are secreted from lysosomes, in contrast to nearly 100% of the substances stored in the other granules [61, 70].

(4) α granules store a variety of proteins such as albumin, which is the protein present at the highest concentration, fibrinogen, vWf and other adhesive molecules (fibronectin, vitronectin, thrombospondin, P selectin), coagulation factors (factor V, factor XI, high molecular weight kininogen, C1 inhibitor, plasminogen activator inhibitor-1, protein S) and growth modulators, such as β thromboglobulin (βTG), platelet factor 4 (PF4), thrombospondin, platelet derived growth factor (PDGF), transforming growth factor β [61, 71]. PF4, transforming growth factor β, PDGF, as well as arachidonic acid metabolites of the lipoxygenase pathway have chemoattractive properties [23] and PF4 stimulates basophils to release histamine [30].
PDGF causes mitogenesis and proliferation of vascular smooth muscle, migration of fibroblasts, migration and proliferaton of monocytes, and superoxide anion generation from eosinophils [23]. PDGF has also been reported to be a mitogen for airway smooth muscle cells *in vitro* [30]. Also platelet themselves respond to PDGF, through an α type PDGF receptor, that causes a feed-back inhibition of aggregation [72].

(5) Dense (or δ) granules. When platelets are observed by electron microscopy, dense granules appear to have a very opaque content. They store non metabolic pools of adenine nucleotides (ATP, ADP), serotonin, vasopressin, pirophosphate and calcium. These granules are absent in patients with storage pool disease that have haemorragic symptoms due to a defective release reaction [4].

Platelet activation

A schematic representation of some of the events that take place during platelet activation is given in Figure 1.

Platelet adhesion

Adhesive interactions between cells are essential for maintaining the structural and functional integrity of the vascular system. Adhesion of platelets to the subendothelial matrix is the first event that takes place in physiological conditions to arrest the blood extravasation from a wounded vessel. Adhesion is mediated by

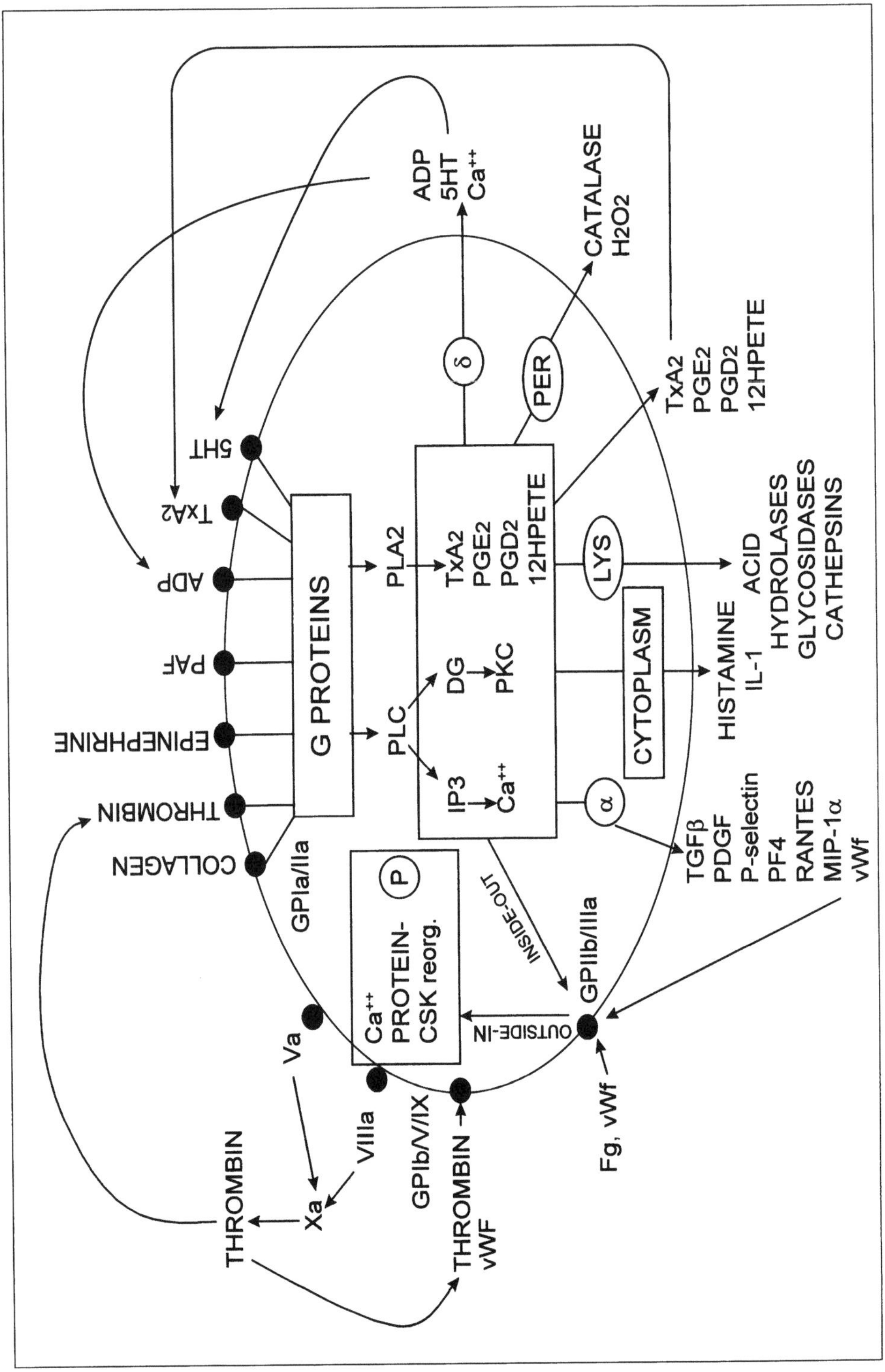
ADP
5HT
Ca++
CATALASE
H2O2
TxA2
PGE2
PGD2
12HPETE
δ
PER
5HT
TxA2
ADP
PAF
EPINEPHRINE
THROMBIN
COLLAGEN
G PROTEINS
PLA2
PLC
DG
PKC
IP3
Ca++
LYS
CYTOPLASM
ACID
HYDROLASES
GLYCOSIDASES
CATHEPSINS
HISTAMINE
IL-1
α
TGFβ
PDGF
P-selectin
PF4
RANTES
MIP-1α
vWf
GPIa/IIa
P
Ca++
PROTEIN-
CSK reorg.
INSIDE-OUT
OUTSIDE-IN
GPIIb/IIIa
Va
VIIIa
Xa
THROMBIN
GPIb/V/IX
THROMBIN
vWF
Fg, vWf

receptors for adhesive molecules which are present in plasma or in the subendothelium. As discussed above, platelet receptors for adhesive molecules are glycoproteins.

When the endothelium is stripped from the vessel, platelets adhere to the denuded extracellular matrix; in particular, platelets adhere to collagen fibers, and fibronectin and vWf are implicated in adhesion to collagen [73]. The initial contact of platelets to subendothelium is mediated by GPIb/IX; in Bernard-Soulier syndrome, because of a GPIb/IX deficiency, platelets do not adhere effectively to the matrix structures in the area of vascular injury [74]. After the initial contact with the subendothelium, platelets spread. Spreading is associated with the change of platelets from a discoidal to a spherical shape (spiny spheres).

Platelet shape change

After the initial adhesion of platelets to the subendothelial matrix, spreading and shape change occur. Resting platelets have a diameter of 2–4 μm and are about 0.5 μm thick; during the shape change phase, platelets become spherical and form many thin philopodia and pseudopodia that can be more than one platelet diameter long. While the platelet volume, during the shape change, remains constant, the platelet surface increases by at least 50% [3]. It has been postulated that the contraction of the actin filaments of the platelet in the early stage of activation causes a relaxation in the membranes that allows the cells to round up. Platelet shape change is associated with myosin phosphorylation: the interaction actin-phosphory-

Figure 1

Schematic representation of platelet structure and activation. The binding of collagen and of soluble platelet agonists to cell surface receptors (close circles) initiates a series of signal transduction events that lead to platelet aggregation and secretion. Most of the platelet receptors are coupled to G proteins that activate, directly or indirectly, PLC and PLA_2, with subsequent activation of PKC, mobilization of calcium (Ca^{2+}), synthesis of TxA_2 and other arachidonic acid metabolites (PGE_2, PGD_2, 12HPETE) that exit from the platelet and act on surrounding cells. Activation of signal transduction mechanisms leads to secretion of the content of α and dense (δ) granules, lysosomes (lys), peroxisomes (per) and to secretion of histamine or IL-1 from the platelet cytoplasm. During platelet activation, GPIIb/IIIa activation occurs (inside-out signaling), with consequent binding of fibrinogen (Fg) and vWf. Activated GPIIb/IIIa, in turn, triggers outside-in events, such as elevation of cytoplasmic calcium, protein phosphorylation (protein-P), reorganization of the cytoskeleton (CSK reorg). Platelets contribute to coagulation, by providing a surface for assembly of activated coagulation factors (Va and VIIIa) that, ultimately, lead to generation of thrombin. vWf and thrombin also bind to GPIb/V/IX complex. For additional abbreviations and details, see text.

lated myosin leads to cellular contraction, organelles centralization and shape change [3].

Platelet aggregation

A number of physiological agonists can induce platelet aggregation (Tab. 2). Platelets can also be activated, *in vitro*, by non-physiological substances, in particular calcium ionophores (e.g. A23187), PKC activators (e.g. phorbol myristate acetate) and non specific G-protein activators (e.g. $AlF4^-$).

The interaction of physiologic agonists with their specific surface receptors triggers a series of signal transduction events that ultimately leads to the activation of the GPIIb/IIIa complex on the platelet surface. As a consequence, in the presence of millimolar concentrations of calcium in the external medium, fibrinogen binds to platelets [58]. Each fibrinogen molecule has two binding sites for GPIIb/IIIa, thus forming bridges between platelet and platelet and allowing aggregation [53].

Receptor-induced GPIIb/IIIa activation is very rapid, and the cell is able to bind fibrinogen within seconds after its initial encounter with the appropriate agonist. The initial fibrinogen binding is reversible, for instance by removal of calcium with chelators, such as EDTA. Following reversible fibrinogen binding, the platelet-platelet interaction undergoes a time-dependent stabilization, that is usually complete in 3–4 min; the irreversible binding of fibrinogen correlates with irreversible platelet aggregation. Once irreversible aggregation has started, removal of calcium or of the agonist is no longer effective in dissociating the aggregates [71].

In certain circumstances, such as under the high shear rates encountered in stenosed atherosclerotic vessels, vWf may substitute for fibrinogen, thus playing a dominant role not only in adhesion, but also in platelet aggregation [75].

Platelet aggregation can be studied *in vitro* in a suspension of platelets in plasma (platelet rich plasma, PRP) or in whole blood. For particular purposes, platelets can be resuspended in buffers at physiological pH and calcium concentrations. In these cases, fibrinogen can be added to the platelet suspension to facilitate aggregation; this is not always necessary, in particular when strong agonists (such as thrombin or TxA_2 analogues) are used because the fibrinogen secreted from activated platelets is sufficient to support aggregation [71].

The most common way of studying platelet aggregation is that of measuring the changes in light transmission through a platelet suspension. At a concentration of $1–3 \times 10^8$/ml platelet suspensions are opalescent. After addition of an agonist, when platelets are stirred at a high-speed, shape change and aggregation occur. In the aggregometer, the shape change phase is recordered as a slight decrease of light transmittance. Although in most cases aggregation is preceded by shape change, this is not always true; for example, epinephrine induces aggregation without shape change. Aggregation is recordered by the aggregometer as an increase in light trans-

Table 2 - A summary of physiological platelet agonists

Agonist	**Comment**
Thrombin	formed by activation of the coagulation cascade
Collagen	present in the subendothelial matrix
ADP	released from platelet dense granules, stressed red blood cells
TxA_2	synthesized by activated platelets
Serotonin	released from platelet dense granules; may sensitize platelets to other stimuli
PAF	synthesized by platelets and other cells
epinephrine	may modulate platelet response to other stimuli

mittance because the more platelets aggregate and the more light will pass through the suspension. With some agonists (e.g. epinephrine or ADP) a first and a second wave of aggregation can be observed [58]. The first wave of aggregation occurs when fibrinogen is bound in a reversible way; if the agonist concentration is high enough, this first wave is followed by a second wave corresponding to an irreversible platelet aggregation. If the agonist is used at maximal concentrations, the first wave of aggregation is not detectable, and only one wave will be observed.

It should be noted that ADP and epinephrine are able to induce irreversible aggregation, *in vitro*, only if low calcium concentrations are present (such as in citrated PRP); thus, it is unlikely that these substances induce secondary aggregation *in vivo* [58].

Release reaction

Irreversible platelet aggregation is triggered and accompanied by secretion of the content of α and dense granules and by the production of mediators, in particular TxA_2, that potentiates aggregation. As discussed above, α and dense granules contain substances that can activate surrounding platelets thus reinforcing the aggregation process. The dense granules contain substances that are rapidly secreted and are listed in Table 3.

The α granules contain especially proteins and peptides that have roles in modulating the growth and gene expression of the cells of the vessel wall. Among these substances there is PDGF (see above) that acts on smooth muscle cells and fibroblasts, and PF4, involved in inflammation. α granules also release coagulation factors, such as factor V and XI, that are taken up by the megakaryocytes and stored in the granules during thrombopoiesis. Factor V is also synthesized by megakary-

Table 3 - A summary of substances released from dense granules

Substance	Comment
ADP	is an agonist for platelets
ATP	may act as an agonist for other blood cells
Serotonin	influences vascular tone and can weakly activate other platelets; contributes to inflammation through vasoconstriction and capacity to increase vascular permeability
Calcium	the physiological role of the secreted calcium is not clear; it can ensure adequate calcium levels for calcium-dependent enzymes of the coagulation cascade

ocytes, since the concentration of this protein is higher than can be accounted for by an uptake from plasma [71]. βTG and PF4 are platelet-specific proteins and their concentration in plasma or in the supernatant of activated platelets is used as a measure of platelet secretion [58].

While platelet dense bodies are released by exocytosis, the mechanism of release of α granules is more complex. Indeed, during secretion, these granules are centralized in the cytoplasm, as a consequence of cytoskeleton reorganization and platelet contraction (see above). Two hypotheses have been proposed for exocytosis when granules are centralized [71].

(1) α granules secrete their content in the open canalicular system, i.e. in the invaginations of the plasma membrane that goes deep into the center of the platelet.
(2) α granules fuse with each other or with another cellular compartment to form a compound granule morphologically distinct from the α granule. This compound granule moves toward the plasma membrane and undergoes exocytosis.

Secretion of the granules is a feature that platelets share with inflammatory cells, such as mast cells and granulocytes, and with neurons. In contrast to neurons, platelet granules do not seem to be pre-docked, and there is a significant lag between activation of the cell and secretion. It has been recently proposed that the key regulatory step in platelet exocytosis is not at the membrane fusion step, as it is in the rapid secretion process of the neuron, but it is at the granule docking step [76]. In addition to transport proteins that mediate the secretory event, low pH within secretory granules, which results from the action of proton pumps and a common characteristic of secretory granules in other cells, may be important in the exocytic event [60].

The molecular mechanisms that regulate platelet secretion can be briefly described as follow. When a stimulatory platelet agonist interacts with its specific receptor, PLC is activated *via* G proteins. PLC cleaves phosphatidylinositol 4,5, biphosphate with the formation of membrane-bound DG and cytosolic IP_3. IP_3 induces Ca^{2+} release from intracellular stores, such as the dense tubular system. In addition to Ca^{2+} release, agonist-receptor interaction also causes a rapid influx of Ca^{2+} from the extracellular medium, through receptor operated Ca^{2+} channels or through cytosolic alkalinization. The Ca^{2+} increase causes activation of myosin light chain kinase and, in turn, phosphorylation of myosin light chain (MLC). This process seems to be involved in platelet shape change, and not in secretion. DG stimulates PKC which phosphorylates pleckstrin (p47). Since the time-course of pleckstrin phosphorylation is the same as that of dense granule secretion and PKC inhibitors inhibit platelet secretion, PKC activation and pleckstrin phosphorylation are considered to be necessary steps in the signal transduction pathways that control secretion [61]. On the other hand, increase in intracellular cyclic AMP inhibits secretion by reducing cytosolic Ca^{2+} levels, although the mechanism for this reduction is unclear [61].

Another substance released from activated platelets is histamine. It is now well established that human, pig or rabbit platelets contain histamine in concentrations similar to those of serotonin. Platelets can both synthesize histamine or sequester it from plasma by an active process. Although it is not clear if histamine is stored in platelet organelles, it can be released following activation of the cells with inflammatory stimuli. In particular, platelets from atopic donors aggregate and release histamine when directly stimulated with anti-IgE antibodies, suggesting that platelets, in this regard, can behave as basophils and mast cells [77]. Released histamine enhances platelet aggregation induced by other agonists (ADP, collagen, arachidonic acid, thrombin and immunological stimuli) through the action on H1 receptors that, in turn, modulate intracellular calcium levels and activate PLA_2 in rabbit platelets [78]. Histamine also induces bronchoconstriction [30].

Platelet migration, parasite killing, particle scavenging

Platelets exert a number of functional activities which appear to be independent and regulated by mechanisms that are different from their well recognized haemostatic function. Platelets can migrate into tissues and have been detected in inflammed tissues or in the bronchoalveolar lavage fluid of asthmatic patients in the absence of red blood cells, thus excluding haemorrage [23, 30, 79]. Several *in vitro* studies have shown that normal platelets migrate in response to non aggregating stimuli such as carbachol, PGE_1 or PGE_2, or to collagen [80–82]. More recently it has been reported that blood platelets from allergic asthmatics migrate upon stimulation with the specific sensitizing allergen *in vitro* [83].

Platelets exert a central role in the defense against parasite invasion, by displaying a cytocidal action on parasite larvae through the production of oxygen radicals (for review see [27]) and may also ingest microparticles, a property that contributes to the scavenging of foreign materials penetrated into the circulation.

Biochemical mechanisms of platelet activation

The functional reactions above described are regulated by a complex series of intracellular events. Indeed, physiologic stimuli do not penetrate the membranes and thus the agonist/receptor interaction evokes a series of signal transduction mechanisms leading to the generation of intracellular messengers that are responsible for the effects of the agonist inside the cell [60].

PLC and PLA_2 are phospholipases activated following platelet stimulation. TxA_2 (formed following PLA_2 activation) and some of the substances released from platelet granules are themselves platelet agonists: they reinforce the activation process by an additional supply of agonist, resulting in the generation of a more sustained signal [36]. In addition to stimulatory pathways triggered by platelet agonists, other signal transduction events take place when receptors for antiaggregatory substances are activated. PGI_2 and PGD_2, in particular, activate adenylate cyclase with consequent increase of intracellular cyclic AMP (cAMP). While an increase of cAMP inhibits platelet activation, the converse is not true: inhibition of adenylate cyclase is not sufficient to promote fibrinogen binding and platelet aggregation [60].

Signal transduction

An activated receptor, belonging to the class of the GPCR, activates an effector (usually an enzyme or an ion channel) through the activation of GTP-binding proteins, also called G proteins. The effector then synthesizes second messengers that are responsible for the cellular response. Although probably not all the intracellular systems regulated by G-proteins have yet been identified, enzymes that are certainly regulated by G proteins are PLC, PLA_2, adenylate cyclase.

The G proteins involved in the activation of these enzymes are heterotrimeric G proteins, formed by three subunits, α, β and γ. In the resting state, the α subunit binds GDP. Agonists whose receptors interact with G proteins promote the release of GDP, which is replaced by the GTP present in the cytosol. This event leads to a conformational change of $G\alpha$, that dissociates from the $\beta\gamma$ complex and activates an effector system. Many evidences exist that demonstrate that not only the α subunit but also the free $\beta\gamma$ complex can activate effector proteins [84]. After a variable length of time, $G\alpha$ hydrolyzes GTP to GDP, goes back to an inactive conformation and reassociates with the $\beta\gamma$ complex, until the next cycle of receptor-mediated activation starts. Several G proteins have been identified in platelets [36, 39, 43, 85] (Tab. 4). The functions of some G proteins in platelets, such as G16 and

Table 4 - G proteins α subunits identified in human platelets

G protein family (α subunits)	Effector	Function	Phosphorylated
Gi			
Gαi2>>Gαi3>Gαi1	Adenylate cyclase	⇓ cAMP	No
	PLC	⇑ IP3, DG	
Gαz	?	?	Yes
Gs			
GαsS, GαsL	Adenylate cyclase	⇑ cAMP	No
Gq			
Gαq	PLC	⇑ IP3, DG	No
Gα16	PLC ?	⇑ IP3, DG ?	No
G12			
Gα12, Gα13	?	?	Yes
Gh			
Gαh	PLC ?	⇑ IP3, DG ?	?

Gh, have not been investigated, although an increase of inositol phosphate upon activation of these G proteins has been observed in overexpression systems [43, 86].

It is interesting to note that phosphorylation of Gzα, G12α and G13α has been observed following platelet activation and shown to be protein kinase C (PKC)-mediated, although the biological effects of this phosphorylation are not well understood [87, 88]. Recently, mice deficient in Gi2 [89], G13 [90] and Gq [91] have been generated. While no platelet defects are described in the Gi2 and G13 knock-outs, major platelet abnormalities are present in the Gq-deficient animals. Indeed, platelets from these mice fail to aggregate and to undergo release reaction induced by several agonists (thrombin, ADP, collagen, thromboxane analogues and arachidonic acid). These abnormalities are accompanied by a defective activation of PLC and thus suggest that stimulation of PLC in platelets occurs mainly through Gq. Platelets from Gq-deficient mice undergo, on the other hand, normal shape change, indicating that other G proteins, such as Gi, G12 or G13, are involved in induction of shape change. Recently, a patient with decreased levels of Gq in platelets and a bleeding diathesis has been described for the first time [92].

PLCβ1 and PLCβ3 are activated predominantly by the members of the Gq family (Gq, G11, G16 and its murine counterpart G15), while PLCβ2 seems to be activated predominantly by the βγ complex released by Gi, although different hierarchies have been reported depending on the system used [36, 93]. The activation of PLC leads to the hydrolysis of membrane inositol phospholipids (in particular phosphatidyl inositol 4,5 biphosphate) with consequent synthesis of IP_3 and DG. IP_3, acting on specific receptors, mobilizes calcium from the dense tubular system, thus promoting an increase of intracellular calcium. Calcium is necessary for activation of other enzymes, such as PLA2, PKC, myosin light chain kinase. DG activates PKC, in synergism with calcium [94], which in turn phosphorylates some proteins, such as pleckstrin (p47) and myosin light chain (MLC, p20) that ultimately lead to secretion and shape change, respectively [60]. MLC can be phosphorylated by both PKC and myosin light chain kinase which is a calcium-calmodulin dependent enzyme [95]. As discussed above, myosin phosphorylation is directly involved in shape change, contraction and granule centralization. In addition to members of the PLCβ family, PLCγ1 has been detected in platelets, and a complex mechanism for its activation, not related to heterotrimeric G proteins but to small G proteins, has been proposed [96].

Phospholipase A_2 is another key enzyme activated following platelet stimulation, and it will be discussed later (see below). Another enzyme involved in platelet activation, although its roles are not yet fully elucidated, is phospholipase D (PLD). PLD cleaves the terminal phosphodiester bond of membrane phospholipids, in particular phosphatidylcholine, causing the release of phosphatidic acid (PA) and a free base. PLD is activated, in platelets, by thrombin [97, 98], collagen [98] and, to a lesser extent, by other agonists [99]. The PLD-derived PA accounts for only 10–20% of the total PA formed in thrombin-stimulated platelets while the majority of the PA pool is formed as a consequence of PLC activation, following the phosphorylation of DG by the enzyme DG kinase [97]. It must be noted that not only DG can be metabolized into PA, but that also PA can be degraded into DG, through the enzyme phosphatidate phosphohydrolase. Recent data, obtained in endothelial cells, show that the PA formed through the activation of PLC and PLD have a different fatty acid composition [100] rising the possibility that PLD-derived PA and PLC-derived PA play distinct roles in signal transduction. It needs to be elucidated if these differences in signaling pathways also occur in platelets.

Adenylate cyclase is activated when platelets encounter antiaggregatory substances, such as PGD_2, PGI_2 and adenosine. Agents that activate adenylate cyclase do so by turning-on Gs and this results in an increase of intraplatelet cAMP that, in turn, activates protein kinase A (PKA). cAMP causes inhibition of both PLC and PLA_2, although a direct PKA-mediated phosphorylation of these enzymes has not been demonstrated [96]. cAMP also alters the binding of fibrinogen to platelets [60] and it can also decrease the binding of certain platelet agonists to their receptor [101]. Little is known about the isoforms of adenylate cyclase present in platelets, but it is known that the type I enzyme is absent; in HEL cells, which share many characteristic with platelets, type III and IV adenylate cyclase have been detected by polymerase chain reaction (PCR) [36].

Adenylate cyclase is also under the control of an inhibitory G protein, Gi. The activation of Gi by several GPCR leads to the inhibition of adenylate cyclase and to a decrease of raised intracellular cAMP.

Arachidonic acid metabolism and PLA_2

As briefly discussed above, TxA_2, an arachidonic acid metabolite, represents a mediator potentially important for both the haemostatic and non haemostatic functions of platelets. Arachidonic acid is cleaved from the 2 position of several membrane phospholipids by PLA_2 although minor amounts can also be released by other routes, such as the release from DG by diacylglycerol lipase [60]. Several PLA2 enzymes exist and the present knowledge on this topic has recently been reviewed [102]. Platelets have at least two PLA_2 isoforms. One is secretable PLA_2 ($sPLA_2$), it has a low molecular weight (13–15 kDa) and, to be active, requires high, supraphysiological, concentrations of calcium (in the millimolar range) [102]. In many cell types $sPLA_2$ is found in secretable granules, in addition to snake and bee venoms, synovial fluid and pancreatic secretions [103] but the exact location of sPLA2 in platelets in not known. Also the functions of platelet $sPLA_2$ are not fully elucidated; secreted $sPLA_2$ does not seem to significantly contribute to the biosynthesis of TxA_2 in stimulated platelets [104].

Platelet cytosolic PLA2 (cPLA2) has been studied more extensively and its role and regulation are better understood. cPLA2 is responsible for the bulk of arachidonic acid release after platelet activation. cPLA2 is active at physiologic calcium concentrations (~ 0.05 μM) and has a molecular weight of ~ 85–100 kDa [102, 103]. $cPLA_2$ is specific for the 2 position of phospholipids; arachidonic acid is the preferred fatty acid in this position, but other polyunsaturated fatty acids can be released as well [103]. The preferred substrate for $cPLA_2$ is phosphatidylcholine, but also phosphatidylethanolamine and phosphatidylserine can be hydrolyzed, while phosphatidylinositol is a poor substrate for this enzyme [103, 105]. Studies in cells different from platelets have demonstrated that $cPLA_2$ binds to the cytoplasmic surface of the endoplasmic reticulum and is associated topologically with cyclooxygenase 1, which is located on the luminal surface [7]; accordingly, in platelets the release of arachidonic acid is thought to occur primarily at the membrane of the dense tubular system [36].

The regulation of $cPLA_2$ in platelets has not been fully elucidated. It has been demonstrated that activation of $cPLA_2$ is associated, at least in thrombin-stimulated platelets, with its phosphorylation [104] and that thrombin also activates a member of MAPK family, called p38 [106]. Although p38 phosphorylates $cPLA_2$, this phosphorylation is not required for $cPLA_2$ catalytic activity: indeed, $cPLA_2$ activity is not attenuated when p38 MAPK-mediated phosphorylation is abrogated [107]. The regulation of $cPLA_2$ by PKC and more in general by phosphorylation/dephosphorylation reactions is complex and probably differently modulated depending on the stimulus leading to the activation of the enzyme [103, 108]. Another issue that is not clear concerning $cPLA_2$ regulation, is if $cPLA_2$ is directly activated by G proteins [103]. Although it has been demonstrated that fluoro-aluminate, an aspecific G proteins activator, is able to induce arachidonic acid release from intact human platelets [109] and many other studies have been performed with platelet membranes, it is not yet known which is the GPCR and the G protein(s) involved in $cPLA_2$ activation and whether the α or the $\beta\gamma$ subunits are important [103].

Once released from membrane phospholipids arachidonic acid is metabolized by cyclooxygenase. This enzyme has a cyclooxygenase activity, which catalyzes PGG_2 formation from arachidonic acid, and a hydroperoxydase activity, that catalyzes the reduction of a hydroperoxy group of PGG_2, resulting in PGH_2 synthesis [28]. PGH_2 is further metabolized by different enzymes, that give TxA_2, PGD_2 and PGE_2 in platelets. Other metabolites, such as PGI_2 and $PGF_{2\alpha}$, can be formed in other cells. While PGD_2, PGE_2 and $PGF_{2\alpha}$ are rather stable, TxA_2 and PGI_2 are very rapidly degraded into TxB_2 and 6-keto $PGF_{1\alpha}$, respectively, that are stable but biologically inactive.

In addition to cyclooxygenase, arachidonic acid in platelets can be metabolized by one of the enzymes of the lipoxygenase family, 12-lipoxygenase. 12-lipoxygenase catalyzes the formation of 12HPETE, which is then converted to 12HETE by a peroxidase. 12HETE can not be further metabolized by platelets, but it can be taken up by neutrophils. Neutrophils possess 5-lipoxygenase that, in activated cells, can convert 12HETE into 5,12 diHETE [28].

Production of oxygen radicals

Oxygen free radicals are reactive chemical species. Among these, superoxide anion (O_2^-), hydrogen peroxide (H_2O_2), peroxyl radicals (ROO•), hydroxyl radicals (OH•) and peroxynitrites ($ONOO^-$) are produced in the vascular system, in particular during ischemia followed by reperfusion of the myocardium. In fact, the reoxygenation that occurs during reperfusion generates oxygen free radicals that react with several cellular targets, resulting in injury of the tissue [110].

It is well established that polymorphonuclear neutrophils release cytotoxic oxygen free radicals [111]. Similarly, platelets can produce oxygen radicals and do so after stimulation with agonists, and following the activation that takes place during ischemia and reperfusion [112]. In particular, reoxygenated anoxic platelets produce O_2^- and OH• and these reactive species are able to induce platelet aggregation. The aggregatory activity of O_2^- and OH• is largely mediated by cyclooxygenase, through the metabolism of arachidonic acid and the synthesis of TxA_2 that, in turn, can cause activation of PLC and PLA_2 [112]. OH• can exit the cell and form H_2O_2 in the external medium. H_2O_2 can react with O_2^- and generate the highly reactive hydroxyl radical OH•. Also superoxide dismutase, presumably by its ability to produce H_2O_2, can activate platelets [110].

Oxygen free radicals have cytotoxic activity because they cause oxidation of membrane phospholipids, disrupting the membrane integrity and fluidity and perhaps also interfering with the functions of receptors on the cell surface [110]. A platelet agonist whose activity may be enhanced by oxygen free radicals is PAF. PAF is inactivated by PAF-acetylhydrolase that can be inhibited irreversibly by oxygen radicals. This phenomenon leads to a more sustained effect of PAF not only on platelets, but also on sites of inflammation, thus worsening the inflammatory effects of this mediator [110].

Oxygen radicals also inhibit other enzymes important for platelet function. In particular, hydroperoxides, such as 15(S)-hydroperoxyeicosatetranoic acid (15(S)HPETE), inhibit cyclooxygenase and thromboxane synthase. In the case of cyclooxygenase, 15(S)HPETE-induced inhibition involves both a modification of the heme group and a modification of the protein itself and both the cyclooxygenase and the peroxidase activity of the enzyme are lost [113].

Cyclooxygenase and thromboxane synthase can also be inhibited by their own substrates, which are PGG_2 and PGH_2, respectively. This particular kind of inactivation is called "suicide" inactivation and, since it occurs during catalysis, can provide an important mechanism to limit prostanoid biosynthesis. The mechanism of inactivation of cyclooxygenase and thromboxane synthase by their substrates is somewhat different from the inactivation caused by other hydroperoxydes. In particular, while 15(S)HPETE or other hydroperoxydes inhibit both the cyclooxygenase and the peroxydase activity of the enzyme cyclooxygenase, during "suicide" inactivation only the cyclooxygenase activity is inhibited. It has been proposed that, during "suicide" inactivation, an activated and unstable cyclooxygenase protein intermediate is formed, that then rearranges irreversibly into an inactive cyclooxygenase, without concomitant loss of peroxidase activity [113].

In the case of thromboxane synthase, "suicide" inactivation is accompanied by a modification of the prostetic heme group and it differs from the inactivation due to hydroperoxydes that seems to result from apoenzyme modification [114].

Role of platelets in inflammation

Functional activities relevant to inflammation

It is now widely accepted that platelets can behave, in particular conditions, as inflammatory cells [23, 30, 115–118]. Historically, the first clues to the inflammatory role of platelets came from the observations that platelets are recovered at inflammatory sites or in inflammatory exudates [119–123]. More recently, with the increasing interest in the participation of platelets to respiratory allergy, several reports have shown the presence of platelets or of abnormal megakaryocytes in lungs or alveolar space of patients with asthma [79, 124, 125].

It is interesting to observe that platelets themselves can elicit inflammatory reactions as shown by the swelling, redness and tenderness lasting several hours reported after the subcutaneous injection of platelet extracts in normal humans, a reaction more evident and more prolonged than that observed after the injection of leukocyte extracts [126].

Platelets display a number of functional activities that are quite typical of inflammatory cells. Indeed, similarly to white blood cells, platelets show rolling and attachment on altered endothelium [22], diapedesis through endothelial cells [125], chemokinesis and chemotaxis [83].

Biochemical properties of platelets relevant to inflammation

Platelets present a number of biochemical properties which may be relevant to inflammation. Indeed, they can release a series of mediators, either stored in their granules or cytoplasm or synthetized upon activation, that may participate in eliciting and maintaining the inflammatory reaction. The series of substances potentially important include [23, 117]:

δ-granules; serotonin is vasoactive, vasopermeabilizing and stimulates fibroblasts and as such acts as an inflammatory mediator [127];

α-granules; PGDF and TGFβ are growth factors which display vasoactive and chemotactic properties [128]; PF4, which stimulates basophils to release histamine and is chemotactic for eosinophils [129, 130]; RANTES, a powerful chemoattractant for eosinophils but also a modulator of chemokine secretion by monocytes, released by activated human blood platelets [131, 132]; MIP-1α, a chemokine able to induce histamine release from basophils and is chemotactic for T lymphocytes [133]; P-selectin, an adhesion molecule expressed on the surface of activated platelets as well as on endothelial cells, which regulates the interactions between platelets and leukocytes as well as the initial attachment and rolling of leukocytes to endothelium. Monoclonal antibodies directed against P-selectin [134] or gene disruption of the P-selectin gene [135], reduces allergic airway responses;

Cytoplasm or anyway in an undefined location within platelets, histamine, a notorious inflammatory mediator which can be released in relevant concentrations from platelets, at least in some species, after stimulation with aggregating agonists or immunologic stimuli [77]; interleukin-1 (IL-1), an important cytokine modulating the interactions between leukocytes and endothelial cells which take place during the inflammation reaction [136]. IL-1 can be released by activated platelets and can lead to the liberation of several cytokines from endothelial and vascular smooth muscle cells [137];

Lysosomes, several acid hydrolases and cathepsins which can be released *in vivo* upon platelet activation [138] and that may participate in inflammation through their cytotoxic and tissue-degrading activities [70];

Substances produced upon metabolic activation, such as TxA_2, several prostanoids (PGE_2, PGD_2), products of the lipoxygenases cascade (12HPETE, LTB_4), PAF and hydrogen peroxide, which may all contribute to the vasomotor, chemotactic and vasopermeabilizing phenomena of inflammation [23, 30].

Platelets and the airways

Functional and biochemical activities relevant to allergic airway responses

Interestingly, FCγRII can be phosphorylated following platelet stimulation with collagen through a α2β1-independent pathway suggesting that this phosphorylation is mediated by binding of collagen to a receptor different from α2β1, such as GPIV [17]. The exact role of FcγRII in collagen signaling remains, to date, unclear. As for collagen, stimulation of platelets through FcγRII causes PLCγ2 phosphorylation [69].

A number of functional activities and biochemical properties of platelets above described for inflammation may be of special relevance to the dynamic and anatomic changes which take place during airway allergic responses.

Platelets can roll on altered endothelium, the first step for margination and subsequent diapedesis [22]. Platelets express IgE receptors which have an affinity similar to the receptors present on macrophages and eosinophils and which are implicated in the cytotoxic response against parasites [30]. Interestingly, while only approximately 25% of platelets from normal subjects bind IgE, more than 35% of platelets of patients with allergic asthma do [27]. Moreover, the cross-linking of surface-bound IgE, with anti-IgE monoclonal antibodies or with the specific sensitizing allergen, induces platelet chemotaxis *in vitro* (Gresele et al., unpublished observations).

Once migrated into the airways [125] platelets may release spasmogenic substances (serotonin, TxA_2, histamine), cytotoxic mediators (H_2O_2, lysosomal content), agents able to induce remodelling (e.g. PDGF or TNFβ, etc.) and, most importantly, a series of powerful chemotactic substances able to recruit eosinophils and other inflammatory cells (PF4, 12HPETE, RANTES, MIP-1α, IL-1, etc.).

Experimental models on the participation of platelets to airway inflammation

The first experimental observations on the potential participation of platelets to bronchoconstiction came from studies showing that the intravenous injection of platelet agonists in animals induces thrombocytopenia associated with severe bronchospasm [139, 140]. Conversely, the challenge of sensitized rodents with allergen induces bronchospasm associated with thrombocytopenia and platelet depletion of the animals prevents allergen-induced bronchospasm [141, 142]. During these reactions platelets accumulate in lungs, as shown by the use of radiolabelled platelets [30] and by the analysis of the broncho-alveolar lavage fluid [79]. Simultaneously, platelet-released products (e.g. PF4) are detected in the bloodstream, as observed in sensitized rabbits challenged with allergen or after stimulation with PAF [143]. Histologic studies show that platelets undergo diapedesis and localize in proximity to bronchial smooth muscle cells and, interestingly, colocalize in lung tissue with eosinophils [144]. It appears that eosinophil recruitment is in some way modulated by platelets as platelet depletion of the animals reduces antigen-induced eosinophil infiltration in lungs [145].

Eosinophils play a central role in the histopathologic changes accompanying asthma (see chapter by Coyle and Gutierrez-Ramos, this volume). We have already mentioned some substances released by platelets and that have been shown to exert strong chemoattractant properties on eosinophils. The converse is also true: eosinophils may release platelet activating substances [166] and it is suggestive that some conditions of hypereosinophilia in humans have been reported to be associated with thrombotic phenomena [147, 148].

One link between platelets and eosinophils may be represented by PAF, as this lipidic mediator induces eosinophil infiltration in lungs which is prevented by platelet depletion [145] and, on the other hand, eosinophils from allergic asthmatics produce large amounts of PAF [149]. Interestingly, PAF antagonists inhibit airway hyperresponsiveness induced by antigen challenge in allergic rabbits [30].

The exact sequence of events leading to platelet and eosinophil localization in lung tissue is presently unknown. It is tempting to speculate that the allergen interacts with IgEs localized on the IgE-receptor of platelets of sensitized subjects provoking platelet diapedesis in lungs and that, subsequently, PAF locally produced by inflammatory cells (macrophages?) induces platelets to release chemotactic substances which recruit eosinophils in lungs. Eosinophils in turn may release cytotoxic, chemotactic and platelet activating substances giving rise to a vicious circle leading to airway hyperreactivity and tissue remodelling.

Observations in humans on the participation of platelets to airway inflammation

Several studies have assessed the involvement of blood platelets in bronchial asthma in humans. These have been previously extensively reviewed [23, 30, 150]. Most of the studies have evaluated platelet aggregation or other parameters related to platelet activation *in vitro* and, more recently, parameters related to *in vivo* platelet activation. Several investigations have shown some degreee of platelet function abnormality *in vitro*, with hypoaggregability to ADP, adrenaline or collagen and reduced release of α- and δ-granule content [23, 30]. Platelet refractoriness has been reported to be particularly evident for PAF [151–153] and this has been considered as an indicator of PAF-release *in vivo* as platelets develop refractoriness to this agonist after exposure. Indeed, the number of freely accessible PAF-receptors on platelets of allergic asthmatics undergoing allergen challenge is significantly reduced, indicating that part of them are occupied by PAF secreted in the circulation [154].

Reduced *in vitro* platelet activation upon stimulation with PAF has been more recently demonstrated by the impaired expression of surface platelet activation antigens, such as CD62P and CD63, by cytofluorimetry in asthmatics [155]. Platelet hypoaggregability *in vitro* is compatible with a partial refractoriness developed as a result of previous *in vivo* platelet activation, and other altered platelet function parameters have been reported in asthmatics, such as increased resting levels of cytoplasmic Ca^{2+}, or increased IP3 [151, 156] which may also reflect previous *in vivo* platelet stimulation. Many attempts have been made to demonstrate an *in vivo* activation of platelets in asthmatic patients, especially by measuring platelet-release markers in plasma (βTG and PF4) or urinary metabolites of TxA_2. Although contrasting results with βTG and/or PF4 have been reported [23], the prevailing view is that, at least in some patients with allergic asthma, allergen challenge induces the release of α-granules markers in the circulation [23, 30, 131, 157–159]. In one study, plasma levels of PAF were also measured and found to correlate with βTG or PF4, suggesting a relationship between PAF release and platelet activation [159].

The use of plasma levels of βTG/PF4 has been criticized because of possible artifacts or lack of sensitivity [160, 161]. However, *in vivo* platelet activation during asthmatic attacks has been detected with other methods which are less prone to methodologic problems, such as the measurement of urinary metabolites of TxA_2 or the expression of surface activation antigens on circulating platelets by cytofluorimetry [162–164].

The main limitations of the studies summarized above are represented by the measurement of *in vivo* platelet activation parameters only during the acute reaction that follows an allergen provocation test and by the use of techniques which measure parameters of platelet activation which are usually adopted for the assessment of *in vivo* thrombus formation. From animal studies and the basic knowledge on platelet biochemistry, it is more likely that platelets may be involved in the genesis of the inflammatory reactions that accompany bronchial asthma and, in addition, it has been shown that several of the non-haemostatic functions of platelets follow mechanisms which are different from those involved in haemostasis and thrombosis [23, 27].

More recent studies have adopted a new approach to the evaluation of platelet activation in asthma. It has been shown that platelets undergo functional changes during exacerbations of nocturnal asthma, a condition which corresponds to airway hyperresponsiveness and is strictly dependent on airway inflammatory changes [152]. In addition, using subsegmental antigen challenge in asthmatics it was shown that βTG and PF4 increase strikingly in bronchoalveolar lavage fluid not immediately but 19 h after allergen challenge and correlates with levels of eosinopil-derived proteins [165] indicating that platelets participate in the late asthmatic response in a way that is strictly linked to eosinophil infiltration. Indeed, RANTES, a powerful chemoattractant, has been found to be increased in patients with asthma during spontaneous attacks in a way that correlates with the rise in plasma βTG, thus suggesting a platelet origin of the chemokine [131]. Platelets from atopic individuals stimulated through their IgE receptors release large amounts of RANTES [166] and histamine [77]. Interestingly, platelets from allergic asthmatics migrate *in vitro* in response to the sensitizing allergen but also to monoclonal antibodies anti human IgE, thus involving platelet sensitization through the IgE receptor in the platelet recruitment in lungs ([83] and Gresele et al., unpublished observations). Indeed, several reports have shown platelets in lung tissue in patients with asthma [79, 124, 167] and platelet migrated through the endothelium have been observed on electron microscopy of the lung tissue [125].

Once penetrated in lung tissue, an increased production of oxygen radicals as a consequence of defective GSH-peroxidase may contribute to tissue damage [168].

Pharmacologic modulation of platelet function: possible relevance to airways inflammation

If platelets are involved in the pathogenesis of allergic bronchocostriction then it is tempting to speculate that platelet-inhibitory drugs might be useful in this clinical condition. Thus, a few studies have tested antiplatelet agents in animal models or in patients with allergic asthma for their effects on bronchoconstriction.

Aspirin and sulphinpyrazone have not been able to inhibit bronchoconstriction or to blunt the *in vivo* platelet activation which follow allergen challenge in humans or PAF administration in animals [169, 170]. Even prostacyclin, a powerful platelet inhibitor and a vasodilator, was unable to affect the bronchoconstriction induced by PAF inhalation, despite inhibition of platelet aggregation [171]. Similarly, indomethacin, at doses suppressing the increase of urinary TxA_2-metabolites induced by allergen challenge, was not able to influence pulmonary function [172]. PAF antagonists too have been administered to asthmatic patients with disappointing results on pulmonary function despite inhibition of *ex vivo* PAF-induced platelet-aggregation [30].

These data may indicate that platelets are not really important for the pathogenesis of allergic bronchoconstriction or else that the mechanisms involved in the expression of platelet proinflammatory properties are insensitive to inhibitors of the platelet prothrombotic activities. The latter hypothesis seems to be supported by a number of observations on the effects of some antiallergic agents on non-haemostatic platelet functions.

Nedocromil sodium, an inhibitor of IgE-mediated-histamine-release from mast cells, reduces the IgE-stimulated parasitocidal and hydrogen peroxide-producing activity of human platelets [173, 174]. Nedocromil sodium was also able to inhibit platelet activation induced by PAF, but not by the calcium ionophore A23187, *in vitro* [175]. Other antiallergic drugs which have shown an action on platelets *in vitro* are: cortisol, cromolyn and albuterol, which were shown to normalize the decreased platelet sodium-potassium adenosine triphosphatase activity of allergic subjects [176] and disodium cromoglycate, that was found to reduce the inhibitory effect exerted by IgE on monoamine uptake in normal platelets [177].

A few studies have also assessed the effect of some antiallergic agents on platelet function *ex vivo* or *in vivo* in allergic subjects: glucocorticoids and ketotifen [178] as well as disodium cromoglycate (40 mg daily for 4 weeks) increased significantly the shortened platelet survival time in patients with stable allergic asthma [177]; terbutaline was reported to reduce the platelet hypereactivity, assessed by platelet clumping on smear or by platelet adhesiveness, observed during acute asthma [179].

These data, although rather preliminary and probably not yet centered on the platelet functions most relevant to airway hypereactivity, suggest that therapeutic interventions aimed at suppressing platelet pro-inflammatory activities may be useful for the treatment of allergic asthma.

Conclusions

This review has tried to give an account of the latest knowledge on platelet physiology and on the mechanisms that regulate the participation of platelets to haemostasis and thrombosis and to non-haemostatic processes. The picture that emerges is that of the platelet as a multifunctional cell, with different pathways regulating on one side platelet haemostatic activities and on the other platelet proinflammatory actions.

While a very large research effort has been spent in understanding the participation of platelets in the pathophysiology of thrombosis, much less attention has been given to the role of platelets in inflammation. A major limitation in the research on the role of platelets in inflammation derives from the application of methodologies used to study platelet haemostatic function, which may be inappropriate in the study of platelets in the context of inflammation. The application of unconventional methodologies to the study of platelets is giving new impetus to the efforts to better understand the mechanisms regulating platelet inflammatory activities.

The identification of the molecular mechanisms regulating platelet inflammatory activities, and in particular of the mechanisms involved in platelet diapedesis in the inflammed tissue, may allow the development of new antinflammatory and anti-asthmatic therapeutic strategies.

Acknowledgments
The authors thank Dr. S. Momi and Dr. A.M. Mezzasoma for their help with the preparation of the manuscript and of the figure.

References

1 Antiplatelet Trialists' Collaboration (1994) Collaborative overview of randomized trials of antiplatelet therapy: 1. Prevention of death, myocardial infraction and stroke by prolonged antiplatelet therapy in various categories of patients. *Brit Med J* 308: 81–106
2 de Gaetano G, Cerletti C, Gresele P (1996) Pathogenesis of arterial thrombosis. *L'Ospedale Maggiore* 90: 290–299
3 Daniel JL (1994) Platelet contractile proteins. In: RW Colman, J Hirsh, VJ Marder, EW Salzman (eds): *Haemostasis and thrombosis: basic principles and clinical practice.* JB Lippincott, Philadelphia, 557–573
4 White JG (1994) Anatomy and structural organization of the platelet. In: RW Colman, J Hirsh, VJ Marder, EW Salzman (eds): *Haemostasis and thrombosis: basic principles and clinical practice.* JB Lippincott, Philadelphia, 397–413
5 Hershman HR (1996) Prostaglandin synthase 2. *Biochim Biophys Acta* 1299: 125–140
6 DeWitt D, Smith WL (1995) Yes, but do they still get headaches? *Cell* 83: 345–348
7 Smith WL, DeWitt DL, Arakawa T, Spencer AG, Thuresson ED, Song I (1997) Independent prostanoid biosynthetic systems associated with prostaglandin endoperoxide synthases-1 and -2. *Thromb Haemost* 77: 627–630
8 Charo IF, Kniffer N, Phillips DR (1994) Platelet membrane glycoproteins. In: RW Colman, J Hirsh, VJ Marder, EW Salzman (eds): *Haemostasis and thrombosis: basic principles and clinical practice.* JB Lippincott, Philadelphia, 489–507
9 Hawiger J (1994) Adhesive interactions of blood cells and the vascular wall. In: RW Colman, J Hirsh, VJ Marder, EW Salzman (eds): *Haemostasis and thrombosis: basic principles and clinical practice.* JB Lippincott, Philadelphia, 762–796
10 Faull RJ, Ginsberg MH (1996) Inside-out signalling through integrins. *J Am Soc Nephrol* 7: 1091–1097
11 Calvete JJ (1994) Clues for understanding the structure and function of a prototypic human integrin: the platelet GPIIb/IIIa complex. *Thromb Haemost* 72: 1–15
12 Du X, Ginsberg MH (1997) Integrin $\alpha IIb\beta 3$ and platelet function. *Thromb Haemost* 77: 96–100
13 van Willigen G, Hers I, Gorter G, Akkerman JWN (1996) Exposure of the ligand-bind-

ing sites on platelet integrin αIIb/β3 by phosphorylation of the β3 subunit. *Biochem J* 314: 768–779
14 Moroi M, Jung SM (1997) Platelet receptors for collagen. *Thromb Haemost* 77: 439–444
15 Watson SP, Reep B, Connell RT, Lapetina EG (1985) Collagen stimulates [^{3}H] inositol triphosphate formation in indomethacin-treated human platelets. *Biochem J* 226: 831–837
16 Shattil SJ, Ginsberg MH, Brugge JS (1994) Adhesive signaling in platelets. *Curr Opin Cell Biol* 6: 695–704
17 Keely PJ, Parise LV (1996) The α2β1 integrin is a necessary co-receptor for collagen-induced activation of Syk and the subsequent phosphorylation of phospholipase Cγ2 in platelets. *J Biol Chem* 271: 26668–26676
18 Clemetson KJ (1997) Platelet GPIb/V/IX complex. *Thromb Haemost* 77: 266–270
19 Jamieson GA (1997) Pathophysiology of platelet thrombin receptor. *Thromb Haemost* 77: 241–245
20 Du X, Fox JE, Pei S (1996) Identification of a binding sequence for the 14-3-3 protein within the cytoplasmic domain of the adhesion receptor, platelet glycoprotein Ibα. *J Biol Chem* 271: 7362–7367
21 Ruggeri ZM (1997) Mechanisms initiating platelet thrombus formation. *Thromb Haemost*as 78: 611–616
22 Frenette PS, Johnson RC, Hynes RO, Wagner DD (1995) Platelets roll on stimulated endothelium *in vivo*: an interaction mediated by endothelial P-selectin. *Proc Natl Acad Sci USA* 92: 7450–54
23 Gresele P (1991) The platelet in asthma. In: CP Page (ed): *The platelet in health and disease*. Blackwell Scientific Publications, Oxford, 132–157
24 Fox JEB (1993) Regulation of platelet function by the cytoskeleton. In: KS Authi, SP Watson, VV Kakkar (eds): *Mechanisms of platelet activation and control*. Plenum Publishing Co., New York, 175–185
25 Fox JEB (1993) The platelet cytoskeleton. *Thromb Haemost* 70: 884–893
26 Fox JEB.(1996) Platelet activation: new aspects. *Haemostasis* 26 (Suppl 4): 102–131
27 Joseph M (1991) The involvement of platelets in the allergic response. In: CP Page (ed): *The platelet in health and disease*. Blackwell Scientific Publications, Oxford, 120–131
28 Marcus AJ (1994) Multicellular eicosanoid and other metabolic interactions of platelets and other cells. In: RW Colman, J Hirsh, VJ Marder, EW Salzman (eds): *Haemostasis and thrombosis: basic principles and clinical practice*. JB Lippincott, Philadelphia, 590–602
29 FitzGerald GA (1991) Mechanisms of platelet activation: thomboxane A_2 as an amplifying signal for other agonists. *Am J Cardiol* 68: 11B–15B
30 Herd CM, Page CP (1994) Pulmonary immune cells in health and disease: platelets. *Eur Resp J* 7: 1145–1160
31 Coleman RA, Smith WL, Narumiya S (1994) VIII. International Union of Pharmacolo-

gy. Classification of prostanoid receptors: properties, distribution, and structure of the receptors and their subtypes. *Pharmacol Rev* 46: 205–229
32 Hirata M, Hayashi Y, Ushikubi F, Yokota Y, Kageyama R, Nakanishi S, Narumiya S (1991) Cloning and expression of cDNA for a human thromboxane A_2 receptor. *Nature* 349: 617–620
33 Raychowdhury MK, Yakawa M, Collins LJ, McGrail SH, Kent C, Ware JA (1994) Alternative splicing produces a divergent cytoplasmic tail in the human endothelial thromboxane A_2 receptor. *J Biol Chem* 269: 19256–19261 and (1995) published erratum *J Biol Chem* 270: 7011
34 Allan CJ, Higashiura K, Martin M, Morinelli TA, Kurtz DT, Geoffroy O, Meier GP, Gettys TW, Halushka PV (1996) Characterization of the cloned HEL thromboxane A_2 receptor: evidence that the affinity state can be altered by the Galpha 13 and Galpha q. *J Pharmacol Exp Ther* 277: 1132–1139
35 Hirata M, Ushikubi F, Kakizuka A, Okuma M, Narumiya S (1996) Two thomboxane A2 receptor isoforms in human platelets. Opposite coupling to adenylyl cyclase with different sensitivity to Arg^{60} to Leu mutation. *J Clin Invest* 97: 949–956
36 Brass LF, Manning DR, Cichowski K, Abrams CS (1997) Signaling through G proteins in platelets: to the integrins and beyond. *Thromb Haemost* 77: 581–589
37 Shenker A, Goldsmith P, Unson CG, Spiegel AM (1991) The G protein coupled to the thromboxane receptor in human platelets in a member of the novel Gq family. *J Biol Chem* 266: 9309–9313
38 Knezevic I, Borg C, Le Breton GC (1993) Identification of Gq as one of the G proteins that copurify with human platelet thromboxane A_2 receptors. *J Biol Chem* 268: 26011–26017
39 Offermanns S, Laugwitz L, Spicher K, Schultz G (1994) G proteins of the G12 family are activated *via* thromboxane A_2 and thrombin receptors in human platelets. *Proc Natl Acad Sci USA* 91: 504–508
40 Offermanns S, Simon MI (1995) $G\alpha_{15}$ and $G\alpha_{16}$ couple to a wide variety of receptors to phospholipase C. *J Biol Chem* 270: 15175–15180
41 Brass LF, Sheller CC, Belmonte EJ (1987) Inositol 1,4,5-triphosphate induced granule secretion in platelets. Evidence that the activation of phospholipase C mediated by thromboxane receptors involves a guanine nucleotide binding protein-dependent mechanism from that of thrombin. *J Clin Invest* 79: 1269–1275
42 Ushikubi F, Nakamura K, Narumiya S (1994) Functional reconstitution of platelet thromboxane A_2 receptor with Gq and Gi2 in phospholipid vesicles. *Mol Pharmacol* 46: 808–816
43 Vezza R, Habib A, Nestor PV, FitzGerald GA (1997) Association of Gh, a novel GTP binding protein, with thromboxane receptors. *Circulation* 96: I547 (Abstr 3058)
44 Vezza R, Roberti R, Nenci GG, Gresele P (1993) Prostaglandin E_2 potentiates platelet aggregation by priming protein kinase C. *Blood* 82: 2704–2713
45 Ushikubi F, Hirata M, Narumiya S (1995) Molecular biology of prostanoid receptors; an overview. *J Lipid Mediat Cell Signal* 12: 343–359

46 Schmid A, Thierauch KH, Schleuning WD, Dinter H (1995) Splice variants of the human EP3 receptor for prostaglandin E_2. *Eur J Biochem* 228: 23–30
47 Kanapuli SP, Fen Mao G, Bastepe M, Liu-Chen LY, Li S, Cheung PP, DeRiel JK, Ashbi B (1994) Cloning and expression of a prostaglandin E receptor EP3 subtype from human erythroleukemia cells. *Biochem J* 298: 263–267
48 Murata T, Ushikubi F, Matsuoka T, Hirata M, Yamasaki A, Sugimoto Y, Ichikawa A, Aze Y, Tanaka T, Yoshida N, Veno A, Oh-ishi S, Narumya S (1997) Altered pain perception and inflammatory response in mice lacking prostacyclin receptor. *Nature* 388: 678–682
49 Gresele P, Deckmyn H, Huybrechts E, Vermylen J (1984) Serum albumin enhances the impairment of platelet aggregation with thromboxane synthase inhibition by increasing the formation of prostaglandin D_2. *Biochem Pharmacol* 33: 2083–2088
50 Sugimoto Y, Yamasaki A, Segi E, Tsuboi K, Aze Y, Nishimura T, Oida H, Yoshida N, Tanaka T, Katsuyama M, Hasumoto K, Murata T, Hirata M, Ushikubi F, Negishi M, Ichikawa A, Narumiya S (1997) Failure of parturition in mice lacking the prostaglandin F receptor. *Science* 277: 681–683
51 Brass LF, Molino M (1997) Protease-activated G protein-coupled receptors on human platelets and endothelial cells. *Thromb Haemost* 77: 233–240
52 Nystedt S, Emilsson K, Larsson AK, Strombeck B, Sundelin J (1995) Molecular cloning and functional expression of the gene encoding the human proteinase-activated receptor 2. *Eur J Biochem* 232: 84–89
53 Brass LF (1995) Molecular basis for platelet activation. In: R Hoffman, EJ Benz, SJ Shattil, B Furie, HJ Cohen, LE Silberstein (eds): *Hematology: basic principles and practice.* Churchill Livingstone, New York, 1536–1552
54 Barr AJ, Brass LF, Manning DR (1997) Reconstitution of receptors and GTP-binding regulatory proteins (G proteins) in Sf9 cells. A direct evaluation of selectivity in receptor-G protein coupling. *J Biol Chem* 272: 2223–2229
55 Gachet C, Hechler B, Leon C, Vial C, Leray C, Ohlmann P, Cazenave JP (1997) Activation of ADP receptors and platelet function. *Thromb Haemost* 77: 271–275
56 Hourani SMO, Hall DA (1996) P2T purinoreceptors: ADP receptors on platelets. *Ciba Foundation Symposium* 198: 53–70
57 Anfossi G, Trovati M (1996) Role of the catecholamines in platelet function: pathophysiological and clinical significance. *Eur J Clin Invest* 26: 353–370
58 Holmsen H (1994) Significance of testing platelet functions *in vitro*. *Eur J Clin Invest* 24 (suppl 1): 3–8
59 MacKinnon AC, Spedding M, Brown CM (1994) α2-adrenoreceptors: more subtypes but fewer functional differences. *Trends Pharmacol Sci* 15: 119–123
60 Hawiger J, Brass LF, Salzman EW (1994) Signal transduction and intracellular regulatory process in platelets. In: RW Colman, J Hirsh, VJ Marder, EW Salzman (eds): *Haemostasis and thrombosis: basic principles and clinical practice.* JB Lippincott, Philadelphia, 603–628
61 Holmsen H (1994) Platelet secretion and energy metabolism. In: RW Colman, J Hirsh,

VJ Marder, EW Salzman (eds): *Haemostasis and thrombosis: basic principles and clinical practice.* JB Lippincott, Philadelphia, 524–545

62 Vezza R, Spina D, Tallarida RJ, Nathan M, Page CP, Gresele P (1997) Antivasoconstrictory and antiaggregatory activities of picotamide unrelated to thromboxane A_2 antagonism. *Thromb Haemost* 78: 1385–91

63 Gyermek L (1996) Pharmacology of serotonin as related to anesthesia. *J Clin Anestesia* 8: 402–425

64 Vanderwel M, Lum DS, Haslam RJ (1983) Vasopressin inhibits the adenylate cyclase activity in human platelet particulate fraction through V1-receptors. *FEBS Lett* 164: 340–344

65 Gresele P, Arnout J, Deckmyn H, Vermylen J (1986) Mechanism of the antiplatelet action of dipyridamole in whole blood: modulation of adenosine concentration and activity. *Thromb Haemost* 55: 12–18

66 Ongini E, Fredholm BB (1996) Pharmacology of adenosine A_{2A} receptors. *Trends Pharmacol Sci* 17: 364–372

67 Ledent C, Vaugeois JM, Schiffmann SN, Pedrazzini T, El Yacoubi M, Vanderhaeghen JJ, Costantin J, Heath JK, Vassart G, Parmentier M (1997) Aggressiveness, hypoalgesia and high blood pressure in mice lacking the adenosine A2a receptor. *Nature* 388: 674–678

68 Anderson CL, Chacko GW, Osborne JM, Brandt JT (1995) The Fc receptor for immunoglobulin G (FcγRII) on human platelets. *Semin Thromb Haemost* 21: 1–9

69 Blake RA, Schieven GL, Watson SP (1994) Collagen stimulates tyrosine phosphorylation of phospholipase Cg2 but not phospholipase Cg1 in human platelets. *FEBS Lett* 353: 212–216

70 Emiliani C, Martino S, Orlacchio A, Vezza R, Nenci GG, Gresele P (1995) Platelet glycohydrolase activities: characterization and release. *Cell Biochem Funct* 13: 31–39

71 Plow EF and Ginsberg MH (1995) Molecular basis of platelet function. In: R Hoffman, EJ Benz, SJ Shattil, B Furie, HJ Cohen, LE Silberstein (eds): *Hematology: basic principles and practice.* Churchill Livingstone, New York, 1524–1535

72 Vassbotn FS, Havnen OK, Heldin CH, Holmsen H (1994) Negative feedback regulation of human platelets *via* autocrine activation of the platelet derived growth factor alpha-receptor. *J Biol Chem* 269: 13874–13879

73 Turitto VT, Baumgartner HR (1994) Initial deposition of platelets and fibrin on vascular surface in flowing blood. In: RW Colman, J Hirsh, VJ Marder, EW Salzman (eds): *Haemostasis and thrombosis: basic principles and clinical practice.* JB Lippincott, Philadelphia, 805–822

74 George JN, Nurden AT (1994) Inherited disorders of the platelet membrane: Glanzmann thrombasthenia, Bernard-Soulier syndrome, and other diseases. In: RW Colman, J Hirsh, VJ Marder, EW Salzman (eds): *Haemostasis and thrombosis: basic principles and clinical practice.* JB Lippincott, Philadelphia, 652–672

75 Ikeda Y, Handa M, Kawano K, Kamata T, Murata M, Araki Y, Anbo H, Kawai Y, Watanabe K, Itagaki I, Sakai K, Ruggeri ZM (1991) The role of von Willebrand factor

and fibrinogen in platelet aggregation under varying shear stress. *J Clin Invest* 87: 1234–1240
76 Lemons PP, Chen D, Bernstein AM, Bennett MK, Whiteheart SW (1997) Regulated secretion in platelets: identification of elements of the platelet exocytosis machinery. *Blood* 90: 1490–1500
77 Masini E, Di Bello MG, Raspanti S, Bacchi Sacchi T, Maggi E, Mannaioni PF (1994) Platelet aggregation and histamine release by immunologic stimuli. *Immunopharmacology* 28: 19–29
78 Murayama T, Kajiyama Y, Nomura Y (1990) Histamine-stimulated and GTP binding protein-mediated phospholipase A_2 activation in rabbit platelets. *J Biol Chem* 265: 4290–4295
79 Metzger WJ, Sjoerdsma K, Richerson HB, Moseley P, Zavala D, Monick M, Hunnighake GW (1987) Platelets in bronchoalveolar lavage from asthmatics patients and allergic rabbits with allergen-induced late phase responses. *Agent Action* 21 (Suppl): 151–59
80 Lowenhaupt RW, Miller MA, Glueck HI (1973) Platelet migration and chemotaxis demonstrated *in vitro*. *Thromb Res* 3: 477–486
81 Valone F, Austen KF, Goetzl EJ (1974) Modulation of the random migration of human platelets. *J Clin Invest* 54: 1100–1104
82 Lowenhaupt RW, Glueck HI, Miller MA, Kline DL (1997) Factors which influence blood platelet migration. *J Lab Clin Med* 90: 37–45
83 Zhang X, Selli ML, Baglioni S, Hauri A, Chiari R, Dottorini M, Todisco T, Nenci GG, Gresele P (1993) Platelets from asthmatics patients migrate *in vitro* in response to allergen stimulation. *Thromb Haemost* 69: 916
84 Simon MI, Strathmann MP, Gautam N (1991) Diversity of G proteins in signal transduction. *Science* 252: 802–808
85 van Willigen G, Donath J, Lapetina EG, Akkerman JWN (1995) Identification of α-subunits of trimeric GTP-binding proteins in human platelets by RT-PCR. *Biochem Biophys Res Commun* 214: 254–262
86 Wu D, Kuang Y, Jiang H (1995) Selective coupling of beta 2-adrenergic receptor to hematopoietic-specific G proteins. *J Biol Chem* 270: 16008–16010
87 Lounsbury KM, Casey PJ, Brass LF, Manning DR (1991) Phosphorylation of Gz in human platelets: selectivity and site of modification. *J Biol Chem* 266: 22051–22056
88 Offermanns S, Hu YH, Simon MI (1996) Gα12 and Gα13 are phosphorylated during platelet activation. *J Biol Chem* 271: 26044–26048
89 Rudolph U, Finegold MJ, Rich SS, Harriman GR, Srinivasan Y, Brabet P, Bradley A, Birnabaumer L (1995) Gi2 protein deficiency: a model for inflammatory bowel disease. *J Clin Immunol* 15: 101S–105S
90 Offermanns S, Mancino V, Revel JP, Simon MI (1997) Vascular system defects and impaired cell chemokinesis as a result of G13 deficiency. *Science* 275: 533–536
91 Offermanns S, Toombs CF, Hu YH, Simon MI (1997) Defective platelet activation in Gq-deficient mice. *Nature* 389: 183–186

92 Gabbeta J, Yang X, Kowalska MA, Sun L, Dhanasekaran N, Rao AK (1997) Platelet signal transduction defect with Gαq subunit dysfunction and diminished Gαq in a patient with abnormal platelet responses. *Proc Natl Acad Sci USA* 94: 8750–8755

93 Lee SB, Rhee SG (1995) Significance of PIP2 hydrolysis and regulation of phospholipase C isozymes. *Current Opinion Cell Biol* 7: 183–189

94 Nishizuka Y (1984) The role of protein kinase C in cell surface signal transduction and tumor promotion. *Nature* 308: 693–698

95 Halbrugge M, Walter U (1993) The regulation of platelet function by protein kinases. In: CK Huang, RI Sha'afi (eds): *Protein kinases in blood cell function.* CRC Press, Boca Raton, 245–298

96 Peterson SN, Lapetina EG (1994) Platelet activation and inhibition. Novel signal transduction mechanisms. *Ann NY Acad Sci* 714: 53–63

97 Huang R, Kucera GL, Rittenhouse SE (1991) Elevated cytosolic Ca^{2+} activates phospholipase D in human platelets. *J Biol Chem* 266: 1652–1655

98 Chiang TM (1994) Activation of phospholipase D in human platelets by collagen and thrombin and its relationship to platelet aggregation. *Biochim Biophys Acta* 1224: 147–155

99 Martinson EA, Scheible S, Greinacher A, Presek P (1995) Platelet phospholipase D is activated by protein kinase C *via* an integrin αIIb/β3-independent mechanism. *Biochem J* 310: 623–628

100 Pettitt TR, Martin A, Horton T, Liossis C, Lord JM, Wakelam MJO (1997) Diacylglycerol and phosphatidate generated by phospholipases C and D, respectively, have distinct fatty acid compositions and functions. Phospholipase D-derived diacylglycerol does not activate protein kinase C in porcine aortic endothelial cells. *J Biol Chem* 272: 17354–17359

101 Lerea KM, Glomset JA, Krebs EG (1987) Agents that elevate cAMP levels in platelets decrease thrombin binding. *J Biol Chem* 262: 252–258

102 Dennis EA (1997) The growing phospholipases A_2 superfamily of signal transduction enzymes. *Trends Biochem Sci* 22: 1–2

103 Exton JH (1994) Phosphatidylcholine breakdown and signal transduction. *Biochim Biophys Acta* 1212: 26–42

104 Kramer RM, Roberts EF, Manetta JV, Hyslop PA, Jakubowski JA (1993) Thrombin-induced phosphorylation and activation of Ca^{++}-sensitive cytosolic PLA_2 in human platelets. *J Biol Chem* 268: 26796–26804

105 Rittenhouse-Simmons S (1981) Differential activation of platelet phospholipases by thrombin and ionophore A23187. *J Biol Chem* 256: 4153–4155

106 Kramer RM, Roberts EF, Strifler BA, Johnstone EM (1995) Thrombin induces activation of p38 MAPK in human platelets. *J Biol Chem* 270: 27395–27398

107 Kramer RM, Roberts EF, Um SL, Borsch-Haubold AG, Watson SP, Fisher MJ, Jakubowski JA (1996) P38 mitogen-activated protein kinase phosphorylates cytosolic PLA_2 ($cPLA_2$) in thrombin-stimulated platelets. Evidence that proline-directed phos-

phorylation is not required for mobilization of arachidonic acid by $cPLA_2$. *J Biol Chem* 271: 27723–27729
108 Iorio P, Gresele P, Stasi M, Nucciarelli F, Vezza R, Nenci GG, Goracci G (1996) Protein kinase C inhibitors enhance G protein induced phospholipase A_2 activation in intact human platelets. *FEBS Lett* 381: 244–248
109. Stasi M, Gresele P, Porcellati S, Quero E, Nenci GG, Goracci G (1992) Activation of phospholipase A_2 and β-thromboglobulin release in human platelets stimulated with thrombin and fluoroaluminate. *Biochim Biophys Acta* 1124: 279–287
110 Forde RC, Fitzgerald DJ (1997) Reactive oxygen species and platelet activation in reperfusion injury. *Circulation* 95: 787–789
111 Siminiak T, Flores NA, Sheridan DJ (1995) Neutrophils interactions with endothelium and platelets: possible role in the development of cardiovascular injury. *Eur Heart J* 16: 160–170
112 Leo R, Pratico D, Iuliano L, Pulcinelli FM, Ghiselli A, Pignatelli P, Colavita AR, FitzGerald GA, Violi F (1997) Platelet activation by superoxide anion and hydroxyl radicals intrinsically generated by platelets that had undergone anoxia and then reoxygenated. *Circulation* 95: 885–891
113 Smith WL, Marnett LJ (1991) Prostaglandin endoperoxide synthase: structure and catalysis. *Biochim Biophys Acta* 1083: 1–17
114 Jones DA, Fitzpatrick FA (1991) Thromboxane A_2 synthase. Modification during "suicide" inactivation. *J Biol Chem* 266: 23510–23514
115 de Gaetano G, Cerletti C, Nanni-Costa MP, Poggi A (1987) Blood platelets as inflammatory cells. In: GVR Born, GG Neri Serneri (eds): *Antiplatelet therapy: twenty years' experience*. Excerpta Medica, Amsterdam, 52–62
116 Collins CE, Rampton DS (1997) Platelets in inflammatory bowel disease – Pathogenetic role and therapeutic implications. *Aliment Pharmacol Ther* 11: 237–247
117 Klinger MH (1997) Platelets and inflammation. *Anat Embryol* 196: 1–11
118 Page CP (1988) The involvement of platelets in non-thrombotic processes. *Trends Pharmacol Sci* 9: 66–71
119 Cotran RS (1965) The delayed and prolonged vascular leakage in inflammation. II. An electron microscopic study of the vascular response after thermal injury. *Am J Pathol* 46: 589–620
120 Zawliska K, Giroud JP, Timsit S, Caen JP (1973) Plaquettes et inflammation. *Pathol Biol* 21 (Suppl): 51–56
121 Schumacher HR (1975) Synovial membrane and fluid morphologic alterations in early rheumatoid arthritis: microvascular injury and virus-like particles. *Ann NY Acad Sci* 256: 39–64
122 Kravis T, Henson PM (1977) Accumulation of platelets at sites of antigen-antibody-mediated injury. *J Immunol* 118: 1569–1573
123 Yaron M, Djaldetti M (1978) Platelets in synovial fluid. *Arthritis Rheum* 21: 607–608
124 Slater DN, Martin JF, Trowbridge EA (1985) The platelet in asthma. *Lancet* 1: 110

125 Page CP (1993) Platelets. In: ST Holgate, MK Church (eds): *Allergy illustrated.* Gower Medical Publishing, London, 8.1–8.8
126 Day RP, Behrmann S, Dolovich J, Hargreawe FE (1975) Inflammatory effects of leukocytes and platelets. *J Allergy Clin Immunol* 55: 87–92
127 Dray A (1995) Inflammatory mediators of pain. *Brit J Anaesth* 75: 125–131
128 Vignola AN, Chiappara G, Chanez P, Merendino AM, Pace E, Spatafora M, Bousquet J, Bonsignore G (1997) Growth factors in asthma. *Monaldi Arch Chest Dis* 52: 159–169
129 Brindley LL, Sweet JM, Goetz EJ (1983) Stimulation of histamine release from human basophils by human platelet factor 4. *J Clin Invest* 72: 1218–1223
130 Chihara J, Fukuda K, Yasuda H, Kishigami N, Sugihara R, Kubo H, Nakajma S (1988) Platelet factor 4 enhances eosinophil IgG and IgEFc receptor and has eosinophil chemotactic activity. *Am Rev Resp Dis* 137: 421–427
131 Chihara J, Yasuba H, Tsuba A, Urayama O, Saito N, Honda K, Kayaba H, Yamashita T, Kurimoto F, Yamada H (1997) Elevation of the plasma level of RANTES during asthma attacks. *J Allergy Clin Immunol* 100: S52–S55
132 Weyrich AS, Eistad MR, Mc Ever RP, Mc Intyre TM, Moore KL, Morrissey JH, Prescott SM, Zimmerman GA (1996) Activated platelets signal chemokine synthesis by human monocytes. *J Clin Invest* 97: 1525–1534
133 Klinger MH, Wilhelm D, Bubel S, Sticherling M, Schröder J-M, Kühnel W (1995) Immunocytochemical localization of the chemokins RANTES and MIP-1α within human platelets and their release during storage. *Int Arch Allergy Immunol* 107: 541–546
134 Symon FA, Walsh GM, Watson S, Wardlaw AJ (1994) Eosinophils adhesion to nasal polyp endothelium is P-selectin dependent. *J Exp Med* 180: 371–376
135 De Sanctis GT, Wolyniec WW, Green FHY, Qui S, Jiao A, Finn PW, Noonan T, Joetham AA, Gelfand E, Doerschuk CM, Drazen JM (1997) Production of allergic airway responses in P-selectin-deficient mice. *J Appl Physiol* 83: 681–687
136 Shanley TP, Worner RL, Ward PA (1995) The role of cytokines and adesion molecules in the development of inflammatory injury. *Mol Med Today* 1: 40–45
137 Loppnow H, Bil R, Hirt S, Schonbeck V, Herzberg M, Werdan K, Riietschel ET, Brandt E, Flad HD (1998) Platelet-derived interleukin-1 induces cytokine production, but not proliferation of human vascular smooth muscle cells. *Blood* 91: 134–141
138 Ciferri S, Emiliani C, Orlacchio A, Nenci GG, Gresele P (1997) Human blood platelets release their lysosomal content "*in vivo*" at a localized site of platelet activation. *Thromb Haemost* 78 (Suppl): 483
139 Vaage J, Havge A (1977) Small airway constriction and closure after induced intravascular platelet aggregation. *Acta Physiol Scand* 100: 221–230
140 Lefort J, Vargaftig BB (1978) Mechanism of collagen-induced bronchoconstriction and thrombocytopenia in the guinea-pig. *Eur J Pharmacol* 62: 422–428
141 Pinckard RN, Halonen M, Palmer JD, Butler C, Shaw JO, Henson PM (1977) Intravascular aggregation and pulmonary sequestration of platelets during IgE-induced systemic

anaphylaxis in the rabbit: abrogation of lethal anaphylactic shock by platelet depletion. *J Immunol* 119: 2185–93

142 Halonen M, Palmer JD, Lohman C, McManus LM, Pinckard RN (1981) Differential effect of platelet depletion on the physiologic alterations of IgE anaphylaxis and acetyl ether phosphorylcholine infusion in the rabbit. *Am Rev Resp Dis* 124: 416–419

143 McManus LM, Morley CA, Levine SP, Pinckard RN (1979) Platelet activating factor (PAF) induced release of platelet factor 4 (PF4) *In vitro* and during IgE anaphylaxis in the rabbit. *J Immunol* 123: 2835–2841

144 Lellouch-Tubiana A, Lefort J, Pirotzky E, Vargafting BB, Pfiisfer A (1985) Ultrastructural evidence for extra-vascular platelet recruitment in the lung upon intravenous injection of platelet activating factor (PAF-acether) to guinea pigs. *Brit J Exp Pathol* 66: 345–355

145 Coyle AJ, Spina D, Page CP (1990) PAF-induced bronchial hyperresponsiveness in the rabbit: contribution of platelets and airway smooth muscle. *Brit J Pharmacol* 101: 31–38

146 Rohrbach MS, Wheatley CL, Slifman NR, Gleich GJ (1990) Activation of platelets by eosinophil granule proteins. *J Exp Med* 172: 1271–1274

147 Waker M (1987) Idiopathic hypereosynophilia associated with epatic vein thrombosis. *Arch Intern Med* 147: 2220–2221

148 Zyllberberg H, Valla D, Viguie F, Casadevall N (1996) Budd-Chiari syndrome associated with 5q deletion and hypereosynophilia. *J Clin Gastroenterol* 23: 66–68

149 Lee T, Lenihan DJ, Malone D, Roddy LL, Wasserman SI (1984) Increased biosynthesis of platelet activating factor in activated human eosinophils. *J Biol Chem* 259: 5526–5530

150 Gresele P, Ribaldi E, Grasselli S, Todisco T, Nenci GG (1986) Evidence for platelet activation in allergic asthma. *Agent Action* 21 (suppl): 119–128

151. Block LH, Imhof E, Emmons LR, Roth M, Perruchoud AP (1990) PAF-dependent phosphatidylinositol turnover in platelets: differences between asthmatics and normal individuals. *Respiration* 57: 372–378

152 Gresele P, Dottorini M, Selli ML, Iannacci L, Canino S, Todisco T, Romano S, Crook P, Page CP, Nenci GG (1993) Altered platelet function associated with the bronchial hyperresponsiveness accompanying nocturnal asthma. *J Allergy Clin Immunol* 91: 894–902

153 Beer JH, Wuthrich B, von Felten A (1995) Allergen exposure in acute asthma causes the release of platelet activating factor (PAF) as demonstrated by the desensitization of platelets to PAF. *Int Arch Allergy Immunol* 106: 291–296

154 Burgers JA, Bruynzeel PL, Mengelers HJ, Kreukinet J, Akkerman JW (1993) Occupancy of platelet receptors for platelet-activating factor in asthmatic patients during an allergen-induced bronchoconstrictive reaction. *J Lipid Mediat* 7: 135–149

155 Taylor ML, Misso NL, Steward GA, Thompson PJ (1996) Differential expression of platelet activation markers in aspirin-sensitive asthmatics and normal subjects. *Clin Exp Allergy* 26: 202–215

156 Kuroda S, Ishikawa K, Hanamitsu H, Komori M, Komiya K, Ichikawa Y, Maejima K,

Hasegawa K, Ninomiya R, Kuroda M (1995) Evidence for an increased intracellular free calcium concentration in platelets of bronchial asthma patients. *Intern Med* 34: 722–727

157 Knauer KA, Lichtestein LM, Adkinson NF, Fish JE (1981) Platelet activation during antigen-induced airway reactions in asthmatic subjects. *New Engl J Med* 304: 1404–1407

158 Gresele P, Todisco T, Merante F, Nenci GG (1982) Platelet activation and allergic asthma. *New Engl J Med* 306: 549

159 Yamamoto H, Nagata M, Tabe K, Kimura I, Kiuchi H, Sakamoto Y, Yamamoto K, Dohi Y (1993) The evidence of platelet activation in bronchial asthma. *J Allergy Clin Immunol* 91: 79–87

160 Kaplan KL, Owen J (1981) Plasma levels of betathromboglobulin and platelet factor 4 as indices of platelet activation *in vivo*. *Blood* 57: 199–202

161 Gresele P, Catalano M, Giammaresi C, Volpato R, Termini R, Ciabattoni G, Nenci GG, Davì G (1997) Platelet activation markers in patients with peripheral arterial disease. A prospective comparison of different platelet function tests. *Throm Haemost* 78: 1434–1437

162 Lupinetti MD, Sheller JR, Catella F, FitzGerald GA (1989) Thromboxane biosynthesis in allergen-induced bronchospasm. *Am Rev Resp Dis* 142: 932–935

163 Wu G, Li F, Li P, Ruan C (1992) Detection of activated platelets using activation-dependent monoclonal antibody (SZ-51) in clinical disorders. *Nouv Rev Fr Hematol* 34: 31–35

164 Kumlin M, Dahlen B, Bjorck T, Zetterstrom O, Granstrom E, Dahlen SE (1992) Urinary excretion of leukotriene E4 and 11-dehydro-thromboxane B2 in response to bronchial provocations with allergen, aspirin, leukotriene D4, and histamine in asthmatics. *Am Rev Resp Dis* 146: 96–103

165 Averill FJ, Hubbard WC, Proud D, Gleich GJ, Liu MC (1992) Platelet activation in the lung after antigen challenge in a model of allergic asthma. *Am Rev Resp Dis* 145: 571–576

166 Klouche M, Klinger MH, Kuhnel W, Wilhelm D (1997) Endocytosis, storage, and release of IgE by human platelets: differences in patients with type I allergy and nonatopic subjects. *J Allergy Clin Immunol* 100: 235–241

167 Jeffrey PK, Wardlaw AJ, Neldon FC, Collins JV, Kay AB (1989) Bronchial biopsies in asthma: an ultrastructural quantitative study and correlation with hyperreactivity. *Am Rev Resp Dis* 140: 1745–1753

168 Misso NL, Powers KA, Gillon RL, Stewart GA, Thompson PJ (1996) Reduced platelet glutathione peroxidase activity and serum selenium concentration in atopic asthmatic subjects. *Clin Exp Allergy* 26: 838–847

169 Vargaftig BB, Lefort J, Wal F, Chignard M, Medeiros MC (1982) Interference of non steroidal anti-inflammatory drugs associated to anti-histamine and anti-serotonin agents with the bronchial and platelet effects of "platelet-activating factor" (PAF-acether). *Eur J Pharmacol* 82: 121–130

170 Gresele P, Grasselli S, Todisco T, Nenci GG (1985) Platelets and asthma. *Lancet* 1: 347
171 Lammers JW, Kioumis I, McCusker M, Chung KF, Barnes PJ (1988) Effect of prostacyclin (PGI2) on bronchoconstriction induced by platelet activating factor (PAF) in man. *Am Rev Resp Dis* 137 (Suppl): A373
172 Sladek K, Dworski R, FitzGerald GA, Buitkus KL, Block FJ, Marney SR, Sheller JR (1990) Allergen-stimulated release of thromboxane A2 and Leukotriene E4 in humans. Effect of indomethacin. *Am Rev Resp Dis* 141: 1441–1445
173 Thorel T, Joseph M, Tsicopoulos A, Tonnel AB, Capron A (1988) Inhibition by nedocromil sodium of IgE mediated activation of human mononuclear phagocytes and platelets in allergy. *Int Arch Allergy Appl Immunol* 85: 232–237
174 Joseph M, Tsicopoulos A, Tonnel AB, Capron A (1993) Modulation by nedocromil sodium of immunologic and non immunologic activation of monocytes, macrophages and platelets. *J Allergy Clin Immunol* 192: 165–170
175 Roth M, Soler M, Lefkowitz H, Emmons LR, Anstine D, Hornung M, Perruchoud AP (1993) Inhibition of receptor-mediated platelet activation by nedocromil sodium. *J Allergy Clin Immunol* 91: 1217–1225
176 Gentile DA, Brown C, Skoner DP (1993) *in vitro* modulation of platelet sodium, potassium adenosine triphosphatase enzyme activity by antiallergy drugs. *J Lab Clin Med* 122: 85–91
177 Tunon de Lara JM, Rio P, Marthan R, Vuillemin L, Ducassou D, Taytard A (1992) The effect of sodium cromoglycate on platelets: an *in vivo* and *in vitro* approach. *J Allergy Clin Immunol* 89: 994–1000
178 Taytard A, Willemin L, Guenarg H, Rio P, Vergeret J, Ducassou D (1987) Platelet kinetics in stable asthma patients: Effect of ketotifen. *Am Rev Resp Dis* 135: 3884–3887
179 Paidhungat AJ, Salgaonkar DS, Nabar ST, Nadkar MY, Chari VI, Khatri DP, Prabhu SR (1994) Effect of inhaled terbutaline on platelet activity in bronchial asthma. *J Assoc Physicians India* 42: 113–115

Neutrophils

Moira Whyte

Respiratory Medicine, Division of Molecular and Genetic Medicine, Royal Hallamshire Hospital, Sheffield S10 2JF, UK

Introduction

Neutrophils are the rapid response cells of acute inflammation and a major component of host defence. Their ability to ingest bacteria and other microbes was recognised by Elie Metchnikoff in the 19th century, but in recent years the double-edged nature of the inflammatory response has been recognised. Despite their beneficial role in host defence, neutrophils and their pro-inflammatory products are increasingly implicated in the pathogenesis of acute and chronic inflammatory diseases. In the lung these include chronic bronchitis and emphysema, asthma, respiratory distress syndrome, bronchiectasis and a number of interstitial lung diseases. Thus, understanding the pro-inflammatory host defence functions of the neutrophil, and the mechanisms by which these are terminated, may yield insights into the pathogenesis of diseases which are a major cause of morbidity and mortality in the developed world.

Cell structure and origin

In numerical terms the neutrophil polymorphonuclear leucocyte is the predominant effector cell of the immune response; 60% of all bone marrow cells belong to the neutrophil lineage. Estimated production is 1–3 × 10^{10} neutrophils per day, rising several fold in serious infections [1]. Neutrophils have a total lifespan of 12–14 days from stem cell to removal in tissues, but a circulating half-life of less than 8 h [2]. Circulating neutrophils are believed to be in dynamic equilibrium with a so-called "marginating" pool of cells. The size of this pool is debated, but the presence of this marginated pool within the lung has been proposed as a rapid-release reservoir of neutrophils for mobilisation in response to injury or stress [3]. The physiological fate of the short-lived neutrophil has recently been an area of considerable interest. Studies with radiolabelled neutrophils suggest they normally meet their fate in the

Cellular Mechanisms in Airways Inflammation, edited by Clive P. Page, Katharine H. Banner and Domenico Spina

liver, spleen and bone marrow, where they are presumed to undergo apoptosis (programmed cell death), leading to their recognition and clearance by specific macrophage populations within these organs. Apoptosis also appears to regulate the removal of neutrophils which have left the circulation and migrated into the tissues (see below).

On electron microscopy, neutrophils have a diameter of about 7 μm and contain a large number of cytoplasmic granules, which are separated on the basis of peroxidase staining into primary or "azurophilic" granules (peroxidase positive) and secondary or "specific" granules (peroxidase negative). A further type of granule, the tertiary or "storage" granule, is also now recognised. Azurophilic granules contain anti-microbial agents, such as proteases (elastase, cathepsins, metalloproteinases), glycosidascs and acid hydrolases, lactoferrin (which chelates iron and participates in hydroxyl radical formation) and defensins (cationic amphipathic proteins which kill pathogens by damage to cytoplasmic membranes) [4]. Sequestration of these agents within the membrane bound granules permits their controlled delivery to the target microbe within the phagolysosome. Although "specific" granules do contain some anti-microbial enzymes (lysozyme, collagenase), their major role is to provide an intracellular reserve of important membrane components, including chemotaxin receptors, adhesion molecules and components of the NADPH (nicotinamide adenine dinucleotide phosphate) oxidase [5] (Tab. 1). Such an arrangement may provide a mechanism for increasing the number of chemotaxin and adhesion receptors at the leading front of a migrating cell [6]. Other cellular organelles, e.g. mitochondria and Golgi apparatus, are relatively scarce, but neutrophils do contain substantial amounts of endoplasmic reticulum (ER). The plasma membrane is of great importance in these highly responsive cells, since it contains receptors which bind pro-inflammatory mediators and transduce these signals into cellular responses. Finally, the complex cytoskeletal network, which links intracellular granule storage pools with the cell membrane and is responsible for cell motility, is composed of both actin and myosin filaments and resides in the submembrane region [7].

The ability to produce large numbers of neutrophils rapidly and with a very short lifespan permits the presence of enormous numbers of these highly effective bacterial killers at a site of infection, but also the subsequent rapid resolution of the inflammatory response; desirable for minimal "bystander" damage to normal tissues. The neutrophil is, however, more than an end-stage cell, programmed to kill bacteria and then disintegrate. Neutrophils generate a limited but important range of cytokines and chemokines, controlling the influx of more neutrophils but also the migration of monocytes which will mature into inflammatory macrophages [8]. Neutrophils' behaviour in the inflammatory response, their migration, subsequent activation and ultimate removal are under tight controls, regulated by signalling pathways whose molecular basis is increasingly understood and which represent powerful therapeutic targets for the modulation of inflammation.

Table 1 - Neutrophil granule contents

Constituent	Azurophilic granules	Specific granules	Tertiary granules
Microbicidal enzymes	Myeloperoxidase Lysozyme	Lysozyme	
Neutral proteases	Elastase Cathepsin G		
Metalloproteinases		Collagenase	Gelatinase
Acid hydrolases	N-acetyl-glucuronidase Cathepsin B Cathepsin D Glucuronidase Glycerophosphatase Mannosidase		
Others	Bactericidal permeability factor (BPI) Defensins Antibacterial cationic protein Kinin-generating enzyme C5a-inactivating factor	Lactoferrin Vitamin B12 binding protein Cytochrome b Histaminase Complement activator Monocyte-chemoattractant Plasminogen PKC inhibitor fMLP receptors C3bi receptors	C3bi receptors Cytochrome b_{558} Alkaline phosphatase Laminin receptors

Mechanisms of neutrophil activation

Neutrophil receptors

The neutrophil surface reveals a number of different groups of receptors: for opsonised particles, destined to be phagocytosed; for chemotactic factors, for cytokines and growth factors and for adhesion molecules (Tab. 2). Structurally, these can be viewed as belonging to four different groups:

(1) G-protein-coupled seven-transmembrane-domain receptors
e.g. for PAF, IL-8, C5a and Substance P

Table 2 - Neutrophil surface receptors

Function	Receptor	Ligand(s)
Chemotaxis	fMLP	f-met peptides
	LTB_4	LTB_4
	C5a	C5a, C5a des-arg
	PAF	PAF
	IL-8	Interleukin-8
Opsonins	C3bi	C3b, C3bi
Phagocytosis	CD32 (FcγRII)	
	CD16 (FcγRIIIb)	IgG_1 and IgG_3
Cytokines	IL-1	Interleukin-1
	IFNγ	Interferon-γ
	CD95 (Fas/APO-1)	CD95L (FasL)
	TNFα (p55 + p75)	Tumour necrosis factor-α
Colony-stimulating factors	GM-CSF	Granulocyte-macrophage-CSF
(CSFs)	G-CSF	Granulocyte-CSF
Adhesion	CD11b/CD18 (Mac-1)	C3bi and ICAM-1
	CD11a/CD18 (LFA-1)	ICAM-1 + 2
	CD66b	Selectins
Others	Adenosine	
	β_2-adrenergic	

(2) Cytokine receptors with a single transmembrane-domain
e.g. for GM-CSF, TNFα
(3) Receptors for adhesion molecules and complement
e.g. for Fc, integrins, CD14
(4) Intracellular receptors
e.g. for steroid hormones

Intracellular events following the binding of a mediator to its receptor on the neutrophil surface have been most extensively studied using the synthetic bacterial peptide, fMLP, which binds to a seven-transmembrane-domain, rhodopsin-like receptor. Seven-transmembrane-domain receptors may be coupled either to effector systems (e.g. actin polymerisation) or to second-messenger generating systems (e.g. phospholipases) within the cell. Receptor occupancy can determine the functional response elicited – maximal superoxide response occurs at maximal receptor occupancy, whereas shape change can occur with only 10% receptor occupancy [9].

Post-receptor mechanisms of neutrophil activation

G-proteins

Guanine nucleotide-binding proteins play a central role in the transduction of receptor signals into effector responses of cells. Adenylate cyclase was the first enzyme shown to be stimulated in a GTP-dependent manner. Chemoattractant receptors, e.g. fMLP, are also G-protein coupled. Gi_2 and Gi_3 are believed to be the predominant G proteins present in the neutrophil. G-protein activation leads to dissociation of the α-$\beta\gamma$ subunits, the α subunit being the predominant effector molecule.

Lipid-derived second messengers

G-protein activation results in recruitment of lipid-derived second messengers such as phospholipase C (PLC) to the cell membrane, where it has access to its membrane-lipid substrate [10]. The seven-transmembrane-domain receptors all activate PLC, resulting in the hydrolysis of phosphatidylinositol 4,5-bisphosphate (PIP_2) to inositol 1,4,5-trisphosphate (IP_3) and diacylglycerol. Other neutrophil receptors have been shown to recruit PLCγ2 to the cell membrane *via* activation of an intrinsic SH2 binding domain (with Src tyrosine kinase homology). This is the proposed mechanism whereby cross-linking of the FcγRI and FcγRII receptors leads to phosphorylation and activation of PLCγ2. Phosphatidylinositol 3-kinase (PI 3-kinase) generates phosphatidylinositol 3,4,5 trisphosphate (PIP_3) from PIP_2, PIP_3 playing a key role both in cytoskeletal functions and in initiation of superoxide generation [11]. Phospholipase D cleaves membrane phosphatidylcholine to generate phosphatidic acid, which has been implicated as an effector both of exocytosis and of the NADPH oxidase [12]. Another important lipid-derived second messenger system is initiated by phospholipase A_2-mediated cleavage of arachidonic acid, generating eicosanoids (prostaglandins, leukotrienes and lipoxins).

Protein phosphorylation

The neutrophil contains two major groups of serine-threonine kinases: protein kinase C (PKC), which is broadly stimulatory of neutrophil functions and the cAMP and cGMP-dependent protein kinases (PKA and PKG), which largely inhibit neutrophil responses. The neutrophil contains multiple isoforms of PKC, with complex functional effects such as stimulation of NADPH oxidase activity but inhibition of chemotaxis. The functional specificities of the various isoforms and their phosphorylation targets are at present mostly unknown. Elevation of cAMP in neutrophils may occur *via* receptor-mediated (e.g. β_2 adrenoreceptor, adenosine receptors) activation of adenylate cyclase or by inhibition of phosphodiesterase activity, PDE4 being the predominant phosphodiesterase isoform in neutrophils. cAMP has been shown to inhibit a wide variety of neutrophil responses [13]. The role of cGMP in neutrophils is less clear, but exogenous nitric oxide (NO), which leads to elevation of cGMP, down-regulates a range of neutrophil functions including degranulation and superoxide generation [14]. Neutrophils can also generate NO and predominantly contain the NOS1 isoform of nitric oxide synthase, at least in unstimulated cells [15].

A number of neutrophil receptors, such as the receptor for the growth factor GM-CSF, have intrinsic tyrosine kinase activity whereas other receptors, e.g. for C5a and Substance P, interact with a family of small cytosolic tyrosine kinases (Lyn, Fyn, Syk). This results in phosphorylation of a number of protein substrates including p125FAK and mitogen-activated protein kinase (MAPK). Tyrosine phosphorylation has also been implicated in neutrophil priming, possibly *via* phosphorylation of MAPK or of a protein component of the NADPH oxidase [16].

Recent data has provided a link between PKC and tyrosine phosphorylation branches of neutrophil signal transduction: PKC has been shown to phosphorylate and thus inhibit tyrosine phosphatase-1 (SHP-1) thus facilitating accumulation of tyrosine phosphorylated proteins following neutrophil activation [17].

Cytosolic calcium

Levels of cytosolic calcium in the neutrophil appear to be determined largely by influx, *via* multiple pathways, but also by release from intracellular stores: the ER and possibly other poorly-defined cytoplasmic organelles, sometimes described as calciosomes. Elevation of $[Ca^{2+}]_i$ in the neutrophil stimulates functions such as degranulation and superoxide generation [18] and may also play a role in regulating the lifespan of neutrophils *via* the inhibition of apoptosis (programmed cell death) [19].

The NADPH oxidase

The NADPH oxidase describes a metabolic path, dormant in resting cells, which underlies all oxygen-dependent killing by phagocytes (Fig. 1). Activation of the oxidase involves translocation of a cytosolic protein complex to the plasma membrane – physical separation of oxidase components in the resting cell may prevent inappropriate activation of the oxidase. The NADPH oxidase is triggered by receptor-mediated binding of soluble agents (fMLP, C5a, etc.) or binding of opsonised organisms to neutrophil Fcγ and C3bi receptors, which can trigger oxidase activity at localised sites of microbial contact. In essence, the NADPH oxidase forms an electron transfer chain, using NADPH as the electron donor to reduce molecular oxygen to superoxide anion [20, 21]. Superoxide (O_2^-) is in turn dismuted to hydrogen peroxide and thereafter metabolised to hydroxyl free radicals and hypochlorous acid. The enzyme complex consists of a unique flavo-cytochrome (cytochrome

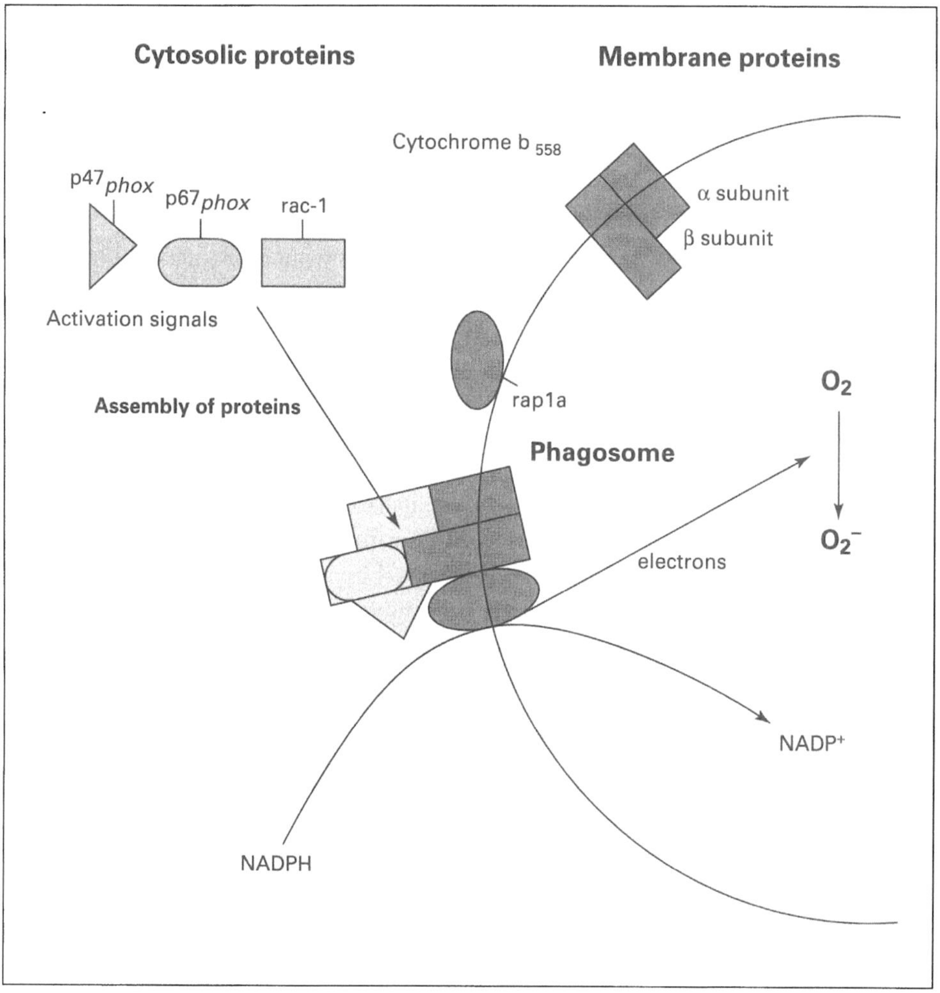

Figure 1
The NADPH oxidase of neutrophils.

b558), a GTP-binding protein (Rap-1A) and two cytosolic proteins (p47phox and p67phox) that bind to b558 following activation or priming of the cell. Finally, the GTP-binding protein Rac-1 must translocate from cytosol, where it is complexed with Rho, to integrate into the oxidase complex. Stimulation of the NADPH oxidase is in part mediated by elevation of cytosolic calcium, but also by PI 3-kinase activation and protein tyrosine phosphorylation [16, 22]. Much of the characterisation of the NADPH oxidase has been achieved using the neutrophils of patients with chronic granulomatous disease (CGD), who have been shown to have defects in b558 (X-linked disease, the commonest form) or of the cytosolic components p47 and p67 (autosomal recessive disease). These patients, as a result of their impaired microbicidal function, develop severe, recurrent infections [20].

Neutrophil priming

Neutrophils are remarkable for their ability to move from a resting state to a state of "priming" or readiness for activation. Priming has been most closely studied in terms of NADPH oxidase function but also affects other cellular functions such as degranulation and phagocytosis. A given mediator, which does not induce a functional response in itself, alters the reactivity of the neutrophil to subsequent stimuli. Thus, in the unprimed state, the neutrophil displays little or no secretory response when incubated with an agent such as fMLP, whereas such a challenge in a fully primed cell would result in a massive increase in respiratory burst activity. This priming-activation axis is believed to be a major determinant of neutrophil behaviour *in vivo* [23]. Priming may be achieved by cytokines (TNFα, IL-8), lipid mediators (LTB_4) or bacterial products (lipopolysaccharide, fMLP). Mechanisms of priming are poorly understood but occur at a post-receptor level and may involve elevations of cytosolic calcium levels [24] and modulation of protein kinases such as PK-C and tyrosine kinases [16, 25]. Some agents, e.g. LPS, GM-CSF, show protracted and possibly irreversible priming but it has recently been shown that priming, e.g. induced by PAF, may also be a transient and reversible phenomenon [26].

Neutrophil migration and function

Migration of neutrophils from the circulation into tissue occurs in response to the generation, by resident tissue cells, of neutrophil chemotaxins (e.g. IL-8, LTB_4). Other pro-inflammatory mediators may indirectly stimulate chemotaxin release from other cell types or may act upon the endothelium to upregulate adhesion molecules required for transmigration (e.g. IL-1β, TNFα). Neutrophil chemotaxins include bacterial peptides (fMLP), complement cleavage products (C5a), LTB_4 and the CXC family of chemokines, notably IL-8. IL-8 can be produced in large quantities in the human lung, and levels correlate with the extent of neutrophilia, e.g. in idiopathic pulmonary fibrosis [27]. In addition to its production by macrophages, fibroblasts and bronchial epithelial cells, neutrophils themselves are a source of IL-8, promoting further neutrophil emigration [28].

Prior to their transmigration, neutrophils must be "sequestered" within blood vessels, typically in the pulmonary capillaries. Neutrophil stiffening or reduction in deformability is believed to be an important early sequestrative event and can be

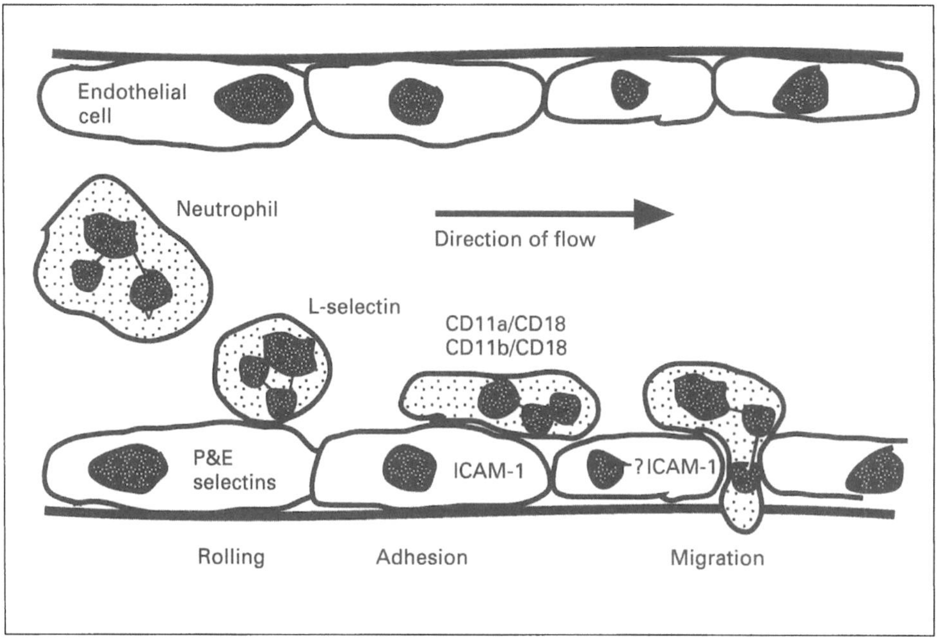

Figure 2
Neutrophil adhesion and migration.

induced by chemotaxins [29]. Ligation of neutrophil surface receptors to counter-receptors on the endothelial cells then occurs, employing similar but not identical receptors to those employed in systemic vascular beds (Fig. 2). Selectins mediate the "rolling" or transient adhesion phase which precedes firm adhesion, which in turn depends upon integrin activation. Neutrophils constitutively express L-selectin, whereas activated but not resting endothelial cells express both E- and P-selectins. Neutrophil L-selectin interacting with endothelial E-selectin is an early adhesive event and may permit integrin activation [30]. Leukocytes express the β_2 subfamily of integrins (LFA-1, Mac-1 and p150,95 or CD11a/CD18, CD11b/CD18 and CD11c/CD18 respectively). These integrins bind to ICAM1-3 receptors on the endothelium [31] but also, in the case of Mac-1, to activated complement (C3bi), implying a role in the phagocytosis of opsonised particles. ICAM-1 is constitutively expressed on the endothelial surface, is strongly upregulated by pro-inflammatory mediators and is believed to be important both in firm adhesion and in subsequent transmigration [32]. CD18 is generally required for neutrophil emigration but inhibition of neutrophil accumulation by anti-CD18 is stimulus and site specific [33]. Mechanisms by which neutrophils then traverse the sub-endothelial basement membrane are unclear, as are mechanisms of their adhesion to and migration past pulmonary epithelial cells. Epithelial cell ICAM-1 is involved in neutrophil adhesion, but with a different cytokine profile of induction of ICAM-1 expression [34].

Neutrophil-mediated tissue injury

The prime function of neutrophils which have emigrated into tissues is the phagocytosis and killing of pathogens, especially bacteria such as *Pneumococcus*. Phagocytosis requires the recognition and subsequent internalisation of the pathogen through invagination of the plasma membrane to form a "phagosome". The phagosome subsequently fuses with both primary and secondary granules to form the phagolysosome. Intracellular killing of the micro-organism requires both activation of the NADPH oxidase and the actions of granule proteases. Interaction of granule contents and NADPH oxidase products within the phagolysosome potentiates their microbicidal effects, e.g. "azurophilic" granules provide myeloperoxidase for the catalysis of hypochlorous acid production from hydrogen peroxide. Granule contents may also be released to the outside of the cell, known as "degranulation", possibly to achieve release of proteases such as elastase leading to basement membrane degradation and thus facilitation of the movement of neutrophils into the tissues. The release of microbicidal products is coupled to specific receptor-mediated events and largely confined to protected intracellular compartments – degradative enzymes are sequestered, predominantly in "azurophilic" granules, until phagocytosis triggers degranulation. Nonetheless, the toxic anti-microbial molecules produced by neutrophils have great potential for damage to normal tissues [35].

The presence of neutrophils in tissue is not *per se* sufficient to cause tissue injury. Neutrophils have been shown to migrate into the lung without causing significant tissue injury in a number of animal models and a recent study of patients with pneumonia and bronchiectasis using positron emission tomography showed large differences in the degree of neutrophil activation between the disease groups, with activation (assessed by uptake of ^{18}FDG) being much greater in patients with pneumonia [36]. Dysregulation of the processes of neutrophil adhesion, transmigration and activation would be predicted to lead to endothelial or epithelial injury as occurs in many forms of inflammatory lung disease.

Tissue clearance of neutrophils: the role of apoptosis

Until recently, neutrophils which had migrated into tissue were assumed to undergo necrosis and disintegrate at the site of inflammation, which would lead to uncontrolled release of toxic neutrophil products. However, a major mechanism for neutrophil clearance may, in fact, be programmed cell death or apoptosis, resulting in the removal of the intact cell, predominantly by ingestion by local macrophages [37,

38]. There is clear evidence that neutrophils undergo apoptosis in the airways in the context of inflammatory lung diseases [39] and in animal models of inflammation [40]. Evidence that apoptosis limits the potential for tissue injury includes the down-regulation of pro-inflammatory functions such as degranulation and superoxide generation with onset of apoptosis [41], clearance of the intact cell, retaining its cytoplasmic granules, by macrophages [38] and the lack of a pro-inflammatory response from the macrophage upon ingestion of apoptotic cells, as opposed to other particulate stimuli [42]. Moreoever, modulation of the rate of apoptosis may be a key determinant of neutrophil survival in tissues. Neutrophil lifespan can be extended *in vitro* by culture with a range of pro-inflammatory mediators such as GM-CSF, C5a and LPS and this is associated with "functional longevity" as evidenced by their ability to undergo chemotaxis and degranulation [43]. Such stimuli may thus have dual pro-inflammatory effects upon the neutrophil, inducing both functional activation and extension of lifespan. Signalling mechanisms which modulate this inhibition of apoptosis and extension of neutrophil lifespan are poorly understood but may include elevation of cytosolic calcium [19] and of cyclic AMP [44]. Induction of neutrophil apoptosis as a therapeutic manoeuvre has the potential to modulate neutrophil survival and thus the "tissue load" of neutrophils in inflammation.

Contribution of the neutrophil to airway inflammation

The role of the neutrophil in the pathogenesis of COPD (chronic obstructive pulmonary disease) is now clearly established [45]. COPD is characterised by airway inflammation, with increased neutrophil numbers in BAL (bronchoalveolar lavage) [46] and in induced sputum [47], together with elevation of neutrophil chemotaxins, including IL-8 and LTB_4 [47, 48]. There is growing support for the concept of protease/anti-protease imbalance as a key pathogenetic mechanism in COPD [45]. Release of proteases results in uncontrolled degradation of elastin and other connective tissue proteins and loss of the alveolar matrix. Key neutrophil proteases implicated in the digestion of elastin and other matrix proteins have been identified, together with a range of endogenous anti-proteases that normally counteract this process. Neutrophil elastase is a major constituent of elastolytic activity, together with cathepsins and matrix metalloproteinases (MMPs) such as collagenase and gelatinase B. The association of emphysema with deficiency of $\alpha 1$ anti-protease implies an important role as an endogenous inhibitor of neutrophil elastase. In addition, a number of tissue inhibitors of MMPs have been identified, together with a serpin SLPI (secretory leukoprotease inhibitor), which is secreted by airway epithelial cells and may be an important inhibitor of elastase activity in the human lung [49].

The contribution of the neutrophil to the pathogenesis of asthma is more controversial [50]. While the eosinophil granulocyte is likely to be the key effector of tissue injury, of bronchial epithelium in particular [51], there have been a number of reports suggesting an additional role for the neutrophil. Recruitment of neutrophils to the asthmatic airway has been demonstrated in BAL studies [52] and in endobronchial biopsies from human subjects 6 h following allergen challenge [53], timings which may imply a role in late asthmatic responses. Neutrophil markers have also been identified in induced sputum from asthmatics [47]. More interestingly, neutrophilic inflammation has been identified in cases of fatal asthma [54] and in acute presentation of status asthmaticus [55]. These findings may suggest the neutrophil is of significance particularly in acute severe asthma. The rapidity of neutrophil influx and potentially short lifespan of these cells may mean that sampling will demonstrate the presence of neutrophils only at very early time points. The role of neutrophils in some forms of occupational asthma, e.g. toluene diisocyanate, is clearer [56] and demonstrates the ability of neutrophil pro-inflammatory functions to induce the clinical syndrome of asthma.

Neutrophils are the primary injurious cells in both adult [57] and neonatal [58] respiratory distress syndromes, with evidence for release of neutrophil elastase being an early event in the development of lung injury [59]. Much of the tissue injury in cystic fibrosis and other forms of bronchiectasis is also attributable to neutrophils and their enzymic products [60].

Pharmacological modulation of neutrophil function

From the above, it is clear that strategies to prevent neutrophil emigration or activation, to prevent release of toxic products or to neutralise their effects may be attractive therapeutic options for the treatment of both acute and chronic neutrophil-mediated pulmonary inflammation. However, concomitant reduction of host defence function may lead to infective complications. Thus anti-neutrophil strategies will need to be applied only during "windows" of opportunity when the injurious consequences outweigh the beneficial effects of neutrophil function. Specificity may be engendered by targetting inhibition of neutrophil emigration only to the lung or by clearance of inflammatory cells direct from the inflamed lung. Further difficulties are posed by the redundancy of mediator pathways, e.g. many signal transduction pathways lead to activation of the NADPH oxidase and to degranulation.

The major current approaches to the limitation of neutrophilic inflammation are summarised in Table 3 and discussed below. Major targets include the chemokines and cytokines which initiate the process of neutrophil migration into the tissues, the adhesion molecules on the neutrophil required for transmigration or their counter-receptors upon the endothelium or epithelium or, once activated neutrophils are present within the lung, pharmacological inhibition of degranulation and NADPH oxidase activity or specific inactivation of potentially deleterious enzymes or reactive

Table 3 - Modulation of neutrophil function

Antagonists to pro-inflammatory receptors and their ligands IL-8 inhibitors Gro-α inhibitors TNF inhibitors LTB_4 antagonists PAF antagonists
Antagonists to adhesion molecules and their receptors
Modulation of signal transduction pathways phosphodiesterase inhibitors MAP kinase cascade inhibitors PI 3-kinase inhibitors PGE_2 analogues corticosteriods
Anti-oxidants
Anti-proteases protease inhibitors (e.g. of elastin, cathepsin, MMPs) endogenous antiproteases (e.g. α_1AP, SLPI, Elafin)
Modulation of apoptosis

oxygen species. Finally, a "whole cell" approach could be taken, with induction of apoptosis or, at least, inhibition of the prolongation of neutrophil lifespan that may occur in inflammation.

Antagonists to pro-inflammatory receptors and their ligands

IL-8 is the predominant neutrophil chemokine in the lung. Anti-IL-8 antibodies have been shown to inhibit neutrophilic inflammation in animal models such as IgG-immune-complex mediated lung injury in the rat [61] and more recently in LPS-induced ARDS in mice [62]. Gro-α, a related CXC chemokine, has also been implicated in studies of human BAL, and blocking antibodies to Gro-α shown to impair neutrophil chemotactic activity [63]. Anti-TNF antibodies have proved effective in other chronic inflammatory diseases with a neutrophilic component, such as rheumatoid arthritis [64]. Studies thus far have employed antibody approaches but these receptors are potential targets for small molecule antagonists.

A leukotriene (LTB_4) antagonist, LY 293 111, has been shown to inhibit neutrophil recruitment in the airways during the late asthmatic response [65]. Both leukotriene receptor antagonists and inhibitors of 5' lipoxygenase, the enzyme synthesising LTB_4, are now available clinically for the treatment of asthma. Intrinsic 5'LO activity appears to be required for neutrophil adherence and chemotaxis, and 5'LO inhibitors were found to attenuate lung injury in a rat model of IL-8 mediated injury [66]. PAF antagonists may also play a role in the amelioration of acute lung injury. PAF is primarily involved in the early adhesion of neutrophils to endothelium and thus in sequestration of neutrophils in the pulmonary vasculature [67].

Adhesion molecule inhibitors

The development of lung injury, at least in rat models, has been shown to require CD11a, CD11b, ICAM-1, L-selectin and P-selectin. Studies have employed monoclonal antibodies to confirm the effects of β2 integrins and selectin function has been confirmed using soluble selectin-Ig chimeras to compete for ligand or by use of a pentasaccharide as a "false substrate", mimicking oligosaccharide binding sites on counter-receptors for selectins [68]. Two models of neutrophil-mediated tissue injury (cobra-venom factor and IgG immune-complex mediated) have confirmed the importance of L-selectin expression on the neutrophil surface for early adhesive events [69]. Concern about adhesion molecule inhibitors arises from the possibility of enhancing susceptibility to infection, as evidenced by the leukocyte adhesion deficiency syndrome (absence of β2 integrins) which is characterised by severe septicemia. However, recent studies examining P-selectin/ICAM-1 double knock-out mice [70] and the CD18-dependence of neutrophilic influx into the lung and skin [33], suggest differences between different sites (and possibly different initiating stimuli) in the adhesion molecule dependency of neutrophil emigration. Further studies may thus identify combination strategies, or even novel alternative adhesion pathways, which will permit pulmonary-specific inhibition of neutrophil influx.

Modulation of neutrophil signal transduction pathways

The predominant phosphodiesterase isoenzyme in human neutrophils is PDE_4 [71]. Inhibition of phosphodiesterase activity leads to increased cAMP levels in neutrophils, and thus to inhibition of pro-inflammatory functions, such as superoxide generation and activation of phospholipase A_2 [13], and also adhesion to bronchial epithelial cells [72]. Selective PDE_4 antagonists are being developed [71]; rolipram inhibits TNF-mediated priming of neutrophil superoxide generation, with a 1000-fold greater potency than the non-specific inhibitor pentoxyfylline [73]. Non-specific phosphodiesterase inhibitors in clinical usage include aminophylline, which has been shown to impair neutrophil chemotaxis *in vitro* [74].

Following exposure of neutrophils to the agonist fMLP, the MAP kinase signalling cascade is rapidly activated. Recent studies with a selective inhibitor (PD098059) to a component of the cascade known as MEK (MAP kinase kinase), demonstrated inhibition of fMLP-induced activation of MEK-1 and MEK-2, the isoforms expressed by neutrophils, and also substantial inhibition of superoxide generation and phagocytosis; degranulation and chemotaxis were unaffected [75].

A PI 3-kinase inhibitor, wortmannin, inhibits neutrophil chemotaxis *in vitro* [76] and may also modulate respiratory burst function and, at higher concentrations, granule secretion [77].

Prostaglandins, notably PGE_2, are potent inhibitors of neutrophil superoxide anion generation, an effect that appears to be mediated *via* the EP2 receptor, with activation of adenylate cyclase leading to elevation of cAMP [78]. However, other PGE_2 effects, such as inhibition of chemotaxis, appear to be independent of cAMP levels [79].

Whether corticosteroids, as a component of their powerful anti-inflammatory functions, specifically modulate neutrophilic inflammation is an area of debate. There is evidence that corticosteroids, probably acting *via* the down-regulation of neutrophil adhesion molecules, prevent the migration of neutrophils from the circulation. Recent evidence suggests that dexamethasone, while not altering expression of Mac-1 or L-selectin on resting neutrophils, may inhibit the up-regulation of CD18 and down-regulation of L-selectin that follows neutrophil priming with PAF [80]. Dexamethasone may also inhibit neutrophil chemotaxis [81]. However, corticosteroids appear to inhibit neutrophil apoptosis, effectively a pro-inflammatory effect of prolongation of inflammatory cell lifespan, in direct contrast to their effects upon eosinophil apoptosis which is markedly accelerated [82].

Anti-oxidants

There is considerable evidence that reactive oxygen species contribute to lung injury, for example in COPD and ARDS. The major source is the neutrophil, although both macrophages and eosinophils also have NADPH oxidase activity [35]. Oxidants may cause tissue injury in a number of ways – by potentiation of elastase activity and activation of matrix metalloproteinases [83], by damage to endogenous anti-proteases [84] and also by activation of NFκB-induced transcription of pro-inflammatory genes such as IL-8 and iNOS [85]. Anti-oxidants such as N-acetyl cysteine have been used in clinical studies [86] and newer anti-oxidants, e.g. spin trap anti-oxidants, have proved effective in animal models of oxidative stress [87].

Anti-protease strategies

The concept of protease/anti-protease imbalance leading to loss of alveolar matrix proteins in emphysema suggests that protease inhibitors or strategies to increase levels of certain anti-proteases may be beneficial. Neutrophils are a major source of proteases within the lung. In addition to their direct elastolytic effects, serine proteases have a number of other modulatory effects: elastase can enhance bronchial epithelial cell mucus production [88] and also the production of the pro-inflammatory chemokine IL-8 [89], while cathepsin G has been shown to be a powerful chemoattractant for both monocytes and neutrophils [90].

Neutrophil elastase, a neutral serine protease, is a major component of neutrophil primary granules. Peptide elastase inhibitors inhibit elastase induced lung injury in animal models [91]. Nebulised human α1 anti-protease reduces elastase activity in patients with cystic fibrosis [92]. Recently, suramin has been shown to be a potent inhibitor of a number of neutrophil serine proteases, including elastase, cathepsin G and proteinase-3 [93].

Matrix metalloproteinases (MMPs) comprise a group of endopeptidases which can, in combination, degrade all extracellular matrix components of the lung. Although MMPs are expressed by other myeloid cells, macrophges and eosinophils, and also by bronchial epithelium, neutrophils are a major source *in vivo*, particularly of collagenase (MMP-1) and gelatinase-B (MMP-9). Endogenous tissue inhibitors of MMPs (TIMPs) exist and enhancement of TIMP secretion or the development of specific MMP inhibitors are possible therapeutic approaches.

A number of serum protease inhibitors (serpins) have been described in addition to α1 anti-protease. These include elafin, an elastase-specific inhibitor, and SLPI (secretory leukoprotease inhibitor), which appears to be a major inhibitor of elastase in the airway and, at least *in vitro*, is more effective in inhibiting neutrophil-mediated proteolysis than α1 anti-protease [94]. Strategies to increase levels of these protective molecules include the use of recombinant proteins, such as rSLPI [95], or perhaps a gene augmentation approach [96].

Acknowledgements
The author would like to thank Samantha Timmons and Stephen Renshaw for their invaluable help in the preparation of this chapter.

References

1 Dancey JT, Deubelbeiss KA, Harker LA, Finch CA (1976) Neutrophil kinetics in man. *J Clin Invest* 58: 705–715
2 Cronkite EP, Fliedner T (1964) Granulocytopoiesis. *New Engl J Med* 270: 1347–1352

3 Peters AM (1997) Just how big is the pulmonary granulocyte pool? *Clin Sci* 94: 7–19
4 Spitznagel JK (1990) Antibiotic proteins of human neutrophils. *J Clin Invest* 86: 1381–1386
5 Smolen JE, Boxer LA (1990) Functions of neutrophils. In: WJ Williams et al (eds): Hematology. Mc Graw Hill, New York, USA, 780–794
6 Gallin JI (1984) Neutrophil specific granules: a fuse that ignites the inflammatory response. *Clin Res* 32: 320–327
7 Ryder MI, Weinreb RN, Niederman R (1984) The organisation of actin filaments in human polymorphonuclear leukocytes. *Anat Rec* 209: 7–20
8 Lloyd AR, Oppenheim JJ (1992) Polys lament – the neglected role of the polymorphonuclear neutrophil in the afferent limb of the immune-response. *Immunol Today* 13: 169–172
9 Sklar LA, Finney DA, Oades ZG, Jesaitis RG, Painter RG, Cochrane CG (1984) The dynamics of ligand-receptor interactions. *J Biol Chem* 259: 5661–5669
10 Smith CD, Cox CC, Synderman R (1986) Receptor-coupled activation of phosphoinositide-specific phospholipase C by an N protein. *Science* 232: 97–99
11 Stephens L, Eguinoa A, Corey S, Jackson T, Hawkins PT (1993) Receptor stimulated accumulation of phosphatidylinositol(3,4,5)-triphosphate by G-protein mediated pathways in human myeloid derived cells. *EMBO J* 12: 2265–2272
12 Erickson RW, Peveri P, Traynorkaplan AE, Curnutte JT (1993) Activation of human neutrophil NADPH oxidase by phosphatidic-acid and diacylglycerol. *FASEB J* 7: A1059
13 Daniels RH, Bird IN, Hill ME, Finnen MJ (1993) Differential regulation of early phase and late phase responses in human neutrophils by cAMP. *Biochem Pharmacol* 45: 1613–1620
14 Moilanen E, Vuorinen P, Kankaanranta H, Metsa-Keteka T, Vapaatalo H (1993) Inhibition by nitric-oxide-donors of polymorphonuclear leucocyte functions. *Br J Pharmacol* 109: 852–858
15 Wallerath T, Gath I, Aulitizky WE, Pollock JS, Kleinert H, Forstermann U (1997) Identification of the NO synthase isoforms expressed in human neutrophil granulocytes, megakaryocytes and platelets. *Thrombosis Haemostasis* 77: 163–167
16 Hallet MB, Lloyds D (1995) Neutrophil priming: the cellular signals that say "amber" but not "green". *Immunol Today* 16: 264–268
17 Brummel JH, Chan CK, Butler J, Borregaard N, Siminovitch KA, Grinstein S, Downey GP (1997) Regulation of Src homology 2-containing tyrosine phosphatase 1 during activation of human neutrophils – Role of protein kinase C. *J Biol Chem* 272: 875–882
18 Pozzan T, Lew CB, Wollheim RY, Tsien RY (1983) Is cystolic ionized calcium regulating neutrophil activation? *Science* 221: 1413–1415
19 Whyte MKB, Hardwick SJ, Meagher LC, Savill JS, Haslett C (1993) Transient elevations of cytosolic free calcium retard subsequent apoptosis in neutrophils *in vitro*. *J Clin Invest* 92: 446–455
20 Segal AW, Abo A (1993) The biochemical basis of the NADPH oxidase of phagocytes. *Trends Biochem Sci* 18: 43–47

21 DeLeo FR, Quinn MT (1996) Assembly of the phagocyte NADPH oxidase: molecular interaction of oxidase proteins. *J Leukoc Biol* 60: 677–691

22 Hallet MB, Davies EV, Campbell AK (1993) Oxidase activation in individual neutrophils is dependent on the onset and magnitude of the Ca^{2+} signal. *Cell Calcium* 11: 655–663

23 Warren JS, Mandel DM, Johnson KJ, Ward PA (1989) Evidence for the role of platelet-activating factor in immune complex vasculitis in the rat. *J Clin Invest* 83: 669–678

24 Forehand JR, Pabst MJ, Phillips WA, Johnston Jr. RB (1989) Lipopolysaccheride priming of human neutrophils for an enhanced respiratory burst. *J Clin Invest* 83: 74–83

25 O'Flaherty JT, Redman JF, Jacobson DP, Rossi AG (1990) Stimulation and priming of protein kinase C translocation by a Ca^{2+} transient-independent mechanism. *J Biol Chem* 265: 21619–21623

26 Kitchen E, Rossi A, Condcliffe AM, Haslett C, Chilvers ER (1996) Demonstration of reversible priming of human neutrophils using platelet-activating factor. *Blood* 88: 4330–4337

27 Carre PC, Mortenson RL, King TE, Noble PW, Sable CL, Riches DWH (1991) Increased expression of the Interleukin-8 gene by alveolar macrophages in idiopathic pulmonary fibrosis – a potential mechanism for the recruitment and activation of neutrophils in lung fibrosis. *J Clin Invest* 88: 1802–1810

28 Kunkel SL, Lukas M, Streiter RM (1995) Expression and biology of neutrophil and endothelial cell-derived cytokines. *Sem Cell Biol* 6: 327–336

29 Worthen GS, Schwab B, Elson EL, Downey GP (1989) Mechanisms of stimulated neutrophils: cell stiffening induces retention in capillaries. *Science* 249: 183–186

30 Tedder TF, Steeber DA, Chen A, Engel P (1995) The selectins: vascular adhesion molecules. *FASEB J* 9: 866–873

31 Springer TA (1990) Adhesion receptors of the immune system. *Nature* 346: 425–434

32 Springer TA (1994) Traffic signals for lymphocyte recirculation and leukocyte emigration: The multistep paradigm. *Cell* 76: 301–314

33 Hellewell PG, Young S, Henson P, Worthen G (1994) Disparate role of the beta 2-integrin CD18 in the local accumulation of neutrophils in pulmonary and cutaneous inflammation in the rabbit. *Am J Respir Cell Mol Biol* 10: 391–398

34 Holtzman MJ, Look DC (1992) Cell adhesion molecules as targets for unravelling the genetic regulation of airway inflammation. *Am J Resp Cell Mol Biol* 7: 246–247

35 Weiss SJ (1989) Tissue destruction by neutropils. *N Engl J Med* 320: 365–376

36 Jones HA, Sriskandan AM, Peters NB, Krausz T, Boobis AR, Haslett C (1997) Dissociation of neutrophil emigration and metabolic activity in lobar pneumonia and bronchiectasis. *Eur Respir J* 10: 795–803

37 Savill JS, Wyllie AH, Henson JE, Henson PM, Haslett C (1989) Macrophage phagocytosis of aging neutrophils in inflammation. Programmed cell death in the neutrophil leads to its recognition by macrophages. *J Clin Invest* 83: 865–875

38 Haslett C (1992) Resolution of acute inflammation and the role of apoptosis in the tissue fate of granulocytes. *Clin Sci* 83: 639–648

39 Grigg JM, Savill JS, Sarraf C, Haslett C, Silverman M (1991) Neutrophil apoptosis and clearance by macrophages in the lungs of neonates with pulmonary inflammation. *Lancet* 338: 720–722
40 Cox G, Crossley J, Xing Z (1995) Macrophage engulfment of apoptotic neutrophils contributes to the resolution of acute pulmonary inflammation *in vivo*. *Am J Resp Cell Mol Biol* 12: 232–237
41 Whyte MKB, Meagher LC, MacDermot J, Haslett C (1993) Impairment of function in aging neutrophils is associated with apoptosis. *J Immunol* 150: 5124–5134
42 Meagher LC, Savill JS, Baker A, Fuller RW, Haslett C (1992) Phagocytosis of apoptotic neutrophils does not induce macrophage release of thromboxane B_2. *J Leukoc Biol* 52: 269–273
43 Lee A, Whyte MKB, Haslett C (1993) Inhibition of apoptosis and prolongation of neutrophil functional longevity by inflammatory mediators. *J Leukoc Biol* 54: 283–288
44 Rossi AG, Cousin JM, Dransfield I, Lawson MF, Chilvers ER, Haslett C (1995) Agents that elevate cAMP inhibit human neutrophil apoptosis. *Biochem Biophys Res Comm* 217: 892–899
45 Stockley RA (1995) The pathogenesis of chronic obstructive lung disease – Implications for therapy. *Q J Med* 88: 141–146
46 Thompson AB, Daughton D, Robbins RA, Ghafouri MA, Oehlerking M, Rennard SI (1989) Intraluminal airway inflammation in chronic bronchitis. Characterisation and correlation with clinical parameters. *Am Rev Resp Dis* 140: 1527–1537
47 Keatings VM, Collins PD, Scott DM, Barnes PJ (1996) Differences in interleukin-8 and tumour necrosis factor in induced sputum from patients with chronic obstructive pulmonary disease or asthma. *Am J Respir Crit Care Med* 153: 530–534
48 Martin TR, Pistorese BP, Chi EY, Goodman RB, Matthay MA (1989) Effects of leukotriene B_4 in the human lung. Recruitment of neutrophils into the alveolar spaces without a change in protein permeability. *J Clin Invest* 84: 1609–1619
49 Bingle L, Tetley TD (1996) Secretory leukoprotease inhibitor: partnering alpha 1-proteinase inhibitor to combat pulmonary inflammation. *Thorax* 51: 1273–1274
50 Busse WW, Calhoun WF, Sedgwick J (1993) Mechanism of airway inflammation in Asthma. *Am Rev Resp Dis* 147: S20–24
51 Laitinen LA, Laitinen A, Haahtela T (1993) Airway mucosal inflammation even in patients with newly diagnosed asthma. *Am Rev Resp Dis* 147: 697–704
52 Frangova V, Sacco O, Silvestri M, Oddera S, Balbo A, Crimi E, Rossi GA (1996) BAL neutrophilia in asthmatic patients. A by-product of eosinophil recruitment? *Chest* 110: 1236–1242
53 Montefort S, Gratziou C, Goulding D, Polosa R, Haskard DO, Howarth PH, Holgate ST, Carroll MP (1994) Bronchial biopsy evidence for leukocyte infiltration and upregulation of leukocyte-endothelial cell adhesion molecules for 6 hours after local allergen challenge in sensitized asthmatic airways. *J Clin Invest* 94: 1411–1421
54 Sur S, Crotty TB, Kephart GM (1993) Sudden-onset fatal asthma. A distant entity with

few eosinophils and relatively more neutrophils in the airway submucosa? *Am Rev Resp Dis* 148: 713–719

55 Lamblin C, Gosset P, TillieLeblond I, Saulnier F, Marquette CH, Wallaert B, Tonnel AB (1998) Bronchial neutrophilia in patients with noninfectious status asthmaticus. *Am J Resp Crit Care Med* 157: 394–402

56 Fabbri LM, Boschetto P, Zocco E, Milani G, Pivirotto F, Plebani M, Burlina A, Licata B, Mapp CE (1987) Bronchoalveolar neutrophilia during late asthmatic reactions induced by toluene diisocyanate. *Am Rev Resp Dis* 136: 36–42

57 Reid PT, Donnelly SC, Haslett C (1995) Inflammatory predictors for the development of the adult respiratory distress syndrome. *Thorax* 50: 1023–1026

58 Brus F, van Oeveren W, Okken A, Oettomo SB (1997) Number and activation of circulating polymorphonuclear leukocytes and platelets are associated with neonatal respiratory distress syndrome severity. *Pediatrics* 99: 672–680

59 Donnelly SC, MacGregor I, Zamani A, Gordon MW, Robertson CE, Steedman DJ, Little K, Haslett C (1995) Plasma elastase levels and the development of the adult respiratory distress syndrome. *Am J Respir Crit Care Med* 151: 1428–1433

60 Elborn JS, McCloskey M (1997) Cystic fibrosis. *Curr Opin Inf Dis* 10: 128–131

61 Mulligan MS, Jones ML, Bolanowski MA, Baganoff MP, Deppeler CL, Meyers DM, Ryan US, Ward PA (1993) Inhibition of lung inflammatory reactions in rats by an anti-human IL-8 antibody. *J Immunol* 150: 5585–5595

62 Matsumoto T, Yokoi K, Mukaida N, Harada A, Yamashita J, Watanabe Y, Matsushima K (1997) Pivotal role of interleukin-8 in the acute respiratory distress syndrome and cerebral reperfusion injury. *J Leukoc Biol* 62: 581–587

63 Villard J, Dayerpastore F, Hamacher J, Aubert JD, Schlegelhaueter S, Nicod LP (1995) Gro-alpha and interleukin-8 in pneumocytosis-carini or bacterial pneumonia and adult-respiratory-distress-syndrome. *Am J Resp Crit Care Med* 152: 1549–1554

64 Elliott MJ, Maini RN, Feldmann M, Longfox A, Charles P, Bijl H, Woody JN (1994) Repeated therapy with monoclonal-antibody to tumour-necrosis-factor-alpha (CA2) in patients with rheumatiod arthritis. *Lancet* 8930: 1125–1127

65 Evans DJ, Barnes PJ, Spaethe SM, Vanalstyne EL, Mitchell MI, O'Connor BJ (1996) Effect of a Leukotriene B-4 receptor antagonist, LY293111, on allergen-induced responses in asthma. *Thorax* 51:1178–1184

66 Guidot DM, Repine MJ, Westcott JY, Repine JE (1994) Intrinsic 5-lipoxygenase activity is required for neutrophil responsivity. *Proc Natl Acad Sci USA* 91: 8156–8159

67 Coughlan AF, Hau H, Dunlop LC, Berndt MC, Hancock WW (1994) P-selectin and platelet-activating-factor mediate initial endotoxin-induced neutropenia. *J Exp Med* 179: 329–334

68 Albelda SM, Smith CW, Ward PA (1994) Adhesion molecules and inflammatory injury. *FASEB J* 8: 504–512

69 Mulligan MS, Miyasaka M, Tamatani T, Jones ML, Ward PA (1994) Requirements for L-selectin in neutrophil-mediated lung injury in rats. *J Immunol* 152: 832–840

70 Bullard DC, Qin L, Lorenzo I, Quinlim WM, Doyle NA, Bosse R, Vestweber D,

Doershuk CM, Beaudet AL (1995) P-selectin ICAM-1 double mutant mice – acute emigration of neutrophils into the peritoneum is completely absent but is normal into pulmonary alveoli. *J Clin Invest* 95: 1782–1788

71 Muller T, Engels P, Fozard J (1996) Subtypes of the type 4 cAMP phosphodiesterase: structure, regulation and selective inhibition. *Trends Pharm Sci* 17: 294–298

72 Bloemem PGM, VandenTweel MC, Henricks PAJ, Engels F, Kester MHA, VandeLoo PGF, Blomjous FJ, Nijkamp FP (1997) Increased cAMP levels in stimulated neutrophils inhibit their adhesion to human bronchial epithelial cells. *Am J Phys-Lung Cell Mol Phys* 16: L580–L587

73 Sullivan GW, Carper HT, Mandell GL (1995) The specific type-IV phosphodiesterase inhibitor rolipram combined with adenosine reduces tumour necrosis factor-alpha-primed neutrophils oxidative activity. *Int J Immunopharm* 17: 793–803

74 Llewellyn Jones CG, Stockley RA (1994) The effects of β_2-agonists and methylxanthines on neutrophil function *in vitro*. *Eur Respir J* 7: 1460–1466

75 Downy GP, Butler JR, Tapper H, Fialkow L, Satiel AR, Rubin BB, Grinstein S (1998) Importance of MEK in neutrophil microbicidal responsiveness. *J Immunol* 160: 434–443

76 Niggli V, Keller H (1997) The phosphatidylinositol 3-kinase inhibitor wortmannin markedly reduces chemotactic peptide-induced locomotion and increases in cytoskeletal actin in human neutrophils. *Eur J Pharm* 335: 43–52

77 SueAQuan AK, Fialkow L, Vlahos CJ, Schlem JA, Grinstein S, Butler J, Downey GP (1997) Inhibition of neutrophil oxidative burst and granule secretion by Wortmannin: Potential role of MAP kinase and renaturable kinases. *J Cell Physiol* 172: 94–108

78 Talpain E, Armstrong RA, Coleman RA, Vardey CJ (1995) Characterization of the PGE receptor subtype mediating inhibition of superoxide production in human neutrophils. *Br J Pharm* 114: 1459–1465

79 Armstrong RA (1995) Investigation of the inhibitory effects of PGE(2) and selective EP agonists on chemotaxis of human neutrophils. *Br J Pharm* 116: 2903–2908

80 Filep JG, Delalandre A, Payette Y, FoldesFilep E (1997) Glucocorticoid receptor regulates expression of L-selectin and CD11/CD18 on human neutrophils. *Circulation* 96: 295–301

81 Lomas DA, Ip M, Chamba A, Stockley RA (1991) The effect of *in vitro* and *in vivo* dexamethasone on human neutrophil function. *Agents Actions* 33: 279–285

82 Meagher LC, Cousin JM, Seckl JR, Haslett C (1996) Opposing effects of glucocorticoids on the rate of apoptosis in neutrophilic and eosinophil granulocytes. *J Immunol* 156: 4422–4428

83 Claesson R, Karlsson M, Zhang YY, Carlsson J (1996) Relative role of chloramines, hypochlorous acid and proteases in the activation of human polymorphonuclear leukocyte collagenase. *J Leukoc Biol* 60: 598–602

84 Ottonello L, Dapino P, Scirocco M, Dallegri F, Sacchetti C (1994) Proteolytic inactivation of alpha-1-antitrypsin by human neutrophils – involvement of multiple and interlinked cell responses to phagocytosable targets. *Eur J Clin Invest* 24: 42–49

85 Barnes PJ, Karin M (1997) Nuclear factor κB: a pivitol transcription factor in chronic inflammatory disease. *N Engl J Med* 336: 1066–1071
86 Boman G, Backer U, Larsson S, Melander B, Wahlander L (1983) Oral acetylcysteine reduces exacerbation rate in chronic bronchitis: a report of a trial organized by the Swedish Society for Pulmonary Diseases. *Eur J Resp Dis* 64: 405–415
87 Miyajima T, Kotake Y (1995) Spin trapping agent, phenyl-N-tert-butyl nitrone, inhibits induction of nitric oxide synthase in endotoxin-induced shock in mice. *Biochem Biophys Res Commun* 215: 114–121
88 Sommerhoff CP, Nadel JA, Basbaum CB, Caughey GH (1990) Neutrophil elastase and cathepsin G stimulate secretion from cultured bovine airway gland serous cells. *J Clin Invest* 85: 682–689
89 Nakamura H, Yoshimura K, McElvaney NG, Crystal RG (1992) Neutrophil elastase in repiratory epithelial lining fluid of individuals with cystic fibrosis induces interleukin-8 gene expression in a human bronchial epithelial cell line. *J Clin Invest* 89: 1478–1484
90 Chertov O, Ueda H, Xu LL, Tani K, Murphy WJ, Wang JM, Howard OMZ, Sayers TJ, Oppenheim JJ (1997) Identification of human neutrophil-derived cathepsin G and azurocidin/CAP37 as chemoattractants for mononuclear cells and neutrophils. *J Exp Med* 186: 739–747
91 Williams JC, Falcone RC, Knee C et al (1991) Biological characterization of ICE 200, 355, novel inhibitors of human neutrophil elastase. *Am Rev Respir Dis* 144: 875–883
92 McElvaney DG, Hubbard RC, Birper P et al (1991) Aerosol α_1-antitrypsin treatment for cystic fibrosis. *Lancet* 337: 392–394
93 Cadene M, Duranton J, North A, SiTahar M, Chignard M, Bieth JG (1997) Inhibition of neutrophil serine proteinases by suramin. *J Biol Chem* 272: 9950–9955
94 Llewellyn Jones CG, Lomas DA, Stockley RA (1994) Potential role of recombinant secretory leucoprotease inhibitor in the prevention of neutrophil mediated matrix degradation. *Thorax* 49: 567–572
95 Tomee JFC, Koeter GH, Hiemstra PS, Kauffman HF (1998) Secretory leukoprotease inhibitor: a native antimicrobial protein presenting a new therapeutic option? *Thorax* 53: 114–116
96 Sallenave JM, Porteous DJ, Haslett C (1997) Gene therapy for inflammatory lung diseases: not so far away? *Thorax* 52: 742–744

Eosinophils in asthma

Anthony J. Coyle and Jose Carlos Gutierrez-Ramos

Dept. of Biology, Inflammation Division, Millennium Pharmaceuticals, Inc., 45-75 Sidney St., Cambridge, MA 02139, USA

Introduction

Bronchial hyperresponsiveness (BHR) to both specific and nonspecific stimuli is a characteristic feature of bronchial asthma. While the mechanisms underlying this exaggerated responsiveness are still unclear, there is a considerable body of evidence to suggest that mucosal inflammation of the airways is of central importance. Perhaps the most common pathological finding is that of an increased number of eosinophils in the lung mucosa. It is currently believed that the secretion of eosinophil derived highly toxic cationic proteins such as major basic protein (MBP) mediates damage to the epithelium. In addition, following the appreciation that eosinophils can secrete a number of cytokines, there is mounting evidence to suggest that eosinophil recruitment and activation may be involved in not only the acute manifestations of the disease, eosinophilic inflammation may contribute to remodeling events in the airways, characterized by subepithelial deposition of collagen types III and V and fibronectin. This review discusses the mechanisms by which the cells are recruited to the airways and discusses the evidence for and against that eosinophilic inflammation is critical to the pathogenesis of asthma.

Eosinophil structure and contents

Our understanding of the structure of the eosinophil dates to 1966 when Palade and colleagues published a detailed report of the granular contents of human peripheral blood eosinophils. Both blood and tissue eosinophils contain crystalloid granules, which develop from immature granules during the promyelocyte stage. The crystalloid granules contain large amounts of peroxidase and β-glucouronidase. These granules have much in common with basophil granules in that when eosinophil granules first form in the marrow they are basophilic in nature, but lose this property as they mature. In addition, both eosinophils and basophils contain large amounts of lysophospholipase or Charcot-Leyden crystals (CLC), which accounts for the characteristic bipyramidal crystals observed at inflammatory lesions. While

Cellular Mechanisms in Airways Inflammation, edited by Clive P. Page, Katharine H. Banner and Domenico Spina

CLC protein makes up to 10% of the total protein in eosinophils, its function is unknown, although it has been speculated that CLC may protect eosinophils from the toxic effects of lysophospholipids. However, the most distinguishing feature of the eosinophils is its high content of highly charged cationic proteins, Major basic Protein (MBP) eosinophil cationic protein (ECP) and eosinophil derived neurotaxin (EDN). These proteins together with eosinophil peroxidase have been implicated as final effector molecules in eosinophil mediated tissue damage. MBP is the predominant protein in the eosinophil and comprises the crystalloid core of the eosinophil granule. MBP is a 117 amino acid protein, rich in arginine and is translated as a slightly acidic preproprotein with an acidic prodomain, which has been reported to inhibit the effects of mature MBP [1]. MBP was initially reported to be highly toxic to schistosomula of *S. Mansoni*, as well as amstigotes and epimastigotes of *Trypanosoma cruzi*. Subsequently, MBP has been shown to be highly toxic to tracheal epithelia at concentrations of 10^{-5} to 10^{-7} M [2]. At lower concentrations, MBP directly inhibits tracheal ciliary axonems [3] and alters fluid dynamics in canine trachea [4]. Unlike MBP, both ECP and EDN exhibit ribonuclease activity. Comparison of the relative toxicity of ECP and MBP for schistosomula death revealed on a molar basis that ECP is ten times more toxic than MBP. However, as levels of secreted MBP are considerably greater than ECP, the relative contribution of the proteins to tissue destruction remains to be determined. EDN has marked homology to ECP, and exhibits 50–100 fold greater ribonuclease activity than ECP, although it has rather weak toxicity against parasitic larvae. EPO is localized to the matrix of the eosinophil crystalloid granule and has the ability to catalyze the formation of HBrO- ions and H_2O_2. It is currently believed that this mechanism provides an efficient mechanism for killing parasites, bacteria, and some tumour cells [5].

Eosinophil derived cationic proteins and asthma

Elevated levels of MBP have been detected in the sputum of individuals with allergic airway disease, the amount of which correlated with the degree of epithelial denudation and severity of airway hyperresponsiveness [6]. Furthermore, MBP has been shown to be localized to damaged epithelial surfaces and in mucus plugs in the airways of individuals who have died from status asthmaticus [7]. MBP leads to enhanced contractile responsiveness of isolated trachealis [8], and *in vivo*, instillation of MBP and EPO results in a transient bronchoconstriction [9]. The mechanism underlying this effect remains unclear, but appears to be independent of the cationic charge as ECP failed to induce these changes. MBP, but not ECP has been demonstrated to induce histamine release from basophils suggesting that MBP may induce bronchoconstriction at least in part by activating resident airway cells [10]. More recently, a highly divergent MBP homologue has been identified [11], although its function remains to be clarified.

MBP however is the only major eosinophil protein that can induce airway hyperresponsiveness *in vivo* in non-human primates [10]. This effect appears to be a charge dependent effect as preproMBP is ineffective. Furthermore, the effect of MBP is neutralized by anionic agents such as heparin sulphate and can be mimicked by other highly charged proteins such as poly-L- arginine [12]. MBP instillation results in activation of the kinin system inducing an increase in both kallikrein like activity (measuring both tissue and plasma kallikein) and immunoreactive kinins (bradykinin and lyslbradykinin) [13]. MBP induced kinin system activation can also be inhibited by heparin suggesting a charge dependent mechanism is involved [13]. Cationic proteins also result in the activation of sensory C-fibres in the airways resulting in the release of substance P and CGRP from isolated rat trachea [14]. In addition, cationic proteins also induce an increase in plasma protein extravasation, which can be inhibited by a selective NK-1 receptor antagonist [14]. As bradykinin is able to stimulate sensory C-fibers [15], it remains to be determined whether MBP and other cationic proteins induce tachykinin release dependent on the generation of kinins in the airways. Nevertheless, in situations where eosinophil degranulation occurs, MBP could stimulate sensory nerve endings resulting in activation of a local axonal reflex and may play an important role in the pathogenesis of airway hyperresponsiveness.

In addition to these mechanisms a series of elegant data has been reported by Jacoby and colleagues suggesting MBP may act as an allosteric modulator of the muscarnic (M2) autoreceptor [16]. MBP interacts with the inhibitory feedback mechanism of acetylcholine release from parasympathetic nerve terminals, resulting in an augmented bronchoconstrictor response. It is fascinating to hypothesize that MBP may function as a connection between the two hypotheses in asthma: namely, neural and cellular basis for airway hyperresponsiveness.

Recent work from Lefort and colleagues have further supported a key role for MBP in experimental allergen induced airway hyperresponsiveness [17]. Administration of a neutralizing MBP antibody inhibited airway hyperresponsiveness induced by aeroallergen provocation in sensitized guinea pigs. It remains to be determined how these findings extrapolate to the finding in human disease.

Eosinophil derived cytokines

While there is a considerable body of evidence to suggest that eosinophils are final effector cells in the pathogenesis of allergic disease and bronchial asthma, mediated largely through the secretion of cationic proteins, these cells also have the capacity to synthesize and release a wide array of cytokines that may perpetuate a cycle of inflammatory events. Human eosinophils can store IL-5 in the granular matrix, which is secreted by either IgA, IgG or IgE dependent mechanisms [18]. Likewise, eosinophils can also produce IL-3 and GM-CSF, and as such, eosinophil activation may provide, in an autocrine fashion, its own survival factors. Stimulation of human eosinophils with calcium ionophore also leads to the production of IL-8 [19], as well as macrophage inhibitory factor (MIF) [20]. Likewise human eosinophils synthesize and secrete IL-6 [21], which is able to facilitate IL-4 dependent IgE production, and can synergize with IL-3 and GM-CSF for the maturation of multipotential granulocyte progenitors. Interestingly, IL-6 can also promote the secretion of IgA in mucosal tissue, which may subsequently "arm" eosinophils to secrete their granular contents following activation. Eosinophils also secrete TGFβ [22] and this may underlie the possible contribution of the eosinophil to the development of fibrosis in the airways. More recently, eosinophils have been demonstrated to produce IL-4 [23] and could theoretically contribute to local IgE production and perhaps more importantly, to facilitate the commitment of antigen specific cells to the Th2 effector phenotype. In this respect, recent work from Pierce and colleagues has shown that eosinophils can provide the first source of IL-4 to prime T cells for subsequent IL-5 production after *S. Mansoni* infection [24].

Eosinophils as immune competent cells

An interesting area of research over the past 5 years has been the possibility that eosinophils may also function as immune competent cells. Eosinophils express CD40 ligand [25] and may facilitate B-cell proliferation. This together with the ability of eosinophils to secrete IL-4 and IL-13, raises the possibility that eosinophils in the airway may contribute to local IgE production. Interestingly, eosinophils also express the high affinity receptor for IgE (FcεRII) [26]. More recently, eosinophils have been reported to express the costimulatory signals B7-1 and B7-2 [27]. It is interesting to speculate that as a consequence of eosinophil mediated B7 dependent costimulation of antigen specific $CD4^+$ T cells in the lungs, T cells are less resistant to apoptosis, less susceptible to being tolerated and would have an increased capacity to secrete cytokines. Eosinophils also express a number of receptors that may be important for the role of the eosinophil in immune responses including TNFα receptors I and II [28] and both the α and β chains of the IFNγ receptor [29]. More recently, GM-CSF treated eosinophils have been shown to bind rhinovirus *via* ICAM-1 which in turn activate virus specific T cells [30]. Finally, eosinophils can express the IL-2 receptor [31]. The functional significance of this observation remains to be determined.

IL-5 and eosinophil accumulation

Over 20 years ago, the development of eosinophilia in nematode infected rodents was demonstrated to be lymphocyte dependent. Subsequently it was shown that the soluble factor from T cells was identical to B cell growth factor 2 (now designated as IL-5). *In vivo*, administration of exogenous IL-5 induces eosinophil recruitment and IL-

5 transgenic mice overexpressing the IL-5 gene under a variety of different tissue specific promoters (CD3ε, metalloprotein), develop peripheral blood, bone marrow and tissue eosinophilia, although overexpression itself failed to result in any overt disease [32, 33]. These data contrast to more recent work where IL-5 was overexpressed on a CC10 promoter resulting in high levels of IL-5 in the BAL fluid, and these transgenic mice exhibited evidence of airway remodeling (subepithelial fibrosis), the formation of BALT and the induction of airway hyperresponsiveness [34]. Administration of neutralizing anti-IL-5 mAbs has been demonstrated to inhibit eosinophilia induced by nematodes or antigen exposure in sensitized animals [35, 36]. Taken together these data initially lead to the widespread belief that IL-5 was the eosinophil chemoattractant. However, there were a number of discrepancies which failed to support this hypothesis. IL-5 itself is a rather poor eosinophil chemoattractant compared to, for example, PAF. In addition, while it is clear that the number of eosinophils in inflammatory lesions is dramatically reduced in the absence of IL-5, this now appears to be due to a failure to generate mature eosinophils in the marrow, thus the eosinophil number in the blood is greatly reduced, as is the number of eosinophils at inflammatory sites. Implicit in this argument is that while IL-5 secretion is essential for eosinophil mobilization, other factors must be required to attract these cells into specific inflammatory lesions. Nevertheless, if IL-5 itself does not directly contribute to the accumulation of eosinophils, it is likely that once these cells accumulate in the airways, IL-5 is required for the survival of the cells and the prevention of apoptosis.

Th2 cytokines and eosinophil recruitment

While clearly IL-5 has an important role to play in eosinophil recruitment, other Th2 cytokines have also been implicated and merit discussion. Data obtained from genetic studies have implicated IL-9 as an important gene in asthma. To further address this issue, IL-9 transgenic mice have been generated, with IL-9 under the control of a lung epithelial cell specific prompter. These mice develop eosinophilic inflammation, mucus cell hyperplasia and airway hyperresponsiveness [37]. Likewise, IL-11 transgenic mice exhibit similar alterations in airway inflammation. However, while there was no evidence of airway hyperresponsiveness, mice exhibited increased basal airway resistance [38]. It remains however to be determined whether these effects are secondary to IL-5, chemokine generation or the upregulation of adhesion molecules.

Transcriptional factor regulation of lung eosinophilic inflammation

The role of various transcriptional events required for the recruitment of eosinophils has recently been investigated by several groups. Mice deficient in

NKκB exhibit attenuated eosinophilic lung inflammation and markedly reduced levels of IL-5 as well as the chemokines eotaxin, MIP-1α and MIP-1β [39]. Similar STAT-6 deficient mice have greatly diminished eosinophil number and attenuated airway hyperresponsiveness [40]. However, while these data lead to useful information concerning transcriptional events underlying changes in airway eosinophilic inflammation, due to the complexity and multiple mechanisms involved, *in vitro* studies of gene regulation are also required. In this respect, GATA-3 [41, 42] and c-Maf [43] have been shown to be overexpressed in Th2 cells, and their activity required for activation of the IL-4 promoter. Further studies are required to determine the contribution of these transcriptional events, however, it is interesting to note that GATA-3 mRNA is increased in the lungs of atopic asthmatics and localized to primarily CD4⁺ T cells, although mast cells and eosinophils also expressed GATA-3 mRNA [44].

Chemokines and eosinophil accumulation

There is now increasing data to suggest that members of the chemokine superfamily family play an important role in eosinophil accumulation. These proteins range in size from 68-120 amino acids and are classified into four families namely C, C-C and C-X-C, C-X-X-X-C on the basis of the variations in a shared cysteine motif, which can in general be associated with distinct biological activities. For example C-X-C chemokines of which IL-8 is a member, are in general neutrophil chemoattractants, whereas C-C chemokines of which RANTES, eotaxin and MIP-1α are members, exert their biological activities on eosinophils (and also lymphocytes and monocytes). Recently, several groups have addressed the profile of expression of chemokines *in vivo* during the induction of an allergic response both in animal models [45, 46] and in clinical studies [47]. Nevertheless, the importance of different chemokines in mediating eosinophil recruitment *in vivo* is however at present contradictory, with reports suggesting that either MCP-1 [46], eotaxin [45, 48], MCP-5 [46], RANTES and/or MIP-1α [49] are important. However, it is important to note that in each of these studies, the degree of inhibition of eosinophilic inflammation was only partial implying a significant redundancy and that multiple chemokines are involved in this process. Conversely, it is possible that chemokines play a distinct non-redundant function, acting as discrete steps in orchestrating inflammatory response [46]. Nevertheless, it is likely that targeting more than one chemokine or inhibiting more than a single chemokine receptor would have more potent effects in inhibiting inflammatory responses. The effects of C-C chemokines are mediated by a family of seven transmembrane G-protein coupled receptors of which nine human receptors and six murine receptors have been cloned and functionally characterized. Eosinophils express CCR3 and to a lesser extent CCR1. Eosinophils migrate to eotaxin *via* CCR3 and to MIP-1α, RANTES *via* CCR1, it remains to be determined if these are the only chemokine receptors on the eosinophil or whether other chemokine receptors are also expressed and are functionally important in eosinophil migration. There is also some question as to the role of chemokine/eosinophil axis in the development of BHR. In this context, neutralizing mAbs to RANTES and MIP-1α have been reported to suppress eosinophil recruitment into the lungs, but not airway hyperresponsiveness. In contrast, while anti-MCP-1 mAbs failed to suppress eosinophilic inflammation, airway hyperresponsiveness was abrogated [49]. Taken together, the possibility remains that chemokines themselves exert a direct action on airway smooth muscle to modify airway responsiveness, although this warrants further study.

Eosinophils as effectors of bronchial hyperresponsiveness

Despite the enormous literature on the relationship between eosinophilic inflammation and bronchial hyperresponsiveness, this may be the most controversial area in asthma research today. While few would argue with the clinical observations that asthma is almost always associated with the presence of eosinophils in the airways, the reverse is not necessary true.

These observations have lead various groups to question the eosinophil dogma is asthma. However, it is important to note that it is not the presence of eosinophils, but rather their activation status which may govern whether the eosinophil accumulation results in alterations in airway hyperresponsivenesss. In addition, given the possibility that different stimuli result in distinct patterns of activation of the eosinophil, it is possible that in diseases such as idiopathic eosinophilic fibrosis, the eosinophil is activated – but not to the phenotype that can result in airway hyperresponsiveness.

To address these issues extensive studies have been performed in animal models in a number of species. These studies have in general supported the relationship between eosinophils and bronchial hyperresponsiveness; there are a number of examples that are in conflict with this data. These studies have traditionally been performed in guinea pigs, which while demonstrating a robust bronchoconstrictor response to inhaled or intravenous agonists, lack the immunological tools to be able to selectively target eosinophils to dissect the mechanisms involved in bronchial hperresponsiveness. The advent of murine immunology and the application to allergic lung disease heralded a new excitement and confidence in this area and it was anticipated that an answer to this question was finally in sight. This, like many other instances in asthma research, has proven to be a naïve concept and demonstrated how the mechanisms underlying this complex disease still evade us. In this respect, murine eosinophils *in vivo* do not appear to undergo degranulation [50] following antigenic challenge, which has led some groups to question the use of these models in asthma for predicting the contribution of the eosinophil [51].

The first report of IL-5 deficient mice was published by Foster and colleagues in 1996 [52]. They demonstrated in IL-5 gene targeted mice that in the virtual absence of eosinophils in the lungs, airway hyperresponsiveness was completely abolished, confirming at last the link between eosinophilic inflammation and BHR. This excitement was short lived, as it was subsequently demonstrated that administration of anti-IL-5 mAbs – which resulted in a complete inhibition of eosinophilic inflammation, did not affect the induction of BHR [53]. In contrast, anti-IL-4 mAbs, which fail to attenuate the eosinophilic inflammation of the airways, reduced the BHR [53]. These differences can now be explained in terms of the generic background of the mice used – thus IL-5 deletion on a C57/B6 background results in an eosinophilic dependent BHR, whereas the same deletion on Balb/C background results in an eosinophil independent BHR. In addition, the nature of the stimuli also plays an important role. Infection of C57/B6 mice with *Nippostrongylus Braziliensis* results in an eosinophil dependent tissue damage characterized by edema, hemorrhage and destruction of the septal walls. However, despite the lack of widespread damage observed in lL-5 deficient mice, airway hyperresponsiveness was not affected [54]. Taken together, these results suggest that under some circumstances eosinophil activation plays an important role in airway pathology in animal models, although their contribution is greatly influenced by genetic factors and the nature of the allergen.

Conclusions

Despite the intense research and huge financial investment by many pharmaceutical companies in trying to inhibit the accumulation of eosinophils, the role of the eosinophil to the development of asthma still remains unknown. Certainly therapeutics agents such as steroids improve asthmatic exacerbations and also reduce eosinophilic inflammation. However, not until the advent of highly selective inhibitors of eosinophil accumulation chemokine receptor antagonists or IL-5 antagonists will the eosinophil hypothesis be finally settled and we will know whether the association of eosinophils with asthma is some epiphenomena or if crucial cells play a central role as final effectors in this life threatening disease.

References

1 Barker RL, Gundel RH, Gleich GJ, Checkel JL, Loegering DA, Pease LR, Hamann KJ (1991) Acidic polyamino acids inhibit human eosinophil granule major basic protein toxicity. Evidence of a functional role for ProMBP. *J Clin Invest* 88: 798–805
2 Motojima S, Frigas E, Loegering DA, Gleich GJ (1989) Toxicity of eosinophil cationic proteins for guinea pig tracheal epithelium *in vitro*. *Am Rev Respir Dis* 139: 801–805

3 Hastie AT, Loegering DA, Gleich GJ, Kueppers (1987) The effect of purified human eosinophil major basic protein on mammalian ciliary activity. *Am Rev Respir Dis* 135 (4): 848–853
4 Jacoby DB, Ueki IF, Widdicombe JH, Loegering DA, Gleich GJ, Nadel JA (1988) Effect of human eosinophil major basic protein on ion transport in dog tracheal epithelium. *Am Rev Respir Dis* 137 (1): 13–16
5 Weiss SJ, Test ST, Eckmann CM, Roos D, Regiani S (1986) Brominating oxidants generated by human eosinophils. *Science* 234 (4773): 200–203
6 Wardlaw AJ, Dunnette S, Gleich GJ, Collins JV, Kay AB (1988) Eosinophils and mast cells in bronchoalveolar lavage in subjects with mild asthma. Relationship to bronchial hyperreactivity. *Am Rev Respir Dis* 137 (1): 62–69
7 Filley WV, Holley KE, Kephart GM, Gleich GJ (1982) Identification by immunofluorescence of eosinophil granule major basic protein in lung tissues of patients with bronchial asthma. *Lancet* 2 (8288): 11–16
8 Brofman JD, White SR, Blake JS, Munoz NM, Gleich GJ, Leff AR (1989) Epithelial augmentation of trachealis contraction caused by major basic protein of eosinophils. *J Appl Physiol* 66 (4): 1867–1873
9 Gundel RH, Letts LG, Gleich GJ (1991) Human eosinophil major basic protein induces airway constriction and airway hyperresponsiveness in primates. *J Clin Invest* 87 (4): 1470–1473
10 Zheutlin LM, Ackerman SJ, Gleich GJ, Thomas LL (1984) Stimulation of basophil and rat mast cell histamine release by eosinophil granule-derived cationic proteins. *J Immunol* 133 (4): 2180–2185
11 Plager DA, Loegering DA, Weiler DA, Checkel JL, Wagner JM, Clarke NJ, Naylor S, Page SM, Thomas LL, Akerblom I, Cocks B, Stuart S, Gleich GJ (1999) A novel and highly divergent homolog of human eosinophil granule major basic protein. *J Biol Chem* 274 (20): 14464–14473
12 Uchida DA, Ackerman SJ, Coyle AJ, Larsen GL, Weller PF, Freed J, Irvin CG (1993) The effect of human eosinophil granule major basic protein on airway responsiveness in the rat *in vivo*. A comparison with polycations. *Am Rev Respir Dis* 147 (4): 982–988
13 Coyle AJ, Ackerman SJ, Burch R, Proud D, Irvin CG (1995) Human eosinophil-granule major basic protein and synthetic polycations induce airway hyperresponsiveness *in vivo* dependent on bradykinin generation. *J Clin Invest* 95 (4): 1735–1740
14 Coyle AJ, Perretti F, Manzini S, Irvin CG (1994) Cationic protein-induced sensory nerve activation: role of substance P in airway hyperresponsiveness and plasma protein extravasation. *J Clin Invest* 94 (6): 2301–2306
15 Miura M, Belvisi MG, Barnes PJ (1994) Modulation of nonadrenergic noncholinergic neural bronchoconstriction by bradykinin in anesthetized guinea pigs *in vivo*. *J Pharmacol Exp Ther* 268 (1): 482–486
16 Jacoby DB, Gleich GJ, Fryer AD (1993) Human eosinophil major basic protein is an endogenous allosteric antagonist at the inhibitory muscarinic M2 receptor. *J Clin Invest* 91 (4): 1314–8

17 Lefort J, Nahori MA, Ruffie C, Vargaftig BB, Pretolani M 8 1996) *In vivo* neutralization of eosinophil-derived major basic protein inhibits antigen-induced bronchial hyperreactivity in sensitized guinea pigs. *J Clin Invest* 97 (4): 1117–1121
18 Dubucquoi S, Desreumaux P, Janin A, Klein O, Goldman M, Tavernier J, Capron A, Capron M (1994) Interleukin 5 synthesis by eosinophils: association with granules and immunoglobulin-dependent secretion. *J Exp Med* 179 (2): 703–708
19 Braun RK, Franchini M, Erard F, Rihs S, De Vries IJ, Blaser K, Hansel TT, Walker C (1993) Human peripheral blood eosinophils produce and release interleukin-8 on stimulation with calcium ionophore. *Eur J Immunol* 23 (4): 956–60
20 Rossi AG, Haslett C, Hirani N, Greening AP, Rahman I, Metz CN, Bucala R, Donnelly SC (1998) Human circulating eosinophils secrete macrophage migration inhibitory factor (MIF). Potential role in asthma. *J Clin Invest* 101 (12): 2869–2874
21 Melani C, Mattia GF, Silvani A, Care A, Rivoltini L, Parmiani G, Colombo MP (1993) Interleukin-6 expression in human neutrophil and eosinophil peripheral blood granulocytes. *Blood* 81 (10): 2744–2749
22 Walz TM, Nishikawa BK, Malm C, Wasteson (1993) Production of transforming growth factor alpha by normal human blood eosinophils. *Leukemia* 7 (10): 1531–1537
23 Bjerke T, Gaustadnes M, Nielsen S, Nielsen LP, Schiotz PO, Rudiger N, Reimert CM, Dahl R, Christensen I, Poulsen LK (1996) Human blood eosinophils produce and secrete interleukin 4. *Respir Med* 90 (5): 271–277
24 Sabin EA, Kopf MA, Pearce EJ (1996) *Schistosoma mansoni* egg-induced early IL-4 production is dependent upon IL-5 and eosinophils. *J Exp Med* 184 (5): 1871–1878
25 Gauchat JF, Henchoz S, Fattah D, Mazzei G, Aubry JP, Jomotte T, Dash L, Page K, Solari R, Aldebert D et al (1995) CD40 ligand is functionally expressed on human eosinophils. *Eur J Immunol* 25 (3): 863–865
26 Rajakulasingam K, Till S, Ying S, Humbert M, Barkans J, Sullivan M, Meng Q, Corrigan CJ, Bungre J, Grant JA, Kay AB, Durham SR (1998) Increased expression of high affinity IgE (FcεRI) receptor-alpha chain mRNA and protein-bearing eosinophils in human allergen-induced atopic asthma. *Am J Respir Crit Care Med* 158 (1): 233–240
27 Tamura N, Ishii N, Nakazawa M, Nagoya M, Yoshinari M, Amano T, Nakazima H, Minami M (1996) Requirement of CD80 and CD86 molecules for antigen presentation by eosinophils. *Scand J Immunol* 44 (3): 229–238
28 Matsuyama G, Ochiai K, Ishihara C, Kagami M, Tomioka H, Koya N (1998) Heterogeneous expression of tumor necrosis factor-alpha receptors I and II on human peripheral eosinophils. *Int Arch Allergy Immunol* 117 (Suppl 1): 28–33
29 Ishiharu C, Ochiai K, Kagami M, Matsuyama G, Koya N, Tomioka H (1998) Interferon-gamma receptor beta-chain expression and formation of alpha- and beta-chain complexes after receptor conjugation on human peripheral eosinophils. *Int Arch Allergy Immunol* 117 (Suppl 1): 72–76
30 Handsel ZT, Busse WW, Sedgwick JB, Vrtis R, Lee WM, Kelly EA, Gern JE (1998) Eosinophils bind rhinovirus and activate virus-specific T cells. *J Immunol* 160 (3): 1279–1284

31 Levi-Schaffer F, Barkans J, Newman TM, Ying S, Wakelin M, Hohenstein R, Barak V, Lacy P, Kay AB, Moqbel R (1996) Identification of interleukin-2 in human peripheral blood eosinophils. *Immunology* 87 (1): 155–161

32 Tominaga A, Takaki S, Koyama N, Katoh S, Matsumoto R, Migita M, Hitoshi Y, Hosoya Y, Yamauchi S, Kanai Y et al (1991) Transgenic mice expressing a B cell growth and differentiation factor gene (interleukin 5) develop eosinophilia and autoantibody production. *J Exp Med* 173 (2): 429–437

33 Dent LA, Strath M, Mellor AL, Sanderson CJ (1990) Eosinophilia in transgenic mice expressing interleukin 5. *J Exp Med* 172 (5): 1425–1431

34 Lee JJ, McGarry MP, Farmer SC, Denzler KL, Larson KA, Carrigan PE, Brenneise IE, Horton MA, Haczku A, Gelfand EW, Leikauf GD, Lee NA (1997) Interleukin-5 expression in the lung epithelium of transgenic mice leads to pulmonary changes pathognomonic of asthma. *J Exp Med* 185 (12): 2143–2156

35 Hamelmann E, Oshiba A, Loader J, Larsen GL, Gleich G, Lee J, Gelfand EW (1997) Antiinterleukin-5 antibody prevents airway hyperresponsiveness in a murine model of airway sensitization. *Am J Respir Crit Care Med* 155 (3): 819–825

36 Van Oosterhout AJ, Ladenius AR, Savelkoul HF, Van Ark I, Delsman KC, Nijkamp FP (1993) Effect of anti-IL-5 and IL-5 on airway hyperreactivity and eosinophils in guinea pigs. *Am Rev Respir Dis* 147 (3): 548–552

37 Temann UA, Geba GP, Rankin JA, Flavell RA (1998) Expression of interleukin 9 in the lungs of transgenic mice causes airway inflammation, mast cell hyperplasia, and bronchial hyperresponsiveness. *J Exp Med* 188 (7): 1307–1320

38 Tang W, Geba GP, Zheng T, Ray P, Homer RJ, Kuhn C 3rd, Flavell RA, Elias JA (1996) Targeted expression of IL-11 in the murine airway causes lymphocytic inflammation, bronchial remodeling, and airways obstruction. *Clin Invest* 98 (12): 2845–2853

39 Yang L, Cohn L, Zhang DH, Homer R, Ray A, Ray P (1998) Essential role of nuclear factor kappaB in the induction of eosinophilia in allergic airway inflammation. *J Exp Med* 188 (9): 1739–1750

40 Akimoto T, Numata F, Tamura M, Takata Y, Higashida N, Takashi T, Takeda K, Akira S (1998) Abrogation of bronchial eosinophilic inflammation and airway hyperreactivity in signal transducers and activators of transcription (STAT)6-deficient mice. *J Exp Med* 187 (9): 1537–1542

41 Zheng W, Flavell RA (1997) The transcription factor GATA-3 is necessary and sufficient for Th2 cytokine gene expression in CD4 T cells. *Cell* 89 (4): 587–596

42 Ranganath S, Ouyang W, Bhattarcharya D, Sha WC, Grupe A, Peltz G, Murphy KM (1998) GATA-3-dependent enhancer activity in IL-4 gene regulation. *J Immunol* 161 (8): 3822–3826

43 Ho IC, Hodge MR, Rooney JW, Glimcher LH (1996) The proto-oncogene c-Maf is responsible for tissue-specific expression of interleukin-4. *Cell* 85 (7): 973–983

44 Nakamura Y, Ghaffar O, Olivenstein R, Taha RA, Soussi-Gounni A, Zhang DH, Ray A, Hamid Q (1999) Gene expression of the GATA-3 transcription factor is increased in atopic asthma. *J Allergy Clin Immunol* 103 (2 Pt 1): 215–222

45 Gonzalo JA, Lloyd CM, Wen D, Albar JP, Wells TN, Proudfoot A, Martinez-A C, Dorf M, Bjerke T, Coyle AJ, Gutierrez-Ramos JC (1998) The coordinated action of CC chemokines in the lung orchestrates allergic inflammation and airway hyperresponsiveness. *J Exp Med* 188 (1): 157–167

46 Gonzalo JA, Jia GQ, Aguirre V, Friend D, Coyle AJ, Jenkins NA, Lin GS, Katz H, Lichtman A, Copeland N, Kopf M, Gutierrez-Ramos JC (1996) Mouse eotaxin expression parallels eosinophil accumulation during lung allergic inflammation but it is not restricted to a Th2-type response. *Immunity* 4 (1): 1–14

47 Ying S, Taborda-Barata L, Meng Q, Humbert M, Kay AB (1995) The kinetics of allergen-induced transcription of messenger RNA for monocyte chemotactic protein-3 and RANTES in the skin of human atopic subjects: relationship to eosinophil, T cell, and macrophage recruitment. *J Exp Med* 181 (6): 2153–2159

48 Rothenberg ME, MacLean JA, Pearlman E, Luster AD, Leder P (1997) Targeted disruption of the chemokine eotaxin partially reduces antigen-induced tissue eosinophilia. *J Exp Med* 185 (4): 785–790

49 Lukacs NW, Strieter RM, Warmington K, Lincoln P, Chensue SW, Kunkel SL (1997) Differential recruitment of leukocyte populations and alteration of airway hyperreactivity by C-C family chemokines in allergic airway inflammation. *J Immunol* 158 (9): 4398–4404

50 Stelts D, Egan RW, Falcone A, Garlisi CG, Gleich GJ, Kreutner W, Kung TT, Nahrebne DK, Chapman RW, Minnicozzi M (1998) Eosinophils retain their granule major basic protein in a murine model of allergic pulmonary inflammation. *Am J Respir Cell Mol Biol* 18 (4): 463–470

51 Persson CG, Erjefalt JS, Korsgren M, Sundler F (1997) The mousetrap. *Trends Pharmacol Sci* 18 (12): 465–467

52 Foster PS, Hogan SP, Ramsay AJ, Matthaei KI, Young IG (1996) Interleukin 5 deficiency abolishes eosinophilia, airways hyperreactivity, and lung damage in a mouse asthma model. *J Exp Med* 183 (1): 195–201

53 Corry DB, Folkesson HG, Warnock ML, Erle DJ, Matthay MA, Wiener-Kronish JP, Locksley RM (1996) Interleukin 4, but not interleukin 5 or eosinophils, is required in a murine model of acute airway hyperreactivity. *J Exp Med* 183 (1): 109–117

54 Coyle AJ, Kohler G, Tsuyuki S, Brombacher F, Kopf M (1998) Eosinophils are not required to induce airway hyperresponsiveness after nematode infection. *Eur J Immunol* 28 (9): 2640–2647

Fibroblasts and myofibroblasts

Ian A. Akers, Robin J. McAnulty and Geoffrey J. Laurent

The Centre for Cardiopulmonary Biochemistry and Respiratory Medicine, Royal Free and University College London Medical School, The Rayne Institute, 5, University Street, London WC1E 6JJ, UK

Introduction

In this chapter we will briefly review the structure of the normal airway and the extracellular matrix components from which it is composed. The role of the fibroblast/myofibroblast in maintaining this structure will be discussed, together with the evidence for their role in remodelling the airway wall in asthma and COPD. Finally we discuss the potential for pharmacological modulation of fibroblast function as a potential means of reversing the changes in airway structure in these diseases.

Structure of the normal airway

The trachea divides into two main bronchi, which further subdivide into segmental bronchi that enter the left and right lungs. The trachea and bronchi are supported by surrounding cartilage, however, as the bronchi subdivide further into bronchioles the cartilage is lost. The terminal bronchioles give rise to respiratory bronchioles and finally the alveoli. As bronchioles normally control airflow in the lung we focus on their structure in the next section.

Structure of the bronchiole and its connective tissue components

The bronchiole wall consists of a mucosal lining (epithelium), a basement membrane, sub-epithelial connective tissue (lamina reticularis), a sub-mucosal layer (smooth muscle) and adventitia (Fig. 1a). The epithelium is mainly of pseudo-stratified, ciliated, columnar epithelial cells, clara cells, goblet (mucus), serous and basal cells. The structure and function of these cells within the mucosal layer are discussed in an accompanying chapter in this book (see Devalia et al.). In this chapter we focus on the extracellular matrix components within the basement membrane, lamina reticularis, sub-mucosal and adventitial layers (Fig. 1b).

Cellular Mechanisms in Airways Inflammation, edited by Clive P. Page, Katharine H. Banner and Domenico Spina

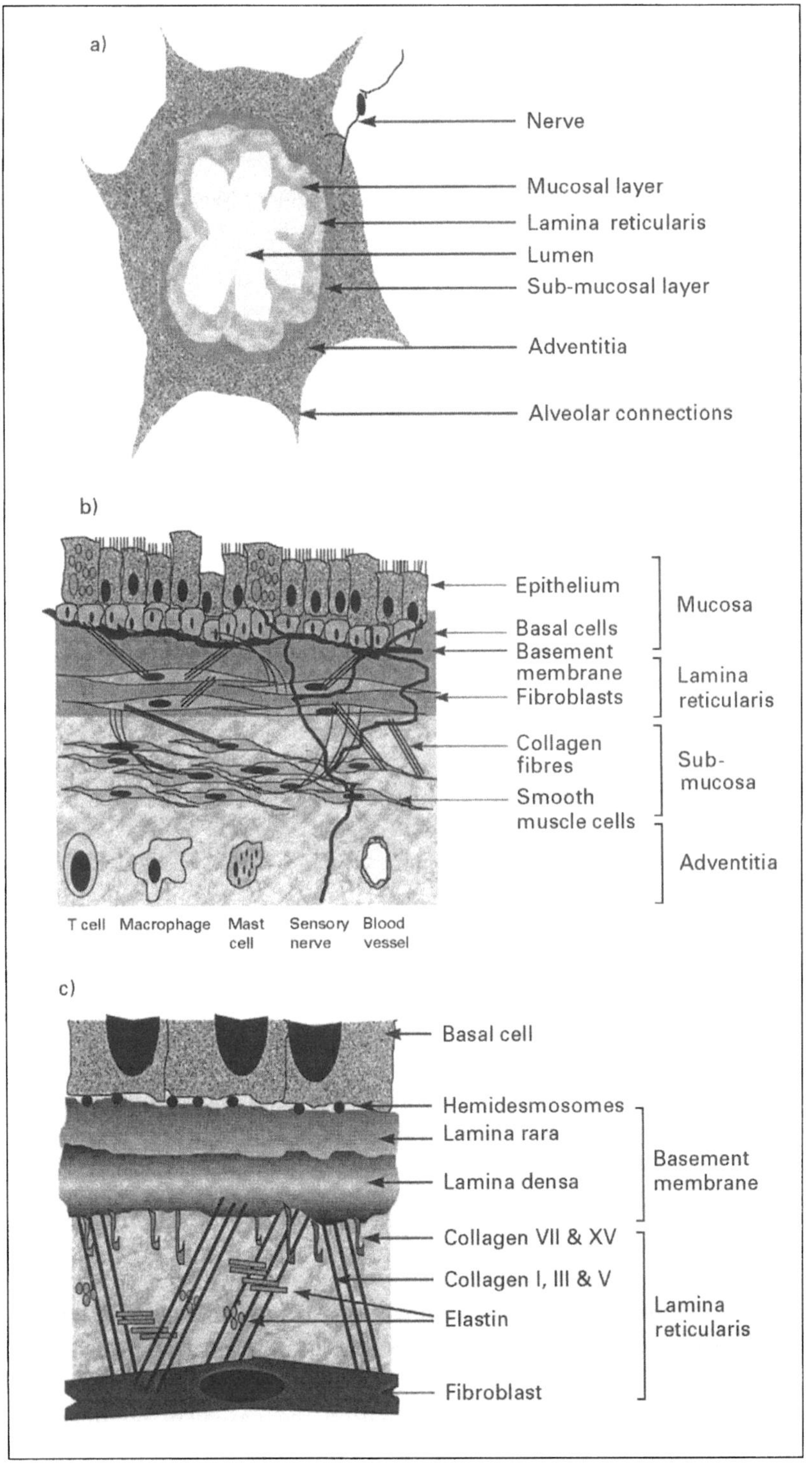
a)
Nerve
Mucosal layer
Lamina reticularis
Lumen
Sub-mucosal layer
Adventitia
Alveolar connections
b)
Epithelium
Basal cells
Basement membrane
Fibroblasts
Collagen fibres
Smooth muscle cells
Mucosa
Lamina reticularis
Sub-mucosa
Adventitia
T cell
Macrophage
Mast cell
Sensory nerve
Blood vessel
c)
Basal cell
Hemidesmosomes
Lamina rara
Lamina densa
Basement membrane
Collagen VII & XV
Collagen I, III & V
Elastin
Fibroblast
Lamina reticularis

The basement membrane is separated into two regions – lamina rara and lamina densa (Fig. 1c) which contain matrix molecules, including collagen types IV, VII and XV, the glycoproteins, laminin, nidogen (entactin), fibronectin, SPARC (BM-40) and proteoglycans. These structures provide a scaffold for attachment of cells and regulate their surrounding milieu by controlling the flux of small and large molecules [1]. It is the distribution and density of these molecules which gives rise to the characteristic features of the lamina rara and lamina densa.

Collagen IV is the most abundant protein in the basement membrane. This molecule is composed of triple helical domains, interrupted by short non-helical regions, providing flexibility. It forms an open-meshed, three-dimensional network (Fig. 2) in close association with laminin, nidogen and the heparan sulphate-linked proteoglycan, perlecan. Collagen type IV in basement membrane is probably produced by epithelial cells [2, 3], although type IV collagen mRNA expression has also been reported in mesenchymal cells [4]. Type V collagen is also found in small amounts within the basement membrane [5].

Collagen XV has recently been demonstrated in basement membrane and it has been suggested this molecule is responsible for the attachment of the basement membrane to the underlying interstitium (Fig. 1c) [6]. Similar roles have been postulated for collagen types V and VII [7, 8].

Laminins are the most abundant non-collagenous protein within the basement membrane. They have a cross-like structure (Fig. 2) and have been reported to mediate cellular attachment to extracellular matrix [9], cell migration, growth and differentiation [10]. A recent study has shown that laminin subtype expression changes during the development of the lung, suggesting that these molecules may play a role in the regulation of airway morphogenesis [11].

The normal basement membrane also contains nidogen, a single polypeptide, composed of three globular domains connected by a flexible link (Fig. 2). It binds to both collagen IV and laminin, *via* one of the globular regions, possibly linking these two molecules [12]. It also binds to cell surface integrins, *via* an Arg-Gly-Asp (RGD) domain [13].

Fibronectin is a high molecular weight glycoprotein present in basement membrane and on cell surfaces. It exists as a disulphide-linked dimer (Fig. 2) which forms

Figure 1
A schematic diagram of the normal bronchiole. (a) shows the overall structure of the bronchiole with the epithelium lining the airway lumen, surrounded by the sub mucosal layer and finally the adventitia extending to the alveolar attachments. (b) shows, in greater detail, the mucosa, lamina reticularis (also called lamina propria), sub mucosa and adventitia with the extensive matrix molecule connections between the cells and the structural components within the bronchiole wall. (c) highlights the matrix molecule connections between the fibroblasts in the lamina reticularis and the basement membrane.

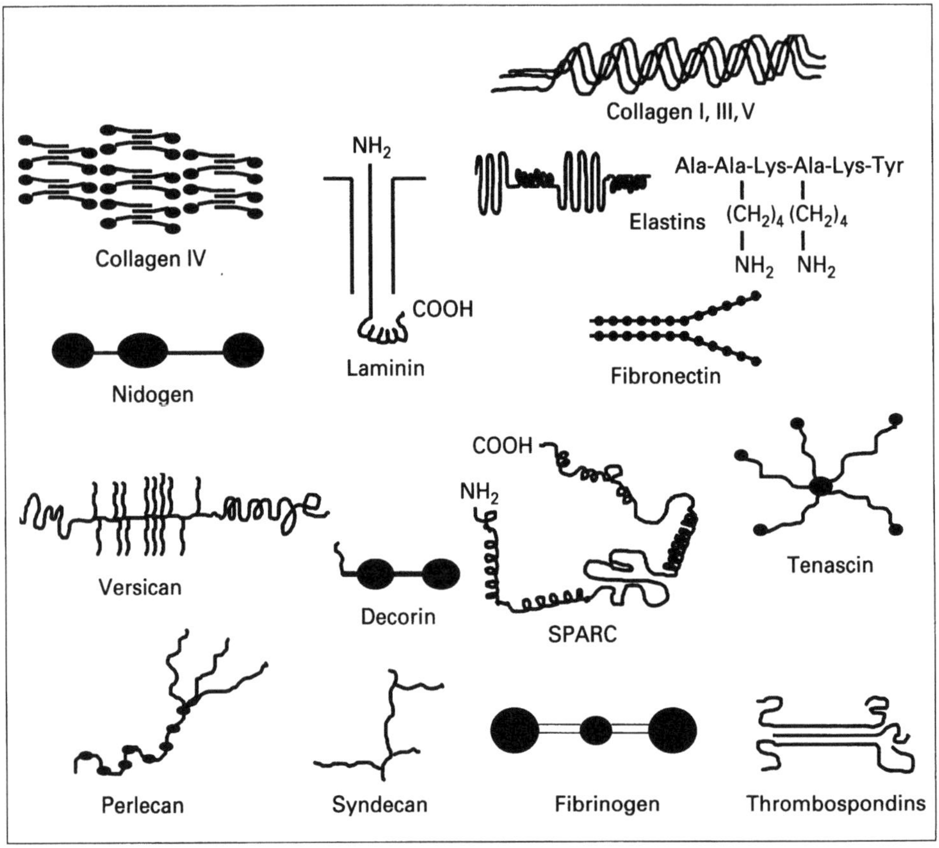

Figure 2
Schematic representations of matrix molecules found within the bronchioles.

high molecular weight insoluble polymers. It contains a variety of binding sites for other extracellular matrix molecules including collagen, heparin/heparan sulphate, hyaluronan and integrins. It has been implicated in a number of processes including cell attachment, migration, proliferation, opsonisation and wound healing (for extensive reviews see [14, 15]).

Another basement membrane component, SPARC (secreted protein, acidic and rich in cysteine) (Fig. 2) is able to bind cell surfaces, collagen types I, II and V and the glycoprotein, thrombospondin. Its exact role is unknown but is associated with morphogenesis, tissue remodelling and inhibits the spreading of a variety of cells, including fibroblasts [16–19].

Heparan sulphate-linked proteoglycans are ubiquitous components of basement membranes [20]. One such proteoglycan is perlecan which has a core protein with 5–7 globular domains and two or three heparan sulphate side chains attached to one end (Fig. 2). It has been associated with cell attachment [21], immobilisation of growth factors, such as FGF-2 [22] and serine proteases [23]. Therefore, in addition to its structural role it may also act as a reservoir for growth factors and metabolic enzymes.

Syndecan is a proteoglycan containing both heparan sulphate and chondroitin sulphate glycosaminoglycan side chains. It is able to bind to extracellular matrix molecules as well as the intracellular actin cytoskeleton. It is mainly associated with epithelial cells and is proposed to regulate their shape and organisation. It is localised to the basolateral surface of epithelial cells, binding these structures to the basement membrane.

In summary, extracellular matrix components of the basement membrane provide a supporting structure for epithelial and basal cells within the airway wall, links to the lamina reticularis and acts as a selective molecular sieve. These components are continuously synthesised and degraded by epithelial and mesenchymal cells. They also influence the behaviour of cells by binding to integrins on cell surfaces, regulating their migration, proliferation and metabolism.

The main components of the lamina reticularis are collagen types I and III, elastin, proteoglycans and glycoproteins, which contribute to the structural and mechanical properties of the airways. The structure and function of these are described below.

Collagens

There are at least 19 different collagens, of which, 11 have been shown to be present in the lung. These collagens are classified into three groups – the fibril-forming types (I, II, III, V, XI), the non-fibril-forming types (IV, VI, VII, VIII) and the FACIT (fibril-associated collagens with interrupted triple helices, XII, XIV). Table 1 shows the collagen types known to be associated with the airways.

Collagen types I and III are produced by fibroblasts [24, 25]. It has been proposed that type I collagen provides the tensile strength to all flexible surfaces of the lung, whilst type III contributes to the tissue compliance [26]. They also provide a structural scaffold to which resident cells attach *via* specific integrins. The α-chains of these collagens have a single triple helical domain which forms 95% of the molecule (Fig. 2). Once secreted into the interstitial space, they form long, thin, cable-like structures covalently bonded to homologous regions of neighbouring fibrils. These fibrils exist as copolymers with common associations between collagens I–V, I–VI, III–VI and III–VII (for review see [27, 28].

Type VI collagen consists of alternating filamentous and beaded regions [29]. The α1 (VI) and α2 (VI) chains contain a number of collagen binding sites and RGD sequences suggesting that collagen type VI participates in matrix-matrix interactions and cell-matrix interactions [29].

Table 1 Collagens known to be present in the airway

Type	Supramolecular structure	Function	Distribution in the airway wall
I	Fibril	Structural component, tensile strength	Lamina reticularis, sub-mucosa, adventitia
II	Fibril	Structural component, tensile strength	Bronchial and tracheal cartilage
III	Fibril	Structural component, compliance	Lamina reticularis, sub-mucosa, adventitia
IV	Non-fibrillar 3-dimensional network	Molecular sieving, cell support	Basement membrane
V	Fibril	Regulation of type I collagen fibrillogenesis	Basement membrane, lamina reticularis
VI	Beaded filament	Cell adhesion to matrix	Associated with type I and III collagen, interstitium
VII	Fibril	Anchors basement membrane to matrix	Basement membrane, lamina reticularis
VIII	Filamentous lattice (short chain)	Mechanical strength	Basement membrane
IX	FACIT	Regulation of type II collagen fibrillogenesis	Cartilage, associated with type II collagen
XI	Fibril	Regulation of type II collagen fibrillogenesis	Cartilage, associated with type II collagen
XV	Multiplexin	Anchors basement membrane to matrix	Basement membrane, lamina reticularis

FACIT, fibril-associated collagens with interrupted triple helix; Multiplexin, multiple triple-helix domains and interruptions

Elastin

Mature elastin is composed of two chemically and morphometrically distinct components – amorphous elastin and a highly structured microfibrillar component. Elastin is formed by the cross-linking of lysine residues in secreted tropoelastin by lysyl oxidase, followed by spontaneous formation of desmosines and isodesmosines, the stable elastin cross-links. The microfibril component acts as a scaffold or template for the development of amorphous elastin which consists of fibrillin, microfibril associated glycoprotein and associated microfibril protein (for a full review see [30]).

Elastin is the second most abundant matrix molecule in the airway representing about 5% of the total protein content [31]. It is produced by fibroblasts [32–34] forming parallel and longitudinal fibres localised to the lamina reticularis and sub-mucosa [35–37].

During both the inflation and deflation cycles of the lung, airway patency is maintained by the radial tension induced by elastin within the wall restricting excessive smooth muscle contraction or relaxation [38].

Proteoglycans and glycoproteins

The core proteins of eighteen different proteoglycan molecules have been reported. Figure 2 shows the structure of four proteoglycan molecules found in airway tissue, perlecan, syndecan, decorin and versican. Each core protein is linked to a variety of glycosaminoglycan side chains which consist of alternating galactosamine and glucuronic/iduronic acid units (chondroitin/dermatan sulphate), alternating glucosamine and glucuronic/iduronic acid units (heparin and heparan sulphate) or alternating glucosamine and galactose units (keratan sulphate). Their functions include matrix hydration, modulation of collagen fibre formation, cell-matrix and cell-cell interactions and the binding of growth factors [39].

Proteoglycans are synthesised by a variety of cell types including fibroblasts [40], type II epithelial cells [41] and pulmonary arterial endothelial cells [42]. Platelet-derived growth factor (PDGF) and transforming growth factor β (TGFβ) are capable of stimulating proteoglycan production by fibroblasts [43, 44].

Decorin and biglycan are two small chondroitin/dermatan sulphated proteoglycans, which are found associated with type I and type VI collagens, the lamina reticularis and smooth muscle bundles of the sub-mucosa within airways [45–47]. These molecules can bind polypeptide growth factors e.g. TGFβ [48] protecting them from denaturation and proteolytic degradation [49, 50]. It has therefore been suggested that these proteoglycans can act as a reservoir for growth factors, storing them until their release by proteases during tissue remodelling.

Versican, a large aggregating chondroitin sulphate proteoglycan is localised around the smooth muscle bundles in the sub-mucosa of the airway wall, in association with hyaluronan [51]. It is thought to change the mechanical properties of the airways in a similar manner to aggrecan in cartilage, by regulating the fluid (osmotic) balance within the airway tissue (see [46]).

Glypican, a glycosyl phosphotidylinositol linked heparan sulphate proteoglycan is expressed on the surface of human lung fibroblasts and bronchiolar epithelial cells. It binds fibronectin, collagen type I and anti-thrombin III *via* the heparan sulphate side chains. The function of glypican is not known, but its binding characteristics suggests a role in cell attachment and control of coagulation. A second heparan sulphate-linked proteoglycan is perlecan. This molecule is found in all basement membranes and gives the structure a fixed negative charge, which is important for the filtration properties of the membrane. It is also able to bind to other extracellular matrix molecules such as laminin and collagen type IV, and is an attachment substrate for cells.

Tenascin

Tenascin is a large disulphide-linked glycoprotein of six identical subunits. In the normal lung it has been localised to both basement membrane and lamina reticularis of proximal airways [52, 53]. It inhibits cell adhesion, migration and causes cell shape changes [54]. Its distribution suggests involvement with tissue morphogenesis and wound healing. These functions and evidence that inflammatory cytokines can increase the secretion of this molecule from cultured epithelial cells [55], suggest a potential role for tenascin in airway remodelling.

Fibroblasts in the normal airways

Fibroblast which possess the greatest capacity to produce extracellular matrix molecules (see [56]), appear flattened and have a stellate appearance, with an average diameter of 28 µm and a thickness of 0.55 µm [57]. They are localised to the lamina reticularis, forming a sheath around the airways (Fig. 1b) [57]. The cells contain prominent rough endoplasmic reticulum, ribosomes and Golgi apparatus, reflecting their high metabolic activity.

A cell of similar phenotype to fibroblasts, but morphologically larger and containing a larger proportion of cytoplasm, is the myofibroblast [58–60]. These cells have been identified within the lamina reticularis of normal airways [61, 62] and can be distinguished from fibroblasts by the prominent amounts of contractile filaments containing α-smooth muscle actin [61, 63]. They are found in multicellular strands and in close apposition with other cells [64]. Myofibroblasts appear in increased numbers subsequent to tissue injury [65, 66].

The source of myofibroblasts at sites of tissue injury is uncertain, both differentiation from fibroblasts and smooth muscle cells have been proposed [67, 68]. TGFβ can induce smooth muscle-actin expression in fibroblasts, thus giving the cell a myofibroblast-like phenotype [69]. Myofibroblasts cultured from granulating wounds are capable of reverting back to a fibroblast phenotype [70].

The role of fibroblasts and myofibroblasts in airway morphogenesis and homeostasis

The fibroblast has been postulated to play an important role in airway morphogenesis and development. The co-culture of human epithelial cells with human foetal lung fibroblasts in collagen gels causes epithelial cell invasion of extracellular matrix, which then develop into groups of cells that resemble primordial sub-mucosal glands, forming tubular structures, which undergo dichotomous branching [71].

The development of the airways occurs during the pseudoglandular phase of lung development, between weeks 5–17 of gestation (for review see [72, 73]. The pattern of airway branching is dependent on the interactions between the developing mesenchyme, epithelial cells, cellular adhesion molecules and the extracellular matrix, in particular, proteoglycans and glycosaminoglycans [74]. In the developing lungs of rats, the differentiation of mesenchymal stem cells into fibroblasts-like and myofibroblast-like cells is associated with the production and deposition of extracellular matrix molecules [75]. The deposition of collagen, syndecan, laminin and fibronectin from these cells is essential for airway morphogenesis, in particular tubule formation and terminal branching [65, 73, 76].

In the mouse, syndecan expression also influences the development of alveolar sacs during the canalicular stages of lung development [77]. The formation of the alveoli is also associated with the synthesis and secretion of elastin, and possibly other extracellular matrix molecules by myofibroblasts at the leading edge of new alveolar buds [33]. Three growth factors produced by mesenchymal and epithelial cells, EGF, IGF-1 and TGFβ_1, also have a role in airway branching and alveolar development [73, 74].

The fibroblast/myofibroblast plays a key role in the maintenance of the airway extracellular matrix. Collagens are continually synthesised and degraded in the normal lung, with average turnover rates estimated to be 10% per day in lungs of young adult rats and rabbits [78–80]. These rates decrease with age, but proceed at relatively rapid rates throughout life [81]. Furthermore, the balance of intracellular and extracellular breakdown pathways also change with age. In young animals about 30% of newly synthesised collagen is degraded intracellularly within minutes of its synthesis [79, 82] but this proportion increases with age to about 80% [81]. In addition, the rates of these processes change when the lung is injured. For example, in experimental models of pulmonary fibrosis the proportion of newly synthesised collagen degraded intercellularly decreases, contributing to the increased collagen deposition in the injured lung [82]. The modulation of these processes could also play an important role in airway remodelling.

The rate of extracellular degradation is thought to depend on the degree of cross-linking and in older animals the mature collagen fibrils may be protected from degradation. Nevertheless, extracellular collagens are susceptible to breakdown and are degraded rapidly both in growing and diseased tissue. This is accomplished by a family of metalloproteinases, which are produced by both resident cells (fibroblasts, epithelial and endothelial cells) and inflammatory cells (activated macrophages and neutrophils) [83].

There are at least fifteen zinc- and calcium-dependent metalloproteinases which have the capacity to breakdown a wide range of extracellular matrix proteins [84–

86]. They are important in embryonic tissue development, cell migration, inflammation and wound healing. The actions of the metalloproteinases is tightly regulated by a diverse group of anti-proteinases including the tissue inhibitors of metalloproteinases (TIMPs), which are synthesised and secreted by activated mesenchymal cells, and circulating anti-proteinases such as α_2-macroglobulin, α_1-antitrypsin, α_2-antiplasmin and secretory leukocyte protease inhibitor. The recent development of synthetic metalloproteinase inhibitors is enabling the characterisation of the role of metalloproteinases in human disease [86].

In summary, fibroblasts and myofibroblast are involved in the morphogenesis and development of the airways. They respond to cytokines and growth factors producing a variety of extracellular matrix molecules, the degradation of which is tightly regulated by both intracellular and extracellular proteinases and their inhibitors. When this tight regulation breaks down, as seen in the collagen diseases (e.g. osteogenous imperfecta) or in inflammatory diseases (e.g. rheumatoid arthritis, asthma, COPD or lung fibrosis) compromised tissue function ensues.

Regulation of fibroblast and myofibroblast extracellular matrix production in normal and diseased airways

As mentioned in the previous section there are several mediators able to influence extracellular matrix production by fibroblasts and myofibroblasts during development, in particular, IGF-1, TGFβ_1 and PDGF. However, mediators regulating extracellular matrix turnover during development or maintenance of the airway wall has not been extensively studied. A variety of cytokines, polypeptide growth factors, lipid mediators and coagulation cascade products are known to activate mesenchymal cells [28, 87]. Many of these mediators are released by both resident and inflammatory cells in the lungs of asthmatics (for review see [88, 89]. We will focus on the effects of the mediators that are currently known to be increased in this group of patients and which have been shown to modulate fibroblast function (Tab. 2).

Cytokines and growth factors

A large number of cytokines and polypeptide mediators released in the inflamed airway can cause fibroblast chemotaxis, proliferation and induce extracellular matrix molecule production (Tab. 2). TGFβ increases procollagen [90–92], fibronectin [91] and proteoglycan [44] production. It is able to regulate procollagen production by direct and indirect mechanisms. In fibroblasts, it increases the synthesis of procollagen, decreases its degradation intracellularly and extracellularly by down-regulation of metalloproteinases and up-regulation of tissue inhibitors of metalloproteinases, thus maximising its effect on collagen deposition [93].

Table 2 - Mediators reported to be increased in asthma which have been shown to promote fibroblast migration, proliferation and matrix production.

Mediator	Likely source	Increased directed migration	Enhanced proliferation	Increased matrix production	Ref.
IL-1	Mϕ, TC, BC, MC Fb, Ep, En, Neut	↑	↑		94, 95
IL-4	TC, MC	↑	↑	↑	96–99
IL-6	Mo, Mϕ, MC, Fb, Ep, En		↑	↑	100, 101
GM-CSF	Mϕ, TC MC, Fb, Ep, Eos	↑			102
TNFα	Mϕ, MC, Eos	↑	↑	↑	103–106
IGF-1	Mϕ, Fb, Ep,		↑	↑	107–109
TGFβ	Mo, Mϕ, Fb, MC, Ep, Eos	↑	↑	↑	44, 90, 92 110–116
FGF-2	Fb, En, SMC	↑	↑		117, 118
ECP	Eos		↑	↑	119–122
Leukotrienes	Mo, Mϕ, Bo, MC Eos, Neut	↑	↑	↑	123–125
ET-1	Mϕ, Fb, Ep, En	↑	↑	↑	126–128
Tryptase	MC	↑	↑	↑	129–132
Thrombin	plasma	↑	↑	↑	133–136
Fibrinogen & fibrinopeptides	plasma		↑		134
Neuropeptides	Sensory nerves	↑	↑		137
Histamine	Bo, MC	↑	↑	↑	138, 139

Mo, monocyte; Mϕ, macrophage; TC, T cell; BC, B cell; Bo, basophil; MC, mast cell; Fb, fibroblast; Ep, epithelial cell; En, endothelial cell; Eos, eosinophil; Neut, neutrophil; SMC, smooth muscle cell; IL, interleukin; GM-CSF, granulocyte-macrophage colony-stimulating factor; IGF-1, insulin-like growth factor 1; TGFβ, transforming growth factor β; TNFα, tumour necrosis factor α; ECP, eosinophil cationic protein, ET-1, endothelin-1, FGF-2, fibroblast growth factor 2, ↑ increased function

TGFβ has been detected in the sputum of patients with asthma [140], in eosinophils infiltrating the epithelium of asthmatic airway [141], in nasal polyps [142] and in eosinophils, macrophages and fibroblasts within the lamina reticularis of airways from asthmatic patients [143, 144]. The latter finding is associated with an increase in the sub-epithelial thickness within the airway and disease severity [143, 144]. In addition, TGFβ has been shown to cause a change in the phenotype of fibroblasts to myofibroblasts [69] and may therefore contribute to the increased numbers of myofibroblasts in asthmatic airways [61, 145]. These data, coupled with the known activity of TGFβ as a potent promoter of procollagen production, suggest that it may have a pivotal role in tissue remodelling within the diseased airway.

Granulocyte macrophage-colony stimulating factor (GM-CSF) secreted by inflammatory cells including lymphocytes, macrophages and fibroblasts [146, 147] prolongs the survival and activation of eosinophils potentiating the deleterious effects of these cells in the airways of asthmatics [146, 148]. Consistent with this, recent studies have demonstrated that transient over-expression of the GM-CSF gene leads to peri-bronchial accumulation of eosinophils, an increased number of macrophages in the lung parenchyma, increases in the levels of TGFβ and irreversible fibrotic lesions [149, 150]. GM-CSF is chemotactic for myofibroblasts [102], suggesting another mechanism by which these cells could accumulate in the lamina reticularis of asthmatic airways [61, 145] with subsequent activation by TGFβ.

Fibroblasts are able to produce inflammatory cytokines such as IL-1, IL-6, chemokines and GM-CSF in response to activation by the acute phase proteins IL-1 and TNFα [56]. These mediators have paracrine effects leading to enhanced inflammatory cell accumulation (Fig. 3). In this way the fibroblast may both activate and prolong the inflammatory response.

A close apposition of eosinophils and fibroblasts was noted by Glynn and Michaels [151] in the airways of asthmatics. Furthermore, activated eosinophils degranulate and release mediators, which include TGFβ, and granule products, eosinophil cationic proteins (ECP) and major basic protein (MBP), into the surrounding tissue or airway lumen. ECP stimulates the proliferation of fibroblasts and increases the synthesis of collagen and proteoglycans [119, 120, 122, 152]. Whereas, MBP, acts synergistically with TGFβ and IL-1 to enhance IL-6 production by fibroblasts, which stimulates fibroblast proliferation and extracellular matrix protein production by both autocrine and paracrine mechanisms [100, 101, 153].

The mast cell has been shown to play a pivotal role in asthma, both in the transient bronchoconstriction and the chronic inflammatory phase of the disease [154]. As shown in Table 2 many of the mediators released by mast cells are able to modulate fibroblast function.

One such mediator is tryptase, a trypsin-like serine protease [155] which is elevated in bronchoalveolar lavage fluid from patients with allergic inflammation [156] and asthma [157]. Tryptase is chemotactic and mitogenic for fibroblasts [129–132, 158], stimulates type I collagen production in human lung fibroblasts [132] and increases procollagen mRNA levels in dermal fibroblasts [129]. With the established role of mast cells and their mediators in allergy and asthma, it is likely that they also play an important role in the activation of fibroblasts and myofibroblasts in the diseased airway.

Other peptides present in the airways of asthmatic patients also have the capacity to activate fibroblasts. Endothelin-1 is found in high concentrations within the airways of asthmatic patients [159–161] and has been demonstrated to be a chemoattractant and mitogen for fibroblasts and also stimulates collagen synthesis [126–128].

Neuropeptide-containing sensory nerves have been localised in human airways and apposed to fibroblasts (Fig. 1b) [162, 163]. The activation of these sensory nerves, with the subsequent release of the neuropeptides, substance P and neurokinin A, in the asthmatic airways may lead to bronchoconstriction and neurogenic inflammation [164]. In addition to these recognised roles both substance P and neurokinin A are capable of stimulating fibroblast proliferation and chemotaxis [137].

Coagulation cascade products

Fibrin has been shown to be deposited within the airway wall [165, 166] demonstrating the activation of the blood coagulation cascade. Several products of this cascade are known to have pro-fibrotic effects.

Thrombin is mitogenic and chemotactic for lung fibroblasts [133, 134] and increases collagen synthesis by these cells at least partly by protease-activated receptor-1 [136]. Thrombin may also activate fibroblasts indirectly by the release of mediators from resident cells, platelets and the extracellular matrix. In addition, recent studies from our laboratory demonstrate Factor Xa stimulation of fibroblast proliferation and collagen synthesis [167].

The generation of fibrin by the actions of thrombin on fibrinogen generates fibrinogen-cleavage products, fibrinopeptides A and B which are mitogenic for fibroblasts [134]. Also, the isolated Aα and Bβ chains from the fibrinogen molecule possess mitogenic activity [168]. Thus products of the coagulation cascade derived from plasma protein exudation observed in the inflamed airway can activate fibroblasts and have the potential to contribute to airway remodelling.

Mechanical load

Mechanical load is now recognised as an important regulator of cell function. The cyclic mechanical stretch of fibroblasts has been shown to cause an increase in cell proliferation [169] and procollagen production [170]. A clinical feature of asthma is repeated, transient bronchoconstriction. This raises the possibility that changes in contractile properties of the airways may influence the activation of the mesenchymal cells to proliferate and secrete increased amounts of matrix proteins.

Hypoxia

Hypoxemia occurs in asthmatic patients which is associated with the degree of airway obstruction [171]. As the bronchioles receive their blood supply *via* the bronchial artery, which is derived from the aorta, this suggests that the airways may be exposed to transient hypoxia. Hypoxia is known to have marked effects on fibroblast function increasing both proliferation and collagen synthesis in-vitro [172], which is mediated, in part, by TGFβ [173]. In addition hypoxic endothelial and epithelial cells release increased amounts of profibrotic cytokines such as PDGF and endothelin-1 [174].

In summary a number of cytokines and structurally diverse polypeptide and lipid mediators are able to cause fibroblast chemotaxis, proliferation and stimulation of extracellular matrix protein production. In addition mechanical load and hypoxia also capable of activating fibroblasts. Current research implicates several cytokines such as TGFβ and endothelin-1 as important agents promoting matrix deposition but many other mediators could be important (see Tab. 2) including proteases generated by the coagulation cascade and released by activated mast cells.

Fibroblasts as antigen presenting and effector cells in the immune response

It has been suggested that fibroblasts can act as antigen presenting cells based on the expression of thymocyte-1 (Thy-1) antigen on their cell surface (Fig. 3) [175–177]. Murine lung fibroblasts not expressing the Thy-1 antigen up-regulate the expression of MHC class II antigen and therefore have the ability to present antigen to T cells (Fig. 3). In contrast, human lung fibroblasts expressing Thy-1 were able to up-regulate MHC class II antigen, but only after stimulation with IFNγ. A subset of these cells demonstrated the ability to cause T-cell proliferation [177].

Fibroblasts could therefore act as accessory antigen presenting cells, in conjunction with dendritic cells and macrophages, to enhance the local immune and inflammatory response (Fig. 3). More studies are needed to establish the extent to which fibroblasts contribute to the overall immune response.

Recent observations have also shown that a soluble mediator secreted by fibroblasts can prevent lymphocyte apoptosis by maintaining or increasing the expression of the Bcl-XL gene [178, 179]. Thus, there would be a persistence of lymphocytes adding to the chronicity of the inflammatory response.

Extracellular matrix molecule deposition within the lamina reticularis

A change in the structure of airways from patients who had died from asthma was first noted by Huber and Koessler [180]. These findings were confirmed in mor-

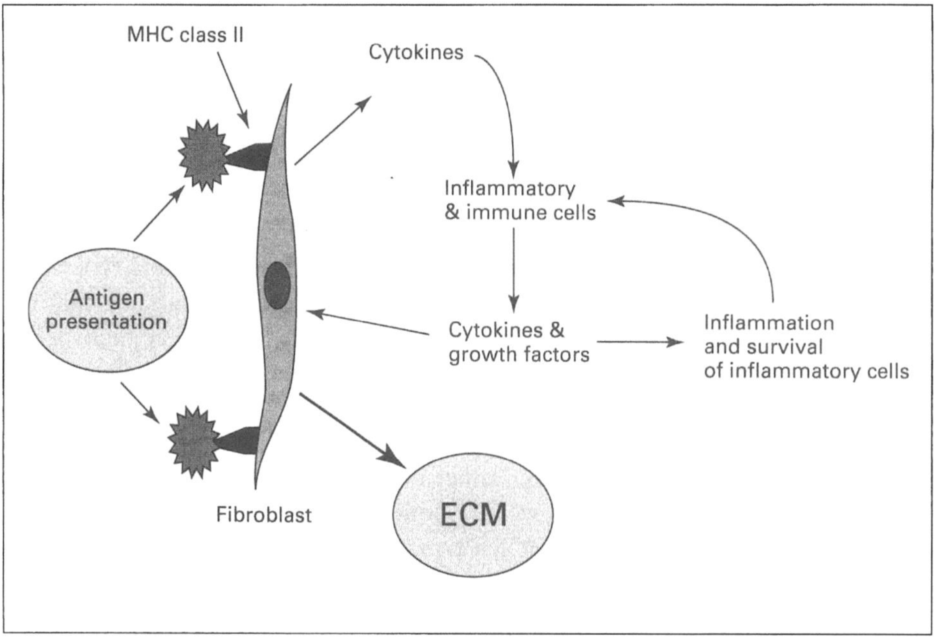

Figure 3
Fibroblasts as antigen presenting and inflammatory cells. Antigen presentation by fibroblasts leads to an enhancement of the immune response, and stimulation of cytokine and extracellular matrix production. The cytokines produced by the fibroblast enhance the inflammatory response by both autocrine and paracrine mechanisms.

phological studies in which the airway wall was found to be significantly thicker in asthmatic compared with non-asthmatic patients [181]. Carroll and colleagues [182] demonstrated increased wall thickness in both the large and small airways in fatal asthma, but only in the small airways in non-fatal asthma.

This increase has also been noted in other airways diseases such as chronic obstructive pulmonary disease [183–185], bronchiectasis, bronchitis, and tuberculosis [183]. The thickening results from increase in the thickness of the mucosa [181, 186], lamina reticularis [5, 166, 187, 188] and sub-mucosal layers of the airway [180, 181, 187, 189, 190]. Changes in the sub-mucosa are likely to involve both smooth muscle hyperplasia [191] and hypertrophy [192].

It was initially thought that the changes in the lamina reticularis were a consequence of the thickening of the epithelial basement membrane, due to increased collagen deposition [151, 180, 189, 193]. However, using ultrastructural techniques, the thickening was localised to the lamina reticularis, with the lamina rara and the lamina densa of the basement membrane remaining unchanged [5, 166, 187]. These changes appear to be an early event in the pathology of asthma, as increases in the sub-epithelial layer are seen in children with asthma [190] and in patients with mild disease [166].

It was postulated that the increased thickness of the lamina reticularis was due to the activation of the epithelial cells [166], which have been shown to secrete collagen *in vitro* [194, 195]. However, the composition of this layer was shown to consist predominantly of collagen types I, III and V, fibronectin [5, 196] and elastin [145], molecules that are generally thought to be produced by fibroblasts, rather than epithelial cells. Also, no laminin was identified within the lamina reticularis, but was found within the "true" basement membrane, again, suggesting that the matrix deposition in the sub-epithelial layer was not associated with epithelium [5].

The increased thickness of the lamina reticularis has been correlated with increased numbers of fibroblasts/myofibroblasts [61, 145, 151]. Furthermore, in a recent study, increased numbers of myofibroblasts were observed in the lamina reticularis of mild asthmatic patients after antigen challenge [62]. From these studies it was suggested that myofibroblasts were responsible for deposition of the increased extracellular matrix. However, other cell types within the airway wall are capable of producing extracellular matrix molecules and are likely to be involved in remodelling. For example, smooth muscle cells are capable of producing similar amounts of procollagen to fibroblasts [197].

In addition to the increase in collagen, amounts of fibronectin, elastin and other extracellular matrix components have been shown to be increased within the lamina reticularis of asthmatic airways. Hyaluronan, versican, biglycan and decorin were increased in the airways of patients with severe asthma [46]. Due to the hydrophilic nature of these molecules, it can be speculated that the airway wall may be further thickened by an increased fluid content within the sub-mucosa. Increased proteoglycans production has been shown from bronchial fibroblast cell lines cultured from asthmatic patients [198] and, increased levels have been demonstrated in the sputum from asthmatic subjects [199]. Currently no data is available for the content of these matrix molecules in bronchial biopsies from mild asthmatics. Fibroblasts may also be involved in the regulation of fluid content of tissues *via* integrin mediated cell-matrix interaction [200–202].

Functional effects of a thickened airway wall

Both the airways and the parenchyma contribute to the elastic recoil of lung tissue. Mead hypothesised that the parenchyma is able to stabilise the alveoli and terminal bronchioles, by generating a recoil force (interdependence), thus preventing airway collapse (Fig. 4a) [203]. A decrease in elastic recoil may have profound effects on the airway contractility. This hypothesis was extended to suggest that the adventitial tissue around the airway is an important determinant of the magnitude of bronchoconstriction (Fig. 4a and b) [204–206]. Several groups have hypothesised that the load exerted by the lung parenchyma in the normal airways must be overcome by the smooth muscle to enable the airway to contract (Fig. 4c) [205–207]. Excessive extracellular matrix deposition outside the smooth muscle layer (peri-bronchial fibrosis) would uncouple these opposing forces allowing the smooth muscle to contract more easily (Fig. 4d) [208].

The increase in the deposition of extracellular matrix within the mucosal layer and lamina reticularis would also have consequences for airway constriction. A thickened mucosal layer, compared to normal, causes an increase in the narrowing of the lumen for any given degree of smooth muscle contraction (Fig. 4c) [209]. An important normal physiological response to smooth muscle contraction is the folding of the mucosa which restricts lumenal narrowing. However, in the inflamed airway, the deposition of the extracellular matrix within the lamina reticularis would limit the number of folds generated, thus allowing a further reduction in lumenal diameter (Fig. 4b and d) [210].

In early stages of disease, the initial deposition of extracellular matrix proteins by fibroblasts and other mesenchymal cells may be beneficial. Extending the hypothesis of Mead and others, the initial deposition of extracellular matrix around the airways, within the lamina reticularis, adventitia and the alveolar connections, may increase the parenchymal load on the airways, increasing interdependence, thus restricting the degree of airway closure.

However, as the disease progresses, excessive deposition of extracellular matrix, along with the thickening of the airway wall due to increased smooth muscle, oedema and epithelial cell hyperplasia, becomes detrimental to airway function. There is now anecdotal evidence that there is a reduction in the number of alveolar connections to the airways of asthmatics, which would reduce interdependence and increase the degree of basal airway tone. Also this reduction in interdependence will allow an increase in airways contractility (airway hyperresponsiveness) to inciting agents (e.g. antigen, cold air, exercise, stress).

In addition to the increase in extracellular matrix deposition, a reduction in the amount of elastin is seen in some patients, while disorganisation of the elastin fibrils is seen in others [35, 211]. This data would support the theory of interdependence, as the force required to overcome the elastic nature of the parenchymal tissue would be less thus increasing the magnitude of the bronchoconstriction. The change in elastin content and structure may partly explain the reduction in lung elasticity seen in asthmatic patients [212, 213]. In contrast, no change in the elastin content of the airways was found by Godfrey and colleagues [214]. Thus no consensus of opinion has been reached regarding the effects on elastin metabolism in the airways during chronic inflammation. However, this is an important feature of remodelling in the inflamed airway and needs further investigation.

A limited number of studies have been performed specifically to examine the interaction of sub-epithelial thickening and airway function. Roche and colleagues found no correlation between sub-epithelial thickness and disease severity or air-

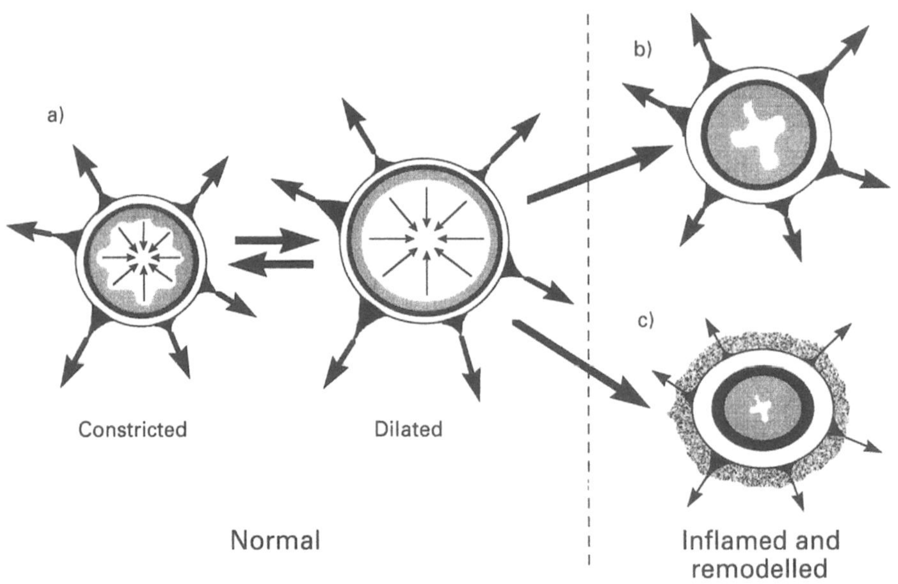

Figure 4
A schematic diagram showing the effect of structural changes on the airway lumen. In the normal airway, constriction and relaxation within this airway is a reversible process.
(a) shows the forces exerted on the normal dilated and constricted airway wall which keeps the lumen open (interdependence). During bronchoconstriction smooth muscle contraction must over come the external forces before the airway is able to constrict. At this point the epithelium folds to compensate for the reduction of the airway lumen, however the external forces restrict the degree of constriction. On smooth muscle relaxation the external elastic forces will allow the airway to relax back to its resting state.
(b) In the inflamed airway constriction is greatly enhanced. The increase in wall thickness due to a thicker epithelium and smooth muscle hypertrophy and hyperplasia, reduces the resting lumen diameter, thus, in the inflamed airway a similar degree of airway constriction to that seen in the normal airways, would result in a greatly reduced lumen diameter. Thus having profound effects of airway function.
(c) In addition to the wall thickening, the increase in matrix deposition within the lamina reticularis reduces the ability of the mucosa to fold. Therefore, in combination with the increased extracellular matrix within the peri-bronchial adventitia, which reduces the load exerted by the parenchyma on the airway wall, this would allow the airway to constrict to a greater extent than in either a) or b). Subsequently, the combination of the thickened airway wall and extracellular matrix deposition also restricts the degree to which the airway can return to its normal resting diameter, potentially leading to a chronic reduction in airflow.

ways hyperresponsiveness [5]. However, the thickness of the sub-epithelial layer or bronchial wall has been correlated to airway hyperresponsiveness by others [166, 215, 216] and in a recent study, Minshall and colleagues were able to demonstrate a correlation between sub-epithelial thickness and lung function (FEV_1) in mild, moderate and severe asthmatic patients [144].

In summary, changes in the structure of the airways in inflammatory diseases, due to changes in key extracellular matrix components such as elastin, collagen and proteoglycans, will have marked effects on the mechanical properties of the lung. This suggests pharmacological agents directed at controlling extracellular matrix deposition may have a place in the treatment of asthma. A reduction of the fibrotic lesions, may lead to the re-establishment of the interdependence between the airway wall and the lung parenchyma, thus returning lung function towards normal. The effects of selected agents on collagen production and degradation will be reviewed in the next section.

Pharmacological modulation of the fibroblast

The current treatment for asthma involves the combination of symptomatic relief with bronchodilators (β-adrenoceptor agonist, theophylline, ipratropium bromide) and anti-inflammatory agents (beclomethasone, budesonide, fluticasone propionate). The steroids are currently the most effective treatment for inflammation in asthma [217]. However, there is a group of patients who are refractive to these agents.

Steroids may inhibit fibroblast function, *in vitro*, either by inhibiting procollagen gene expression [218] or by inhibiting the release of pro-fibrotic cytokines from inflammatory cells. *In vivo* studies are more controversial but there is evidence that steroids can inhibit collagen production and block fibrosis [219]. The effects of inhaled budesonide on extracellular matrix deposition in a number of studies in asthmatic patients, have been unable to show a reduction in the thickening of the sub-epithelial layer [188, 220, 221] or a reduction in the levels of extracellular matrix molecules within this layer [222]. In contrast, in two studies of short-term treatment with either beclomethasone or fluticasone propionate a reduction in sub-epithelial thickening was noted [223, 224]. A similar decrease in sub-epithelial thickening was seen after the removal of inciting agents in occupational asthma [225, 226] suggesting that it is possible to reduce extracellular matrix deposition in chronically inflamed tissue.

The conflicting results obtained with these steroids may be due to the type and dose of steroid used, patient compliance or even a reflection of disease severity. Alternatively, these discrepancies could be accounted for by differing techniques associated with sampling, cutting and analysis of the bronchial biopsies. Further studies are required to determine the effects of steroids on extracellular matrix deposition.

Table 3 - Agents which modulate collagen metabolism

Likely mechanisms of action	Agent	Evaluation	Ref.
Transcription			
Reduction in procollagen	Tranilast	Clinical	230
mRNA levels	Minoxidil; pirfenidone		231, 232
Decrease transcription or	Glucocorticoids	Animal models	233–241
procollagen mRNA stability	INFγ; PGE_1; PGE_2	Clinical	
Translation			
Incorporated to form un-stable collagen chains	Proline analogues	*In vitro* Animal models	242–250
Feedback inhibition	Procollagen peptides		
Blocks chain elongation	Thiaproline; D-α-methyl-proline		251
Hydroxylation			
Removal of cofactors for hydroxylation	Bivalent cations, e.g. Zn^{2+}; ascorbate analogues	*In vitro*; animal models, clinical	252–259
Inhibition of prolyl 4-hydroxylase	Proline analogues; Safironil		
Inhibition of lysyl hydroxylase	Minoxidil		
Microtubular systems/Secretion			
Disruption of microtubules, Golgi and endoplasmic reticulum system	Colchicine; Cytochalasin B; Taxol; Nocodazole; Vincristine; Vinblastine; Brefeldin A	*In vitro* Animal models Clinical	260–262
Cleavage of procollagen peptides			
Inhibition of procollagen proteinases	Amino acids and polyamines	*In vitro*	263
Polymerisation			
Prevention of cross-linking Inhibition of lysyl oxidase	D-Penicillamine; β-Aminopropionitrile	*In vitro*; animal studies; clinical	264–266
Extracellular degradation			
Increases production of collagenase	Colchicine; Relaxin; Pentoxifylline	*In vitro*; animal models; clinical	267–269

Table 4 - Agents which modulate fibroblast activation and proliferation mechanisms

Likely mechanisms of action	Agent	Evaluation	Ref.
Growth factor mediators			
Inhibition of mediator release	Tranilast (MK341)	Clinical	230
Inhibition of TGFβ, PDGF, FGF	Pirfenidone	*In vitro* Animal studies	270–274
Binds and inactivates TGFβ	Decorin		
Growth factor receptors			
Inhibition of TGFβ activation	Mannose-6-phosphate		
Inactivation of growth factors	TGFβ antisense; TGFβ and TNFα antibodies	Animal models	275–278
Inhibition of both proliferation and procollagen synthesis	Receptor antagonists, e.g. endothelin; angiotensin II	*In vitro* Animal models	279–281
Fibroblast proliferation			
Inhibition of proliferation and matrix synthesis	Retinoids	*In vitro* Animal models	282, 283
Inhibits fibroblast proliferation	5-fluorouracil; mitomycin-C,	Clinical	261, 262
Decrease in matrix production	Minoxidil; Taxol		

As steroids have a number of side effects [227] alternative approaches have been investigated, including inhibition of procollagen DNA transcription, mRNA translation or post-translational packaging of the procollagen molecules [87, 228, 229]. These, and other strategies for inhibiting collagen deposition and fibroblast proliferation are shown in Tables 3 and 4 along with other agents which are currently under investigation for a number of fibrotic conditions, including lung fibrosis. These new compounds are now beginning to be evaluated in experimental models and man.

Summary

There is now strong evidence that fibroblasts and myofibroblasts play key roles in airway morphogenesis, maintenance of airway inflammation and tissue repair. They are metabolically active cells, continuously producing extracellular matrix components and are responsible for the maintenance of the structural framework of the airway. Through cell-matrix interactions they can also regulate the three-dimensional structure and mechanical properties of the airways. In asthmatic airways the number of fibroblasts/myofibroblasts and the amount of extracellular matrix increases profoundly affecting airway mechanics and cell function. The mechanisms for this increase in extracellular matrix deposition are uncertain. We propose that structurally diverse mediators from resident cells, inflammatory cells and blood derived proteins modulate the function of fibroblasts and myofibroblasts, increasing mesenchymal cell numbers locally within the airway tissue and enhancing extracellular matrix protein deposition. In addition, with the recently ascribed role of fibroblasts in antigen presentation, the production of pro-inflammatory cytokines and enhancement of inflammatory cell survival, suggests that these cells could also enhance and perpetuate the inflammatory response in the airway. A better understanding of the mechanisms by which fibroblast and myofibroblast functions are modulated, will identify new targets for the development of therapeutic agents for use in diseases associated with inflammation and airway remodelling such as asthma, chronic obstructive pulmonary disease (COPD) and bronchitis.

References

1 Yurchenco PD, Schittny JC (1990) Molecular architecture of basement membranes. *FASEB J* 4: 1577–1590
2 Simon RH, Scott MJ, Reza MM, Killen PD (1993) Type IV collagen production by rat pulmonary alveolar epithelial cell. *Am J Respir Cell Mol Biol* 8: 640–646
3 Bornstein P, Sage H (1980) Structurally distinct collagen types. *Ann Rev Biochem* 49: 957–1003
4 Simon-Assmann P, Bouziges F, Freund JN, Perrin-Schmitt F, Kedinger M (1990) Type IV collagen mRNA accumulates in the mesenchymal compartment at early stages of murine developing intestine. *J Cell Biol* 110 8: 49–857
5 Roche WR, Beasley R, Williams JH, Holgate ST (1989) Subepithelial fibrosis in the bronchi of asthmatics. *Lancet* I: 520–524
6 Myers JC, Dion AS, Abraham V, Amenta PS (1996) Type XV collagen exhibits a widespread distribution in human tissues but a distinct localization in basement membrane zones. *Cell Tissue Res* 286: 493–505
7 Martinez-Hernandez A, Amenta PS (1983) The basement membrane in pathology. *Lab Invest* 48: 656–677
8 Burgeson RE, Lungstrum GP, Rokosova B, Rimberg CS, Rosenbaum LM, Keene DR (1990) The structure and function of type VII collagen. *Ann NY Acad Sci* 580: 32–43
9 Henry MD, Campbell KP (1996) Dystroglycan – an extracellular matrix receptor linked to the cytoskeleton. *Curr Opin Cell Biol* 8: 625–631

10 Timpl R, Engel J, Martin GR (1983) Laminin – a multifunctional protein of basement membrane. *Trends Biochem Sci* 8: 207–209

11 Virtanen I, Laitinen A, Tani T, Pääkkö P, Laitinen LA, Burgeson RE and Lehto V-P (1996) Differential expression of laminins and their integrin receptors in developing and adult human lung. *Am J Respir Cell Mol Biol* 15: 184–196

12 Paulsson M (1992) Basement membrane proteins: structure, assembly, and cellular interactions. *Crit Rev Biochem Mol Biol* 27: 93–127

13 Mann K, Deutzmann R, Aumailley M, Timpl R, Raimondi L, Yamada Y, Pan T-C, Conway D, Chu M-L (1989) Amino acid sequence of mouse nidogen, a multidomain basement membrane protein with binding activity for laminin, collagen IV and cells. *EMBO J* 8: 65–72

14 Hynes RO (1990) Fibronectins. Springer-Verlag, New York

15 Johansson S (1996) Non-collagenous matrix proteins. In: WD Comper (ed): *Extracellular matrix, vol. 2: Molecular components and interactions.* Harwood Academic Publishers GMbH, Netherlands, 68–94

16 Sage H, Vernon RB, Funk SE, Everitt EA, Angello J (1989) SPARC, a secreted protein associated with cellular proliferation, inhibits cell spreading *in vitro* and exhibits Ca^{2+}-dependent binding to the extracellular matrix. *J Cell Biol* 109: 341–356

17 Goldblum SE, Ding X, Funk SE, Sage EH (1994) SPARC (secreted protein acidic and rich in cysteine) regulates endothelial cell shape and barrier function. *Proc Natl Acad Sci USA* 91: 3448–3452

18 Lane TF, Sage EH (1990) Functional mapping of SPARC: peptides from two distinct Ca^{2+}-binding sites modulate cell shape. *J Cell Biol* 111: 3065–3076

19 Lane TF, Sage EH (1994) The biology of SPARC, a protein that modulates cell-matrix interactions. *FASEB J* 8: 163–173

20 Sannes PL, Burch KK, Khosla J, McCarthy KJ, Couchman JR (1993) Immunohistochemical localization of chondroitin sulfate, chondroitin sulfate proteoglycan, heparan sulphate proteoglycan, entactin and laminin in basement membrane of postnatal developing and adult rat lung. *Am J Respir Cell Mol Biol* 8: 245–251

21 Clement B, Segui-Real B, Hassell JR, Martin GR, Yamada Y (1989) Identification of a cell surface-binding protein for the core protein of the basement membrane proteoglycan. *J Biol Chem* 264: 12467–12471

22 Vlodavsky I, Bar-shavit R, Ishai-michaeli R, Bashkin P, Fuks Z (1991) Extracellular sequestration and release of fibroblast growth factor: a regulatory mechanism. *Trends Biochem Sci* 16: 268–271

23 Pejler G, Bäckstöm G, Lindahl U, Paulsson M, Dziadek M Fujiwara S, Timpl R (1987) Structure and affinity for antithrombin for heparin sulfate chains derived from basement membrane proteoglycans. *J Biol Chem* 262: 5036–5043

24 Hance AJ, Bradley K, Crystal RG (1976) Lung collagen heterogeneity. Synthesis of type I and type III collagen by rabbit and human lung cells in culture. *J Clin Invest* 57: 102–111

25 Sage H, Crouch E, Bornstein P (1979) Collagen synthesis by bovine aortic endothelial cells in culture. *Biochemistry* 24: 5433–5442
26 Burgeson RE (1987) The collagens in the skin. *Curr Probl Dermatol* 17: 61–75
27 Amenta PS, Gil J, Martinez-Hernandez A. (1988) Connective tissue of rat lung II: ultrastructural localisation of collagen types III, IV and VI. *J Histochem Cytochem* 36: 1167–1173
28 Chambers RC, Laurent GJ (1997) Collagens. In: RG Crystal, JB West (eds): *The lung. Scientific foundations*, 2nd edition. Lippincott-Raven Publ., Philadelphia, 709–727
29 Timpl R, Engel E (1987) Type VI collagen. In: R Mayne, RE Burgeson (eds): *Structure and function of collagen types*. Academic Press, New York, 105–140
30 Cleary EG, Gibson MA (1996) Elastic Tissue, elastin and elastin associated microfibrils. In: WD Comper (ed): *Extracellular matrix, volume 2: Molecular components and interactions*. Harwood Academic Publishers, Netherlands, 95–140
31 Pierce JA, Ebert RV (1965) Fibrous network of the lung and its change with age. *Thorax* 20: 469–476
32 Ross R (1973) Connective tissue cells, cell proliferation and synthesis of extracellular matrix – a review. *Philos Trans R Soc Lond B Biol Sci* 271: 247–259
33 Brody JS, Vaccaro C (1979) Postnatal formation of alveoli: interstitial events and physiologic consequences. *Fed Proc* 38: 215–223
34 Mecham RP, Lange G, Madaras J, Starcher B (1981) Elastin synthesis by ligamentum nuchae fibroblasts: effects of culture conditions and extracellular matrix on elastin production. *J Cell Biol* 90:332–338
35 Bousquet J, Lacoste J-Y, Chanez P, Vic P, Godard P, Michel FB (1996) Bronchial elastic fibers in normal subjects and asthmatic patients. *Am J Respir Crit Care Med* 153: 1648–1654
36 Van den Steen P, Van Lommel A, Lauweryns JM (1996) Elastogensis is linked to epithelial-stromal interactions in postnatal hamster bronchioles. *Cell Tissue Res* 284: 467–471
37 Böck P, Stockinger L (1984) Light and electron microscopic identification of elastic, elaunin and oxytalan fibers in human tracheal and bronchial mucosa. *Anat Embryol* 170: 145–153
38 Wright RR (1961) Elastic tissue of normal and emphysematous lungs. A tridimensional histologic study. *Am J Pathol* 39: 355–367
39 Fosang AJ, Hardingham TE (1996) Matrix Proteoglycans. In: WD Comper (ed): *Extracellular matrix, volume 2: Molecular components and interactions*. Harwood Academic Publishers, Netherlands, 200–229
40 Lories V, David G, Cassiman J-J, van den Berghe H (1986) Heparan sulfate proteoglycans of human lung fibroblasts. *Eur J Biochem* 158: 351–360
41 Sahu SC, Tanswell AK, Lynn WS (1980) Isolation and characterization of glycosaminoglycans secreted by human foetal lung type II pneumocytes in culture. *J Cell Sci* 42: 183–188
42 Benitz WE, Bernfield M (1990) Endothelial cell proteoglycans: possible mediators of vascular responses to injury. *Am J Respir Cell Mol Biol* 2: 407–408

43 Castor CW, Fremuth TD, Furlong AM, Jourdian GW (1983) Hyaluronic acid and proteoglycan synthesis by lung fibroblasts in basal and activated states. *In vitro* 19: 462–470

44 Tiedemann K, Malström A, Westergren-Thorsson G (1997) Cytokine regulation of proteoglycan production in fibroblasts: Separate and synergistic effects. *Matrix Biol* 15: 469–478

45 Roberts CR, Paramo JI (1992) Localization of decorin and biglycan in the human lung *FASEB J* 6: A3453

46 Roberts CR (1995) Is asthma a fibrotic disease? *Chest* 107: 111S–117S

47 Bidanset DL, Guildry C, Rosenberg LC, Choi HU, Timpl R, Hook M (1992) Binding of the proteoglycan decorin to collagen type VI. *J Biol Chem* 267: 5250–5256

48 Yamaguchi Y, Mann DM, Ruoslahti E (1987) Negative regulation of transforming growth factor-β by the proteoglycan decorin. *Nature* 346: 281–284

49 Sommer A, Rifkin DB (1989) Interaction of heparin with human basic fibroblast growth factor: Protection of the angiogenic protein from proteolytic degradation by a glycosaminoglycan. *J Cell Physiol* 138: 215–220

50 Moscatelli D (1988) Metabolism of receptor-bound and matrix-bound basic fibroblast growth factor by bovine capillary endothelial cells. *J Cell Biol* 107: 753–759

51 Roberts CR, Burke A (1994) Proteoglycans and hyaluronan in human lung fibrosis. *FASEB J* 8: A690

52 Weinacker A, Ferrando R, Elliott M, Hogg J, Balmes J, Sheppard D (1995) Distribution of integrins αvβ6 and α9β1 and their known ligands, fibronectin and tenascin, in human airways. *Am J Respir Cell Biol* 12: 547–557

53 Kuhn C, Mason RJ (1996) Immunolocalization of SPARC, tenascin, and thrombospondin in pulmonary fibrosis. *Am J Pathol* 147: 1759–1769

54 Chiquet-Ehrismann R (1990) What distinguishes tenascin from fibronectin? *FASEB J* 4: 2598–2604

55 Harkonen E, Virtanen I, Linnala A, Laitinen LL, Kinnula VL (1995) Modulation of fibronectin and tenascin production in human bronchial epithelial cells by inflammatory cytokines *in vitro*. *Am J Respir Cell Mol Biol* 13: 109–115

56 Tremblay GM, Jordana M, Gauldie J, Särnstrand B (1995) Fibroblasts as effector cells in fibrosis. In: SH Phan, RS Thrall (eds): *Pulmonary fibrosis*. Series: Lung biology in health and disease, vol. 80. Marchel Dekker, New York, 541–577

57 Evans MJ, Guha SC, Cox RA, Moller PC (1993) Attenuated fibroblast sheath around the basement membrane zone in the trachea. *Am J Respir Cell Mol Biol* 8: 188–192

58 Gabbiani G, Ryan GR, Majne G (1971) Presence of modified fibroblasts in granulation tissue and their possible role in wound contraction. *Experientia* 27: 549–550

59 Skalli O, Schürch W, Seemayer T, Lagace R, Montandon D, Pittet B, Gabbiani G (1989) Myofibroblast from diverse pathologic settings are heterogenous in their content of actin isoforms and intermediate filament proteins. *Lab Invest* 60: 275–285

60 Schürch W, Seemayer TA, Gabbiani G (1992) Myofibroblasts. In: SS Sternberg (ed): *Histology for pathologists*. Raven Press, New York, 109–144

61 Brewster CEP, Howarth PH, Djukanovic R, Wilson J, Holgate ST Roche WR (1990) Myofibroblasts and subepithelial fibrosis in bronchial asthma. *Am J Respir Cell Mol Biol* 3: 507–511
62 Gizycki MJ, Ädelroth E, Rogers AV, O'Byrne PM, Jeffery PK (1997) Myofibroblast involvement in the allergen-induced late response in mild atopic asthma. *Am J Respir Cell Mol Biol* 16: 664–673
63 Sappino AP, Schürch W, Gabbiani G (1990) Differentiation repertoire of fibroblastic cells: expression of cytoskeletal proteins as marker of phenotypic modulations *Lab Invest* 63: 144–161
64 Ryan GB, Cliff WJ, Gabbiani G, Irlé C, Montandon D, Statkov PR, Majno G (1974) Myofibroblasts in human granulation tissue. *Human Pathol* 5: 55–67
65 Mitchell JJ, Reynolds SE, Leslie KO, Low RB, Woodcock-Mitchell J (1990) Smooth muscle cell markers in developing rat lung. *Am J Respir Cell Mol Biol* 3: 515–523
66 Darby I, Skalli O, Gabbiani G (1990) α-smooth muscle actin is transiently expressed by myofibroblasts during experimental wound healing. *Lab Invest* 63: 21–29
67 Phan SE (1996) Role of the myofibroblast in pulmonary fibrosis. *Kid Int* 49 (suppl 54) S46–S48
68 Gabbiani G (1996) The cellular derivation and the life span of the myofibroblast. *Pathol Res Pract* 192: 708–711
69 Desmoulière A, Geinoz A, Gabbiani F, Gabbiani G (1993) Transforming growth factor β1 induces α-smooth muscle actin expression in granulation tissue myofibroblasts and in quiescent and growing cultured fibroblasts. *J Cell Biol* 122: 103–111
70 Oda D, Gown AM, Vande Berg JS, Stern R (1990) Instability of the myofibroblast phenotype in culture. *Exp Mol Pathol* 52: 221–234
71 Infeld MD, Brennan JA, Davies PB (1993) Human fetal lung fibroblasts promote invasion of extracellular matrix by normal human tracheobronchial epithelial cells *in vitro*: a model of early airway gland development. *Am J Respir Cell Mol Biol* 8: 69–76
72 Jeffery PK, (1998) The development of large and small airways. *Am J Respir Crit Care Med* 157: S174–S180
73 McGowan SE (1992) Extracellular matrix and the regulation of lung development and repair. *FASEB J* 6: 2895–2904
74 Minoo P, King RJ (1994) Epithelial-mesenchymal interactions in lung development. *Ann Rev Physiol* 56: 13–45
75 Collet AJ, Des Biens G (1975) Evolution of mesenchymal cells in fetal rat lung. *Anat Embryol* 147: 273–292
76 Leslie KO, Mitchell JJ, Woodcock-Mitchell JL, Low RB (1990) Alpha smooth muscle actin expression in developing and adult human lung. *Differentiation* 44: 143–149
77 Brauker JH, Trautman MS, Bernfield M (1991) Syndecan, a cell surface proteoglycan, exhibits a molecular polymorphism during lung development. *Dev Biol* 147: 285–292
78 Laurent GJ (1982) Rates of collagen synthesis in lung, skin and muscle obtained *in vivo* by a simplified method using [^{3}H] proline. *Biochem J* 206: 535–544
79 McAnulty RJ, Laurent GJ (1987) Collagen synthesis and degradation *in vivo*. Evidence

for rapid rates of collagen turnover with extensive degradation of newly synthesised collagen in tissues of the adult rat. *Collagen Rel Res* 7: 93–104
80 Laurent GJ, Harrison NK, McAnulty RJ (1988) The regulation of collagen production in normal lung and during interstitial lung disease. *Postgrad Med J* 64: 26–34
81 Mays PK, McAnulty RJ, Laurent GJ (1991) Age-related changes in rates of protein synthesis and degradation in rat tissues. *Mechanisms of Age and Develop* 59: 229–241
82 Laurent GJ, McAnulty RJ (1983) Protein metabolism during bleomycin-induced pulmonary fibrosis in rabbits: *In vivo* evidence for collagen accumulation because of increased synthesis and decreased degradation of the newly synthesized collagen. *Am Rev Respir Dis* 128: 82–88
83 O'Conner CM, Fitzgerald MX (1994) Matrix metalloproteinases and lung disease. *Thorax* 49: 602–609
84 Woessner Jr JF (1991) Matrix Metalloproteinases and their inhibitors in connective tissue remodeling. *FASEB J* 5: 2145–2154
85 Murphy G, Docherty AJP (1992) The matrix metalloproteinases and their inhibitors. *Am J Respir Cell Mol Biol* 7: 120–125
86 Wojtowicz-Praga SM, Dickson RB, Hawkins MJ (1997) Matrix metalloproteinase inhibitors. *Invest New Drugs* 15: 61–75
87 McAnulty RJ, Laurent GJ (1995) Pathogenesis of lung fibrosis and potential new therapeutic strategies. *Exp Nephrol* 3: 96–107
88 Holgate ST (1993) Asthma: past, present and future. *Eur Resp J* 6: 1507–1520
89 Barnes PJ (1996) Pathophysiology of asthma. *Br J Clin Pharmacol* 42: 3–10
90 Fine A, Goldstein RH (1987) The effect of transforming growth factor-β on cell proliferation and collagen formation by lung fibroblasts. *J Biol Chem* 262: 3897–3902
91 Rhagow R, Postlethwaite AE, Keski-Oja J, Moses HL, Kang AH (1887) Transforming growth factor-β increases steady state levels of type I procollagen and fibronectin messenger RNA's posttranscriptionally in cultured human dermal fibroblasts. *J Clin Invest* 79: 1285–1288
92 McAnulty RJ, Campa, JS, Cambrey AD, Laurent GJ (1991) The effect of transforming growth factor β on rates of procollagen synthesis and degradation *in vitro*. *Biochimica et Biophysica Acta* 1091: 231–235
93 McAnulty RJ, Chambers RC, Laurent GJ (1995) Regulation of fibroblast procollagen production. Transforming growth factor-β_1 induces prostaglandin E_2 but not procollagen synthesis *via* a pertussis toxin-sensitive G-protein. *Biochem J* 307: 63–68
94 Libby P, Wyler DJ, Janicka MW, Dinarello CA (1995) Differential effects of human interleukin-1 on growth of human fibroblast and vascular smooth muscle cells. *Arteriosclerosis* 5: 186–191
95 Goldring MB, Krane SM (1987) Modulation of recombinant interleukin 1 of synthesis of types I and III collagens and associated procollagen mRNA levels in cultured human cells. *J Biol Chem* 262: 16724–16729
96 Postlethwaite AE, Holness MA, Katai H, Raghow R (1992) Human fibroblasts synthe-

size elevated levels of extracellular matrix proteins in response to interleukin 4. *J Clin Invest* 90: 1479–1485
97 Feghali CA, Bost KL, Bouleware DW, Levy LS (1992) Human recombinant interleukin-4 induces proliferation and interluekin-6 production by cultured human skin fibroblasts. *Clin Immunol Immunopathol* 63: 182–187
98 Sempowski GD, Beckmann MP, Derdak S, Phipps RP (1994) Subsets of murine lung fibroblasts express membrane-bound and soluble IL-4 receptors. Role of IL-4 in enhancing fibroblast proliferation and collagen synthesis. *J Immunol* 152: 3606–3614
99 Monroe JG, Haldar S, Prystowsky MB, Lammie P (1988) Lymphokine regulation of inflammatory processes: Interleukin-4 stimulates fibroblast proliferation. *Clin Immunol Immunpathol* 49: 292–298
100 Grossman RM, Kreuger J, Yourish D, Granelli-Piperno A, Murphy DP, May LT, Kupper TS, Sehgal PB, Gottlieb AB (1989) Interleukin 6 is expressed at high levels in psoriatic skin and stimulates proliferation of cultured human keratinocytes. *Proc Natl Acad Sci USA* 86: 6367–6371
101 Duncan MR, Berman B (1991) Stimulation of collagen and glycosaminoglycan production in cultured human adult dermal fibroblasts by recombinant human interleukin 6. *J Invest Dermatol* 97: 686–692
102 Rubbia-Brandt L, Sappino A-P, Gabbiani G (1991) Locally applied GM-CSF induces the accumulation of α-smooth muscle actin containing myofibroblasts. *Virchows Archiv [B] Cell Pathol* 60: 73–82
103 Postlethwaite AE, Seyer JM (1990) Stimulation of fibroblast chemotaxis by human recombinant tumour necrosis factor α (TNFα) and a synthetic TNFα 31-68 peptide. *J Exp Med* 172: 1749–1756
104 Leibovich SJ, Polverini PJ, Shepard MH, Wiseman DM, Shively V, Nuseir N (1987) Macrophage-induced angiogenesis is mediated by tumour necrosis factor-α. *Nature* 329: 630–632
105 Duncan MR, Berman B (1989) Differential regulation of collagen, glycosaminoglycan, fibronectin and collagenase activity production in cultured human adult dermal fibroblasts by interleukin-1-alpha and beta and tumour necrosis factor-alpha and beta. *J Invest Dermatol* 92: 699–706
106 Solis-Herruzo JA, Brenner DA, Chojkier M (1988) Tumour necrosis factor alpha inhibits collagen gene transcription and collagen synthesis in cultured human fibroblasts. *J Biol Chem* 263: 5841–5845
107 McAnulty RJ, Guerreiro D, Cambrey AD, Laurent GJ (1992) Growth factor activity in the lung during compensatory growth after pneumonectomy: evidence of a role for IGF-1. *Eur Resp J* 5: 739–747
108 Cambrey AD, Kwon OJ, Gray AJ, Harrison NK, Yacoub M, Barnes PJ, Laurent GJ, Chung KF (1995) Insulin-like growth factor I is a major fibroblast mitogen produced by primary cultures of human airway epithelial cells. *Clin Sci* 89: 611–617
109 Goldstein RH, Polgar P (1982) The effect and interaction of bradykinin and prosta-

glandins on protein and collagen production by lung fibroblasts. *J Biol Chem* 257: 8630–8633

110 Postlethwaite AE, Keski-Oja J, Moses HL, Kang AH (1987) Stimulation of the chemotactic migration of human fibroblasts by transforming growth factor β. *J Exp Med* 165: 251–256

111 Penttinen RP, Kobayashi S, Bornstein P (1988) Transforming growth factor β increases mRNA for matrix proteins both in the presence and in the absence of changes in mRNA stability. Proc Natl Acad Sci USA 85: 1105–1108

112 Khalil N, Greenberg AH (1991) The role of TGFβ in pulmonary fibrosis. In: GR Bock, J Marsh (eds): Clinical applications of TGFβ. *Ciba Foundation Symposium* 157: 194–211

113 Lyons RM, Moses HL (1990) Transforming growth factor and the regulation of cell proliferation. *Eur J Biochem* 187: 467–473

114 Ignotz RA, Massague J (1986) Transforming growth factor-β stimulates the expression of fibronectin and collagen and their incorporation into the extracellular matrix. *J Biol Chem* 261: 4337–4345

115 Westergren-Thorsson G, Särnstrand B, Fransson L-A, Malmström A (1990) TGF-beta enhances the production of hyaluronan in human lung but not in skin fibroblasts. *Exp Cell Res* 186: 192–195

116 Westergren-Thorsson G, Hernnäs J Särnstrand B, Oldberg A, Heinegård D, Malström A (1993) Altered expression of small proteoglycan, collagen and transforming growth factor-β_1 in developing bleomycin-induced pulmonary fibrosis in rats. *J Clin Invest* 92: 632–637

117 Kondo H, Matsuda R, Yonezawa Y (1992) Autonomous migration of human fetal skin fibroblasts into a denuded area in a cell monolayer is mediated by basic fibroblast growth factor and collagen. *In Vitro Cell Dev Biol Anim* 29A: 929–935

118 Butt RP, Laurent GJ, Bishop JE (1995) Mechanical load and polypeptide growth factors stimulate cardiac fibroblast activity. *Ann NY Acad Sci* 752: 387–393

119 Pincus SH, Ramesh KS, Wyler DJ (1987) Eosinophils stimulate fibroblast DNA synthesis. *Blood* 70: 572–574

120 Birkland TP, Cheavens MD, Pincus SH (1994) Human eosinophils stimulate DNA synthesis and matrix production in dermal fibroblasts. *Arch Dermatol Res* 286: 312–318

121 Shock A, Rabe KF, Dent G, Chambers RC, Gray AJ, Chung KF, Barnes PJ, Laurent GJ (1991) Eosinophils adhere to and stimulate replication of lung fibroblasts "*in vitro*". *Clin Exp Immunol* 86: 185–190

122 Hernnäs J, Särnstrand B, Lindroth P, Peterson CG, Venge P, Malmström A (1992) Eosinophil cationic protein alters proteoglycan metabolism in human lung fibroblast cultures. *Eur J Cell Biol* 59: 352–363

123 Mensing H, Czarnetzki BM (1984) Leukotriene B_4 induces *in vitro* fibroblast chemotaxis. *J Invest Dermatol* 82: 9–12

124 Rieger GM, Hein R, Adelmann-Grill BC, Ruzicka T, Krieg T (1990) Influence of

eicosanoids on fibroblast chemotaxis and protein synthesis *in vitro*. *J Dermatol Sci* 1: 347–354
125 Phan SH, McGarry BM, Loeffler KM, Kunkel SL (1988) Binding of leukotriene C_4 to rat lung fibroblasts and stimulation of collagen synthesis *in vitro*. *Biochem* 27: 2846–2853
126 Peacock AJ, Dawes KE, Shock A, Gray AJ, Reeves JT, Laurent GJ (1992) Endothelin-1 and endothelin-3 induce chemotaxis and replication of pulmonary artery fibroblasts. *Am J Respir Cell Mol Biol* 7: 492–499
127 Dawes KE, Cambrey AD, Campa JS, Bishop JE, McAnulty RJ, Peacock AJ, Laurent GJ (1996) Changes in collagen metabolism in response to endothelin-1: Evidence for fibroblast heterogeneity. *Int J Biochem Cell Biol* 28: 229–238
128 Kahaleh MB (1991) Endothelin, and endothelial-dependent vasoconstrictor in scleroderma. *Arthritis Rheum* 34: 978–983
129 Gruber BL, Kew RR, Jelaska A, Marchese MJ, Garlick J, Ren S, Schwartz LB & Korn JH (1997) Human mast cells activate fibroblasts. Tryptase is a fibrogenic factor stimulating collagen messenger ribonucleic acid synthesis and fibroblast chemotaxis. *J Immunol* 158: 2310–2317
130 Ruoss SJ, Hartmann T, Caughey GH (1991) Mast cell tryptase is a mitogen for cultured fibroblasts. *J Clin Invest* 88: 493–499
131 Hartmann T, Ruoss SJ, Raymond WW, Seuwen K, Caughey GH (1992) Human tryptase as a potent, cell specific mitogen: role of signalling pathways in synergistic responses. *Am J Physiol* 262: L528–L534
132 Cairns JA, Walls AF (1997) Mast cell tryptase stimulates synthesis of type I collagen in human lung fibroblasts. *J Clin Invest* 99: 1313–1321
133 Dawes KE, Gray AJ, Laurent GJ (1993) Thrombin stimulates fibroblast chemotaxis and replication. *Eur J Cell Biol* 61: 126–130
134 Gray AJ, Reeves JT, Harrison NK, Winlove P, Laurent GJ (1990) Growth factors for human fibroblasts in the solute remaining after clot formation. *J Cell Sci* 96: 271–274
135 Chen LB, Buchanan JM (1975) Mitogenic activity of blood components, I. Thrombin and prothrombin. *Proc Natl Acad Sci USA* 72: 131–135
136 Chambers RC, Dabbagh K, McAnulty RJ, Gray AJ, Blanc-Brude OP, Laurent GJ. (1998) Thrombin stimulates fibroblast procollagen production *via* proteolytic activation of protease-activated receptor-1. *Biochem J* 333: 121–127
137 Harrison NK, Dawes KE, Kwon OJ, Barnes PJ, Laurent GJ, Chung KF (1995) Effects of neuropeptides on human lung fibroblast proliferation and chemotaxis. *Am J Physiol* 268: L278–L283
138 Jordana M, Schulman J, McSharry C, Iring LB, Newhouse MT, Jordana G, Gauldie J (1988) Heterogeneous proliferative characteristics of human adult lung fibroblast lines and clonally derived fibroblasts from control and fibrotic tissue. *Am Rev Respir Dis* 137: 579–584
139 Hatamochi A, Ueki H, Mauch C, Krieg T (1991) Effect of histamine on collagen and collagen m-RNA production in human skin fibroblasts. *J Dermatol Sci* 2: 407–412

140 Adachi T, Motojima S, Hirata A, Fukuda T, Kihara N, Makino S (1995) Detection of transforming growth factor-beta in sputum from patients with bronchial asthma by eosinophil survival assay and enzyme-linked immunosorbent assay. *Clin Exp Allergy* 26: 557–562
141 Ohno I, Nitta Y, Yamauchi K, Hoshi H, Honma M, Woolley K, O'Byrne P, Tamura G, Jordana M, Shirato K (1996) Transforming growth factor β_1 (TGFβ_1) gene expression by eosinophils in asthmatic airway inflammation *Am J Respir Cell Mol Biol* 15: 404–409
142 Ohno I, Nitta Y, Yamauchi K, Hoshi H, Honma M, Woolley K, O'Byrne P, Dolovich J, Jordana M, Tamura G, Tanno Y, Shirato K (1995) Eosinophils as a potential source of platelet-derived growth factor B-chain (PDGF-B) in nasal polyposis and bronchial asthma. *Am J Respir Cell Mol Biol* 13: 639–647
143 Vignola AM, Chanez P, Chiappara G, Merendino A, Pace E, Rizzo A, la Rocca AM, Bellia V, Bonsignore G, Bousquet J (1997) Transforming growth factor-β expression in mucosal biopsies in asthma and chronic bronchitis. *Am J Respir Crit Care Med* 156: 591–599
144 Minshall EM, Leung DYM, Martin RJ, Song YL, Cameron L, Ernst P, Hamid Q (1997) Eosinophil-associated TGF-β_1 mRNA expression and airways fibrosis in bronchial asthma. *Am J Respir Cell Mol Biol* 17: 326–333
145 Gabbrielli S, Di Lollo S, Stanflin N, Romagnoli P (1994) Myofibroblasts and elastic and collagen fiber hyperplasia in the bronchial mucosa: a possible basis for the progressive irreversibility of airway obstruction in chronic asthma. *Pathologica* 86: 157–160
146 Vancheri C, Gauldie J, Bienenstock J, Cox G, Scicchitano R, Stanisz A, Jordana M (1989) Human lung fibroblast-derived granulocyte-macrophage colony stimulating (GM-CSF) mediates eosinophil survival *in vitro*. *Am J Respir Cell Mol Biol* 1:289–295
147 Kaushansky K (1987) The molecular biology of the colony-stimulating factors. *Blood* Cells 13: 2–15
148 Zhang S, Mohammed Q, Burbridge A, Morland CM, Roche WR (1996) Cell cultures from bronchial subepithelial myofibroblasts enhance eosinophil survival *in vitro*. *Eur Respir J* 9: 1839–1846
149 Xing Z, Ohkawara Y, Jordana M, Graham F, Gauldie J (1996) Transfer of granulocyte-macrophage colony-stimulating factor gene to rat lung induces eosinophilia, monocytosis and fibrotic reactions. *J Clin Invest* 97: 1102–1110
150 Xing Z, Tremblay GM, Sime PJ, Gauldie J (1997) Overexpression of granulocyte-macrophage colony-stimulating factor induces pulmonary granulation tissue formation and fibrosis by induction of transforming growth factor-β_1 and myofibroblast accumulation. *Am J Pathol* 150: 59–66
151 Glynn AA, Michaels L (1960) Bronchial biopsy in chronic bronchitis and asthma. *Thorax* 15: 142–153
152 Venge P, Bystrom J (1998) Eosinophil cationic protein (ECP). *Int J Biochem Cell Biol* 30: 433–437
153 Rochester CL, Ackerman SJ, Zheng T, Elias JA (1996) Eosinophil-fibroblast interac-

tions. Granule major basic protein interacts with IL-1 and transforming growth factor-β in the stimulation of lung fibroblast IL-6 type cytokine production. *J Immunol* 156: 4449–4456
154 Schulman ES (1993) The role of mast cells in inflammatory responses in the lung. *Crit Rev Immunol* 13: 35–70
155 Schwartz LB (1990) Tryptase, a mediator of human mast cells. *J Allergy Clin Immunol* 86: 594–598
156 Walls AF, Bennett AR, Godfrey RC, Holgate ST, Church MK (1991) Mast cell tryptase and histamine concentrations in bronchoalveolar lavage fluid from patients with interstitial lung disease. *Clin Sci* 81: 183–188
157 Wenzel SE, Fowler AA, Schwartz, LB (1988) Activation of pulmonary mast cells by bronchoalveolar allergen challenge. *In vivo* release of histamine and tryptase in atopic subjects with and without asthma. *Am Rev Respir Dis* 137: 1002–1008
158 Akers IA, Parsons M, Hollenberg MD, Sanjar S, Laurent GJ, McAnulty RJ (2000) Mast cell tryptase stimulates human lung fibroblast proliferation *via* activation of protease-activated receptor-2 (PAR-2). *Am J Physiol Lung Cell Mol Physiol* 278: L193–201
159 Springall DR, Howarth PH, Counihan H, Djukanovic R, Holgate ST, Polak JM (1991) Endothelin immunoreactivity of airway epithelium in asthmatic patients. *Lancet* 337: 697–701
160 Redington AE, Springall DR, Ghatei MA, Lau LCK, Bloom SR, Holgate ST, Polak JM, Howarth PH (1995) Endothelin in bronchoalveolar lavage fluid and its relation to airflow obstruction in asthma. *Am J Respir Crit Care Med* 151: 1034–1039
161 Redington AE, Springall DR, Meng QH, Tuck AB, Holgate ST, Polak JM, Howarth PH (1997) Immunoreactive endothelin in bronchial biopsy specimens: increased expression in asthma and modulation by corticosteroid therapy. *J Allergy Clin Immunol* 100: 544–52
162 Lundberg JM, Hokfelt T, Martling CR, Saria A, Cuello C (1984) Substance P-immunoreactive sensory nerves in the lower respiratory tract of various mammals including man. *Cell Tiss Res* 235: 251–261
163 Uddman R, Sundler F (1987) Neuropeptides in the airways: a review. *Am Rev Respir Dis* 136: S3–S8
164 Barnes PJ (1986) Asthma as an axon reflex. *Lancet* 1: 242–245
165 Molina C, Brun J, Coulet M, Betail G, Delage J (1977) Immunopathology of the bronchial mucosa in "late onset" asthma. *Clin Allergy* 7: 137–145
166 Jeffery PK, Wardlaw AJ, Nelson FC, Collins JV, Kay AB (1989) Bronchial biopsies in asthma. An ultrastructural, quantitative study and correlation with hyperreactivity. *Am Rev Respir Dis* 140: 1745–1753
167 Blanc-Brude O, Chambers RC (1999) Factor Xa-induced human lung fibroblast proliferation. *Personal Communications*
168 Gray AJ, Bishop JE, Reeves JT, Laurent GJ (1993) Aα and Bβ chains of fibrinogen stimulate proliferation of human fibroblasts. *J Cell Sci* 104: 409–413
169 Bishop JE, Mitchell JJ, Absher PM, Baldor L, Geller HA, Woodcock-Mitchell J, Ham-

blin MJ, Vacek P, Low RB (1993) Cyclic mechanical deformation stimulates human lung fibroblast proliferation and autocrine growth factor activity. *Am J Respir Cell Mol Biol* 9: 126–133
170 Butt RP, Bishop JE (1997) Mechanical load enhances the stimulatory effect of serum growth factors on cardiac fibroblast procollagen synthesis. *J Mol Cell Cardiol* 29: 1141–1151
171 McFadden ER, Lyons HA (1968) Arterial blood gas tension in asthma. *N Engl J Med* 278: 1027–1032
172 Chvapil M, Hurych J (1968) Control of collagen biosynthesis. *Int Rev Connect Tiss Res* 4: 67–196
173 Falanga V, Martin TA, Takagi H, Kirsner RS, Helfman T, Pardes J, Ochoa MS (1993) Low oxygen tension increases mRNA levels of alpha 1 (I) procollagen in human dermal fibroblasts. *J Cell Physiol* 157: 408–412
174 Dawes KE, Peacock AJ, Gray AJ, Bishop JE, Laurent GJ (1994) Characterization of fibroblast mitogens and chemoattractants produced by endothelial cells exposed to hypoxia. *Am J Respir Cell Mol Biol* 10: 552–559
175 Phipps RP, Roper RL, Stein SH (1989) Alternative antigen presentation pathways: accessory cells which down-regulate immune response. *Regional Immunology* 2: 326–339
176 Phipps RP, Penney DP, Keng P, Silvera M, Harkins S, Derdak S (1990) Immune functions of subpopulations of lung fibroblasts. *Immunol Res* 9: 275–286
177 Fries KM, Blieden T, Looney RJ, Sempowski GD, Silvera MR, Willis RA, Phipps RP (1994) Evidence of fibroblast heterogeneity and the role of fibroblast subpopulations in fibrosis. *Clin Immunol Immunopathol* 72: 283–292
178 Gombert W, Borthwick NJ, Wallace DL, Hyde H, Bofill M, Pilling D, Beverley PC, Janossy G, Salmon M, Akbar AN (1996) Fibroblasts prevent apoptosis of IL-2-deprived T cells without inducing proliferation: a selection effect on Bcl-XL expression. *Immunol* 89: 397–404
179 Crowston JG, Salmon M, Khaw PT, Akbar AN (1997) T-lymphocytes-fibroblast interactions. *Biochem Soc Trans* 25: 529–531
180 Huber HL, Koessler KK (1922) The pathology of bronchial asthma. *Arch Intern Med* 30: 689–760
181 James AL, Paré PD, Hogg JC (1989) The mechanics of airway narrowing in asthma. *Am Rev Respir Dis* 139: 242–246
182 Carroll N, Elliot J, Morton A, James A (1993) The structure of large and small airways in nonfatal and fatal asthma. *Am Rev Respir Dis* 147: 405–410
183 Crepea SB, Harman JW (1955) The pathology of bronchial asthma: I. The significance of membrane changes in asthmatic and non-allergic pulmonary disease. *J Allergy* 26: 453–460
184 Bosken CH, Wiggs BR, Paré PD, Hogg JC (1990) Small airways dimensions in smokers with obstruction to airflow. *Am Rev Respir Dis* 142: 563–570
185 Paré PD, Wiggs BR, James A, Hogg JC, Bosken C (1991) The comparative mechanics

and morphology of airways in asthma and in chronic obstructive pulmonary disease. *Am Rev Respir Dis* 143: 1189–1193
186 Laitinen LA, Heino M, Laitinen A, Kava T, Haahtela T (1985) Damage of the airway epithelium and bronchial reactivity in patients with asthma. *Am Rev Respir Dis* 131: 599–606
187 Jeffery PK (1991) Morphology of the airway wall in asthma and in chronic obstructive pulmonary disease. *Am Rev Respir Dis* 143: 1152–1158
188 Jeffery PK, Godfrey RW, Ädelroth E, Nelson F, Rogers A, Johansson S-A (1992) Effects of treatment on airway inflammation and thickening of basement membrane reticular collagen in asthma *Am Rev Respir Dis* 145: 890–899
189 Dunnill MS (1960) The pathology of asthma, with special reference to changes in bronchial mucosa. *J Clin Pathol* 13: 27–33
190 Cutz E, Levison H, Cooper DM (1978) Ultrastructure of airways in children with asthma. *Histopathology* 2: 407–421
191 Heard BE, Hossain S (1973) Hyperplasia of bronchial smooth muscle in asthma. *J Pathol* 101: 171–184
192 Ebina M, Yaegashi H, Chiba R, Takahashi T, Motomiya M, Tanemura M (1990) Hyperreactive site in the airway tree of asthmatic patients revealed by thickening of bronchial muscles. A morphometric study. *Am Rev Respir Dis* 141: 1327–1332
193 Houston JC, De Navasquez S, Trounce JR (1953) A clinical and pathological study of fatal cases of status asthmaticus. *Thorax* 8: 207–213
194 Dodson JW, Hay ED (1971) Secretion of collagenous stroma by isolated epithelium grown *in vitro*. *Exp Cell Res* 65: 215–220
195 Simon RH, Scott MJ, Reza MM, Killen PD (1993) Type IV collagen production by rat pulmonary alveolar epithelial cells. *Am J Respir Cell Mol Biol* 8: 640–646
196 Wilson JW, Li X (1997) The measurement of reticular basement membrane and submucosal collagen in the asthmatic airway. *Clin Exp Allergy* 27: 363–371
197 Dabbagh K, Laurent GJ, McAnulty RJ, Chambers RC (1998) Thrombin stimulates smooth muscle cell procollagen synthesis and mRNA *via* a PAR-1 mediated mechanism. *Thromb Haemost* 79: 405–409
198 Tremblay GM, Lafrenière-Allard M-J, Westergren-Thorsson G, Malmström A, Chakir J, Dubé J, Boulet L-P (1998) *In vitro* production of proteoglycans by asthmatic bronchial fibroblasts correlates with airway hyperresponsiveness. *Am J Respir Crit Care Med* 157: A247
199 Shute JK, Criss J, Hockey P, Howarth PH (1998) Increased proteoglycans in sputum in asthma and cystic fibrosis (CF) and increased GAG levels in CF. *Am J Respir Crit Care Med* 157: A607
200 Reed RK, Rubin K, Wiig H, Rodt SA (1992) Blockade of beta 1-integrins in skin causes edema through lowering of interstitial fluid pressure. *Circ Res* 71: 978–983
201 Rodt SA, Ahlen K, Berg A, Rubin K, Reed RK (1996) A novel physiological function for platelet-derived growth factor-BB in rat dermis. *J Physiol* 495: 193–200
202 Berg A, Ekwall AK, Rubin K, Stjernschantz J, Reed RK (1998) Effect of PGE_1, PGI_2 and

PGF_2 alpha analogs on collagen gel compaction *in vitro* and interstitial pressure *in vivo*. *Am J Physiol* 274: H663–H671
203 Mead J (1961) Mechanical properties of lungs. *Physiol Rev* 41: 281–330
204 Mead J, Takishima T, Leith D (1970) Stress distribution in lungs: a model of pulmonary elasticity. *J Appl Physiol* 28: 596–608
205 Robinson P, Okazawa M, Bai T, Paré P (1992) *In vivo* loads on airway smooth muscle: the role of noncontractile airway structures. *Can J Physiol Pharmacol* 70: 602–606
206 Hoppin FG (1995) Parenchymal mechanics and asthma. *Chest* 107 140S–144S
207 Macklem PT (1995) Theoretical basis of airway instability. *Chest* 107 87S–88S
208 Bramley AM, Thomson RJ, Roberts CR, Schellenberg RR (1994) Hypothesis: excessive bronchoconstriction in asthma is due to decreased airway elastance. *Eur Respir J* 7: 337–341
209 Paré PD, Bai TR (1996) Airway wall remodelling in chronic obstructive pulmonary disease. *Eur Respir Rev* 6: 259–263
210 Lambert RK (1991) Role of bronchial basement membrane in airway collapse. *J Appl Physiol* 71: 666–673
211 Durieu I, Peyrol S, Gindre D, Bellon G, Durand DV, Pacheco Y (1998) Subepithelial fibrosis and degradation of the bronchial extracellular matrix in cystic fibrosis. *Am J Respir Crit Care Med* 158: 580–588
212 Woolcock A, Read J (1968) The static elastic properties of the lung in asthma. *Am Rev Respir Dis* 98: 788–794
213 McCarthy DS, Sigurdson M (1980) Lung elastic recoil and reduced airflow in clinically stable asthma. *Thorax* 35: 298–302
214 Godfrey RW, Lorimer S, Majuridar S, Ädelroth E, Johnston PW, Rogers AV, Johansson SA, Jeffery PK (1995) Airway and lung elastic fibre is not reduced in asthma nor in asthmatics following corticosteroid treatment. *Eur Respir J* 8: 922–927
215 Chetta A, Foresi A, Del Donno M, Consigli GF, Bertorelli G, Pesci A, Barbee RA, Olivieri D (1996) Bronchial responsiveness to distilled water and methacholine and its relationship to inflammation and remodeling of the airways in asthma. *Am J Respir Crit Care Med* 153: 910–917
216 Boulet L-P, Bélanger M, Carrier G (1995) Airway hyperresponsiveness and bronchial wall thickness in asthma with and without fixed airflow obstruction. *Am J Respir Crit Care Med* 152: 865–871
217 Barnes PJ (1997) Current therapies for asthma. Promises and limitations. *Chest* 111: 17S–26S
218 Weiner FR, Czaja MJ, Jefferson DM, Giambrone MA, Tur-Kaspa R, Reid LM, Zern MA (1987) The effects of dexamethasone on *in vitro* collagen gene expression. *J Biol Chem* 262: 6955–6958
219 Weiner FR, Czaja MJ, Giambrone MA, Takahashi S, Biempica L, Zern MA (1987) Transcriptional and posttranscriptional effects of dexamethasone on albumin and procollagen messenger RNAs in murine schistosomiasis. *Biochem* 26: 1557–1562
220 Laursen LC, Taudorf E, Borgeskov S, Kobayasi T, Jensen H, Weeke B (1988) Fiberoptic

bronchoscopy and bronchial mucosal biopsies in asthmatics undergoing long-term high-dose budesonide aerosol treatment. *Allergy* 43: 284–288
221 Lundgren R, Söderberg M, Hörstedt P, Stenling R (1988) Morphological studies of bronchial mucosal biopsies from asthmatics before and after ten years of treatment with inhaled steroids. *Eur Respir J* 1: 883–889
222 Laitinen A, Altraja A, Linden M, Stallenheim G, Venge P, Häkansson L, Virtanen I, Laitinen LA (1994) Treatment with inhaled budesonide and tenascin expression in bronchial mucosa of allergic asthmatics. *Am J Respir Crit Care Med* 149: A942
223 Trigg CJ, Manolitsas ND, Wang J, Calderón MA, McAulay A, Jordan SE, Herdman MJ, Jhalli N, Duddle JM, Hamilton SA, Devalia JL, Davies RJ (1994) Placebo-controlled immunopathologic study of four months of inhaled corticosteroids in asthma. *Am J Respir Crit Care Med* 150: 17–22
224 Olivieri D, Chetta A, Del Donno M, Bertorelli G, Casalini A, Pesci A, Testi R, Foresi A (1997) Effect of short-term treatment with low-dose inhaled fluticasone propionate on airway inflammation and remodeling in mild asthma: A placebo controlled study. *Am J Respir Crit Care Med* 155: 1864–1871
225 Saetta M, Maestrelli P, Di Stefano A, De Marzo N, Milani GF, Pivirotto F, Mapp CE, Fabbri LM (1992) Effect of cessation of exposure to toluene diisocyanate (TDI) on bronchial mucosa of subjects with TDI-induced asthma. *Am Rev Respir Dis* 145: 169–174
226 Saetta M, Maestrelli P, Turato G, Mapp CE, Milani G, Pivirotto F, Fabbri LM, Di Stefano A (1995) Airway wall remodeling after cessation of exposure to isocyanates in sensitized asthmatic subjects. *Am J Respir Crit Care Med* 151: 489–494
227 Barnes PJ and Pedersen S (1993) Efficacy and safety of inhaled corticosteroids in asthma. *Am Rev Resp Dis* 148 (4) S1–S26
228 Coker RK, Laurent GJ (1995) Pathogenesis of pulmonary fibrosis: Implications for Pharmacological intervention. In: EH Walters, RM du Bois (eds): *Immunology and management of interstitial lung diseases.* Chapman & Hall, London, 19–36
229 Coker RK, Laurent GJ (1997) Anticytokine approaches in pulmonary fibrosis bringing factors into focus. *Thorax* 52: 294–296
230 Yamada H, Tajima S, Nishikawa T, Murad S, Pinnell SR (1994) Tranilast, a selective inhibitor of collagen synthesis in human skin fibroblasts. *J Biochem* 116: 892–897
231 Hautala T, Heikkinen J, Kivirikko KI, Myllyla R (1992) Minoxidil specifically decreases the expression of lysine hydroxylase in cultured human skin fibroblasts. *Biochem J* 283: 51–54
232 Yeowell HN, Ha V, Walker LC, Murad S, Pinnell SR (1992) Characterization of a partial cDNA for lysyl hydroxylase from human skin fibroblasts; lysyl hydroxylase mRNAs are regulated differently by minoxidil derivatives and hydralazine. *J Invest Dermatol* 99: 864–869
233 Cutroneo KR, Robowoski R, Counts DF (1981) Glucocorticoids and collagen synthesis: comparison of *in vivo* and cell culture studies. *Coll Relat Res* 1: 557–568
234 Cockayne D, Sterling KM, Shull S, Mintz KP, Illeyne S, Cutroneo KR (1986) Glucocor-

ticosteroids decrease the synthesis of type I procollagen mRNAs. *Biochemistry* 25: 3202–3209
235 Jimenez SA, Freudlich B, Rosenbloom J (1984) Selective inhibition of human diploid fibroblast collagen synthesis by interferons. *J Clin Invest* 74: 1112–1116
236 Baum BJ, Moss J, Breul SD, Crystal RG (1978) Association in normal human fibroblasts of elevated levels of adenosine 3': 5'-monophosphate with a selective decrease in collagen production. *J Biol Chem* 253: 3391–3394
237 Rennard S, Saltzmann L, Moss J (1981) Modulation of fibroblast production of collagen types I and III. Effects of PGE_1 and isoproterenol. *Fed Proc* 40: 1813
238 Baum BJ, Moss J, Breul SD, Berg RA, Crystal RG (1980) Effect of cyclic AMP on the intracellular degradation of newly synthesized collagen. *J Biol Chem* 255: 2843–2847
239 Varga J, Diaz-Perez A, Rosenbloom J, Jimenez SA (1987) PGE_2 causes a coordinate decrease in the steady state levels of fibronectin and types I and III procollagen mRNAs in normal human dermal fibroblasts. *Biochem Biophys Res Commun* 147: 1282–1288
240 Czaja MJ, Weiner FR, Eghbali M, Giambrone MA, Eghbali M, Zern MA (1987) Differential effects of gamma-interferon on collagen and fibronectin gene expression. *J Biol Chem* 262: 13348–13351
241 Haapasaari K-M, Risteli J, Karvonen J, Oikarinen A. (1997) Effect of hydrocortisone, methylprednisolone aceponate and momethasone furoate on collagen synthesis in human skin *in vivo*. *Skin Pharmacol* 10: 261–264
242 Uitto J, Prockop DJ (1975) Inhibition of collagen accumulation by proline analogues: the mechanism of their action. In: H Poppu, K Becker (eds): *Collagen metabolism in the liver, vol. 1*. Stratton Intercontinental, New York, 139–148
243 Riley DJ, Kerr JS Berg RA, Ianni BD, Pietra GG, Edelman NH, Prockop DJ (1981) Prevention of bleomycin-induced pulmonary fibrosis in the hamster by cis-4-hydroxyl-L-proline *Am Rev Respir Dis* 123: 388–393
244 Tan EM, Ryhänen L, Uitto J (1983) Proline analogues inhibit human skin fibroblast growth and collagen production in culture. *J Invest Dermatol* 80: 261–267
245 Wiestner M, Krieg T, Hörlein D, Glanville RW, Fietzek P, Müller PK (1979) Inhibiting effect of procollagen peptides on collagen biosynthesis in fibroblast cultures. *J Biol Chem* 254: 7016 7023
246 Aycock RS, Raghow R, Stricklin GP, Eyer JM, Kang AH (1986) Post-translational inhibition of collagen and fibronectin synthesis by a synthetic homolog of a portion of the carboxyl-terminal propeptide of human type I collagen J Biol Chem 261: 14355–14360
247 Fouser L, Sage EH, Clark J, Bornstein P (1991) Feedback regulation of collagen gene expression: a trojan horse approach *Proc Natl Acad Sci USA* 88: 10158–10162
248 Greco MJ, Kemnitzer JE, Fox JD, Choe JK, Kohn J, Riley DJ, Poiani GJ (1997) Polymer of proline analogue with sustained antifibrotic activity in lung fibrosis. *Am J Respir Crit Care Med* 155: 1391–1397
249 Wu CH, Walton CM, Wu GY (1991) Propeptide-mediated regulation of procollagen synthesis in IMR-90 human lung fibroblast cell cultures. Evidence for transcritional control. *J Biol Chem* 266: 2983–2987

250 Katayama K, Seyer JM, Raghow R, Kang AH (1991) Regulation of extracellular matrix production by chemically synthesized subfragments of type I collagen carboxy propeptide. *Biochemistry* 30: 7097–7104
251 Lubec B, Rokitansky A, Hayde M, Aufricht C, Wagner U, Mallinger WR, Hoger H, Lubec G (1994) Thiaproline reduces glomerular basement membrane thickness and collagen accumulation in the db/db mouse. *Nephron* 66: 333–336
252 Vistica DT, Ahrens FA, Ellison WR (1977) The effects of lead upon collagen synthesis and proline hydroxylation in the Swiss mouse 3T6 fibroblast. *Arch Biochem Biophys* 179: 15–23
253 Anttinen H, Ryhanen L, Puistola U, Arranto A, Oikarinen A (1984) Decrease in liver collagen accumulation in carbon tetrachloride-injured and normal growing rats upon administration of zinc. *Gastroenterology* 86: 532–539
254 Anttinen H, Oikarinen A, Puistola U, Pääkko P, Ryhanen L (1985) Prevention by zinc of rat lung collagen accumulation in carbon tetrachloride injury. *Am Rev Respir Dis* 132: 536–540
255 Franklin TJ, Hales NJ, Johnstone D, Morris WB, Cuncliffe CJ, Millest AJ, Hill GB (1991) Approaches to the design of anti-fibrotic drugs. *Biochem Soc Trans* 19: 812–815
256 Tschank G, Brocks DG, Engelbart K, ohr J, Baader E, Gunzler V, Hanauske-Abel HM (1991) Inhibition of prolyl hydroxylation and procollagen processing in chick embryo calvaria by a derivative of pyridine-2,4-dicarboxylate. Characterization of the diethyl ester as a proinhibitor. *Biochem J* 275: 469–476
257 Carrington MJ, Fornieri C, Bartlet CP, Heale G, Levene CI (1985) Biochemical and ultrastructural study of the effects of proline analogues on collagen synthesis in 3T6 fibroblasts. *J Pharm Pharmacol* 37: 794–801
258 Uitto J, Ryhänen L, Tan EML, Oikarinen AI, Zaragoza EJ (1984) Pharmacological inhibition of excessive collagen deposition in fibrotic diseases. *Fed Proc* 43: 2815–2820
259 Murad S, Walker LC, Tajima S, Pinnell SR (1994) Minimum structural requirements for minoxidil inhibition of lysyl hydroxylase in cultured fibroblasts. *Arch Biochem Biophys* 208: 42–47
260 Dehm P, Prockop DJ (1972) Time lag in the secretion of collagen by matrix-free tendon cells and inhibition of the secretory process by colchicine and vinblastine. *Biochem Biophys Acta* 264: 375–382
261 Khaw PT, Occleston NL, Schultz G, Grierson I, Sherwood MB, Larkin G (1994) Activation and suppression of fibroblast function. *Eye* 8: 188–195
262 Wu J, Danielsson Å (1994) Inhibition of hepatic fibrogenesis: A review of pharmacological candidates. *Scand J Gastroenterol* 29: 385–391
263 Uitto J, Tan EML, Ryhänen L (1982) Inhibition of collagen accumulation in fibrotic processes: review of pharmacological agents and new approaches with amino acids and their analogues. *J Invest Dermatol* 79: 113s–120s
264 Deshmukh K, Nimni ME (1969) A defect in the intramolecular and intermolecular cross-linking of collagen caused by penicillamine. II. Functional groups involved in the interaction process. *J Biol Chem* 244: 1787–1795

265 Siegel RC (1977) Collagen cross-linking. Effect of D-penicillamine on cross-linking *in vitro*. *J Biol Chem* 252: 254 -259
266 Ledwozyw A (1995) The effect of β-aminopropionitrile on bleomycin-induced lung injury in rats. *Acta Physiologica Hungarica* 83: 91–99
267 Harris ED, Werb Z, Cartwright E, Reynolds JJ (1975) Stimulation of collagenase release from synovial fibroblasts in monolayer cultures of colchicine and related compounds *Scand J Rheum* 8 (suppl): 15–24
268 Romanelli RG, Caligiuri A, Carloni V, DeFranco R, Montalto P, Ceni E, Casini A, Gentilini P, Pinzani M (1997) Effect of pentoxifylline on the degradation of procollagen type I produced by human hepatic stellate cells in response to transforming growth factor-β_1. *Brit J Pharmacol* 122: 1047–1054
269 Unemori EN, Pickford LB, Salles AL, Piercy CE, Grove BH, Erikson ME, Amento EP (1996) Relaxin induces an extracellular matrix-degrading phenotype in human lung fibroblasts *in vitro* and inhibits lung fibrosis in a murine model *in vivo*. *J Clin Invest* 98: 2739–2745
270 Lee BS, Margolin SB, Nowak RA (1998) Pirfenidone: a novel pharmacological agent that inhibits leiomyoma cell proliferation and collagen production. *J Clin Endocrinol Metab* 83: 219–223
271 Iyer SN, Wild JS, Schiedt MJ, Hyde DM, Margolin SB, Giri SN (1995) Dietary intake of pirfenidone ameliorates bleomycin-induced lung fibrosis in hamsters. *J Lab Clin Med* 125: 779–785
272 Border WA, Noble NA, Yamamoto T, Harper JR, Yamaguchi Y, Pierschbacher MD, Ruoslahti E (1992) Natural inhibitor of transforming growth factor β protects against scarring in experimental kidney disease. *Nature* 360: 361–364
273 Isaka Y, Brees DK, Ikegaya K, Kaneda Y, Imai E, Noble NA, Border WA (1996) Gene therapy by skeletal muscle expression of decorin prevents fibrotic disease in rat kidney. *Nature Med* 2: 418–423
274 Mietz H, Chévez-Barrios P, Lieberman MW, Wendt M, Gross R, Basinger SF (1997) Decorin and suramin inhibit ocular fibroblast collagen production. *Graefe's Arch Clin Exp Ophthalmol* 235: 399–403
275 Helene C, Toulme J-J (1990) Specific regulation of gene expression by antisense, sense and antigene nucleic acids. *Biochim Biophys Acta* 1049: 99–125
276 Piguet PF, Collart MA, Grau GE, Kapanci Y, Vassali P (1989) Tumour necrosis factor/cachectin plays a key role in bleomycin-induced pneumopathy and fibrosis. *J Exp Med* 170: 655–663
277 Border WA, Okuda S, Languino LR, Sporn MB, Ruoslahti E (1990) Suppression of experimental glomerulonephritis by antiserum against transforming growth factor β1. *Nature* 346: 371–374
278 Giri SN, Hyde DM, Hollinger MA (1993) Effect of antibody to transforming growth factor β on bleomycin-induced accumulation of lung collagen in mice. *Thorax* 48: 959–966
279 Mutsaers SE, Foster ML, Chambers RC, Laurent GJ, McAnulty RJ (1997) Increased

endothelin-1 and its location during the development of bleomycin-induced pulmonary fibrosis in rats. *Am J Respir Cell Mol Biol* 18: 611–619

280 Sun Y, Zhang JQ, Zhang J, Ramires FJA (1998) Angiotensin II, transforming growth factor-beta 1 and repair in the infarcted heart. *J Mol Cell Cardiol* 30: 1559–1569

281 Kawaguchi H, Kitabatake A (1996) Altered signal transduction system in hypertrophied myocardium: angiotensin II stimulates collagen synthesis in hypertrophied hearts. *J Card Fail* 2: S13–19

282 Nelson DL, Balian G (1984) The effects of retinoic acid on collagen synthesis by human dermal fibroblasts. *Collagen Rel Res* 4: 119–128

283 Oikarinen H, Oikarinen AI, Tan EM, Abergel RP, Meeker CA, Chu ML, Prockop DJ, Uitto J (1985) Modulation of procollagen gene expression by retinoids. Inhibition of collagen production by retinoic acid accompanied by reduced type I procollagen messenger ribonucleic acid levels in human skin fibroblast cultures. *J Clin Invest* 75: 1545–1553

Airway macrophages and dendritic cells

Elaine Lee and Stephen A. Kilfeather

School of Health Sciences, University of Sunderland, Sunderland SR1 3SD, UK

Introduction

This chapter concentrates on mediator release from, and interaction with macrophages, and factors that influence antigen presenting activity of the dendritic cell (DC).

Within the monocytic-type cell lineages present in the airways, alveolar macrophages (AM) have received disproportionately more attention due to their accessibility in human and animal studies compared to interstitial macrophages (IM) and DCs. Despite the accessibility of alveolar macrophages (AM), much pharmacological investigation has been conducted using peripheral blood monocytes as a model of effects on airway macrophages. Immunologists in parallel have charted many aspects of the DC, which has the emerging status of the professional antigen presenting cell. At a relatively early stage, however, certain groups also recognised the existence and importance of DCs as related, but distinct from macrophages in the airway [1]. They also demonstrated a fundamental clinically relevant pharmacological event, that corticosteroids reduce the number of DCs in the airways of asthmatics [2, 3].

Undifferentiated monocytes can be observed in the airway, but their function apart from replenishing the more differentiated cell types, dendrites and macrophages, is not known. Monocytic cells produce a range of cytokines and mediators, and could therefore become involved in defence on arrival at tissues and following diapedesis.

Cells within the macrophage and dendritic types can be derived from the bone marrow-drived monocytic lineage arising from the $CD34^+$ myeloid stem cell in bone marrow [4, 5]. Circulating MHC II negative (Ia^-) precursors can also be made to differentiate into DCs. DCs form <2% of circulating mononuclear cells and comprise subsets differing in phenotype and function [6].

The chameleon nature of cells of the monocytic lineage is demonstrated by the capacity of blood-derived monocytic cells to form cells with fibroblastic, dendritic and macrophage characteristics, all with a range of differentiation states. Airway lumen, mucosal and submucosal regions contain several types of bone marrow-

Cellular Mechanisms in Airways Inflammation, edited by Clive P. Page, Katharine H. Banner and Domenico Spina

derived cells of monocytic lineage at various stages of maturation, differentiation and in relatively discrete groupings in relation to surface marker phenotypic characteristics. Macrophages comprise approximately 80–90% of airway lumen leukocytes under normal conditions and provide a large phagocytic capacity. DCs occupy less than 1% of airway lumen cells [7]. DCs are present throughout the peribronchial connective tissue and bronchus-associated lymphoid tissue (BALT) housing T cells. A network of DCs exists within and below the epithelium, with a higher cell concentration in upper airways. The DC network provides antigen presentation as opposed to phagocytosis and is responsible for transfer of antigenic signals to lymphoid regions for activation of naïve T cells.

The differences between monocyte, macrophage and DC behaviour suggest that the relatively extensive pharmacological analysis of monocytes may not be automatically extrapolated to airway macrophages or DCs. At this stage it is more valuable to assimilate the consolidated findings concerning mediator release from AMs and DCs, and the consistent, but limited pharmacological findings relating to those cells.

Airway macrophages

It is clear that while bone-marrow-derived monocytes are recruited during escalation of an inflammatory response [8] and then divide and differentiate into macrophages [9, 10], there is a resident population of macrophages that provide a scavenging role in detecting pathogens, apoptotic cells and cell debris.

AMs influence airway immunology and inflammation through mediator release, including reactive oxygen intermediates, lipid-derived mediators, cytokines and proteases. Interstitial macrophages below the epithelium also provide an immunomodulatory role in facilitation of DC behaviour and are possibly the cells with the professional responsibility for removal of apoptotic cells in this region.

Pharmacological agents have been used to examine the biochemistry of macrophages *en route* to understanding cytokine expression. The high profile that the alveolar macrophage has sustained as a potential target in immunomodulatory drug development has lead to examination of the potential for current therapeutic agents used in treatment of asthma to influence macrophage activity. In this context, blood-derived monocytes have been examined extensively for investigation of the role of phosphodiesterases 4 (PDE4) as potential drug targets in the context of development of immunomodulatory PDE4 inhibitors.

Cells of the monocytic lineage exhibit considerable size range between cell types. Circulating monocytes do not differ greatly from other circulating leukocytes in size, but on differentiating to macrophages can increase in volume by one to two orders of magnitude. Macrophages cultured for prolonged periods can eventually form multinucleated giant cells resulting from cytokine-induced fusion of macrophages [11, 12].

Turnover rates

Airway AM and DC turnover rates differ markedly and reflect their roles in maintenance of airway defence. AM turnover has been reported to be 16–18 days [13]; longer turnover times for pulmonary macrophages have been recorded at approximately 80 days in humans. Airway mucosal epithelial DC turnover has been demonstrated to be in the region of 2 days [14]. It is noteworthy in this context that the turnover rate of tissue DCs in the iris, airway and intestine have similar rapid turnover rates that are much higher than that of macrophages in the same tissues. Clearly, in view of the rapid DC population turnover and continuity of the DC network in the epithelial region, a constant supply of afferent information from the mucosal surface to lymphoid tissue (BALT) can be sustained by DCs migrating between these sites. Macrophages also have the capacity for migration to lymphoid tissue [15], but lack the potency of DCs in initiating primary immune responses at lymphoid tissue. Their slow turnover in relation to that of DCs could reflect the redundancy of this function. Their established role together with epithelia as effectors in secondary immune responses is discussed below (reviewed in [5]).

Attraction of macrophages into the airway

T-cell derived cytokines and chemokines can recruit monocytic cells to the airway. CD4 cells are the primary instigators of monocyte macrophage recruitment demonstrated by the greater impact of removal of CD-4 cells on macrophage number [16]. Thus, the CC chemokines macrophage inflammatory protein-1α (MIP-1α) and RANTES [17, 18] are potent monocyte chemoattractants. In addition T cell-derived interferon γ (IFNγ), tumour necrosis factor α (TNFα), IL-4 and GM-CSF all are potent inducers of chemokine and adhesion molecule expression to assist in recruitment.

Macrophage activation

Several cell types are engaged in activation of macrophages following initiation of inflammatory responses. These include lymphocytes [19–21], neutrophils [22, 23], eosinophil [24–26] and mast cells [24, 27]. This brings into context the presence of binding sites involved in adhesion with other leukocytes and the consequences of close proximity in mediation of complex autocrine/paracrine interactions.

Intracellular messenger pathways involved with activation

CD14 is a binding site for LPS in monocytes and macrophages [28], but not in DCs, where the lack of expression assists in identity of DCs. CD14 is phosphatidylinositol-linked indicating second messenger pathways involved in transduction of LPS-CD14 interaction signals involved in activation of monocyte macrophages by LPS. This reflects the ubiquitous cell activation pathways provided by phosphatidyl inositol hydrolysis, Ca^{2+} mobilisation and activation of protein kinases. The events relating to control of cytokine expression that are triggered by exposure to major stimulants such as LPS are of relevance to inhibitory effects of corticosteroids. LPS in nanogram/ml concentrations can activate nuclear factor κB (NFκB) [29] and thus induce TNFα production in addition to a host of other mediators. The activation of NFκB by LPS is dependent upon production of reactive oxygen intermediates, especially OH^- [30]. Reactive oxygen intermediates also appear to be a requirement for activation of cycloxygenase-2 (COX2) in macrophages [31]. Macrophages will respond to lower than nanogram/ml levels of LPS by priming of subsequent stimuli, in the absence of an apparent release response to the primary exposure to LPS. Many of the inhibitory effects of corticosteroids on macrophages [32] could be achieved through the inhibitory effects of corticosteroids on NFκB.

Interleukin-1 (IL-1) and TNFα

IL-1 and TNFα are cytokines released from macrophages during primary inflammatory responses and are termed early response cytokines [33]. In common with TNFα, IL-1 stimulates the lymphocyte responses and upregulates the expression of adhesion molecules in endothelial cells to mediate cell recruitment [34]. There is a significant correlation between circulating Il-1 and TNFα and mortality in septisemia and acute lung injury [35]. This is endorsed by the prevention of septic shock by administration of antibodies to TNFα during bacteremia [36]. Following initial rises, LPS-induced TNFα levels *in vitro* and *in vivo* in humans fall following following low level endotoxin administration [37]. This reflects the tight regulation of TNFα production that could involve autocrine/paracrine regulation by factors including prostaglandin E_2 (PGE_2) and interleukin-10 (IL-10) [38]. PGE_2 released from macrophages also inhibits T cell IFNγ production in addition to proliferation. PGE_2 does have a significant influence over the nature of DC antigen presentation as described below.

Interferons

IFNγ is a major macrophage priming cytokine facilitating TNFα, IL-1β and interleukin-6 (IL-6) release in addition to enhancing antimicrobial activity [39]. IFNγ can enhance monocyte TNFα responses to LPS [40].

Transforming growth factor β (TGFβ) and IL-10

TGFβ and IL-10 are released from macrophages and inhibit macrophage activity

[41], thereby restricting lung damage from excessive macrophage activity once the response to pathogen is complete. An example is the protection by IL-10 and IL-4 against immune complex induced lung injury [42]. IL-10 is also potent at blocking antigen presentation by DCs and could contribute to the now recognised inhibitory effects of macrophages on DC-mediated antigen presentation observed *in vivo*.

IL-4/IL-13

These cytokines have also been observed to inhibit macrophage activity [41] and promote a macrophage in which mannose receptor mediated endocytosis predominates with elevated MHC II expression for mediation of humoral immunity [43].

Granulocyte-macrophage colony stimulating factor (GM-CSF)

Granulocyte-macrophage colony stimulating factor (GM-CSF) is non activating, but essential for survival of macrophages and promotes growth and differentiation of both macrophages and DCs, discussed in section II. GM-CSF can also enhance responses to IFNγ [44].

The range of mediators, cytokines, enzymes and growth factors released from macrophages suggest the potential for significant influence on airway disease associated inflammation and remodelling [45]. The pro-inflammatory cytokines and other release products have the capacity to contribute to the airway hyperresponsiveness associated with asthma involving persistent macrophage activation in their aetiology. Much of the evidence for this has been gained in the context of asthma [46]. In the context of COPD on the other hand, persistent production of neutrophil chemoattractants IL-8 [47] and LTB_4 [48] would facilitate the neutrophilia and associated edema and elastase-mediated remodelling associated with this condition [49]. The macrophage-derived growth factors TGFβ and platelet-derived growth factor (PDGF) also present the possibility that macrophages contribute to remodelling through growth factor coupled with metalloproteinase activity [50].

Macrophage recruitment

A range of adhesion molecules are already known to contribute to their migration. The macrophage adhesion molecule profile classified so far includes the following CR3, VLA (1, 2, 4–6), CD31, CD44, CD36, L-selectin, LFA-1, p150,95. Mononuclear cell recruitment is facilitated in response to the CC chemokines, monocyte chemoattractant protein-1 (MCP-1), -2 (MCP-2) and -3 (MCP-3), RANTES, MIP-1α and MIP-1β, I-309 and eotaxin. The CXC chemokines (predominantly attracting neutrophils) include IL-8, ENA-78, IP-10, MIP-2, PF-4, NAP-2, MGSA/gro-α, and gro-β/γ.

MCP-1 can be produced ubiquitously in all tissues and a range of cell types in the airway. MCP-1 also upregulates phagocytic activity [51] and MCP-1 exhibits higher expression in the airways of asthmatics [52] and patients with idiopathic pulmonary fibrosis [53]. RANTES production by airway epithelial cells is promoted by cytokines IL-1 and TNFα [54], LPS exposure [55], and viral infection. MIP-1α is predominantly released from leukocytes and release from macrophage type cells is stimulated by LPS exposure. As with MCP-1, MIP-1α levels are elevated in the airways of patients with IPF and asthma [56].

Macrophages produce the CXC chemokine interleukin-8 (IL-8) demonstrating a potentially major role in recruitment of neutrophils; particularly in view of the significant macrophage leukotriene B_4 (LTB_4) release on activation, which would further facilitate neutrophil chemotaxis.

Lipid products

Leukotrienes are released from macrophages and activate them [24]. The mole percentage of arachidonic acid (AA) in macrophage membranes is of the order of 20–25% whereas in most cells it is approximately 3%. AMs metabolise AA through the 5-LO pathway preferentially as opposed to the cyclooxygenase (COX) pathways [57] and have a large capacity for release of leukotriene products. This is underpinned by the greater quantity of 5-LO and FLAP in AM compared to PBM [58]. Activation of leukotriene production in alveolar macrophages is however 5–10-fold less sensitive to stimulation with Ca^{2+} ionophore compared to neutrophils [59], possibly reflecting a down regulation of responses to external stimuli to prevent excessive activation. Macrophages produce a range of leukotrienes (LTB_4, LTC_4, LTD_4, LTE_4) in addition to platelet activating factor (PAF). LTB_4 is the predominant leukotriene produced by human and rat AMs. The potential excessive production of leukotrienes could assist the development of disease aspects mediated by leukotrienes and opposed by prostaglandins. These could include acute bronchoconstriction and mesenchymal cell hyperplasia leading to increased smooth muscle mass or fibroplasia. One of the more obvious actions of LTB_4 is in chemoattraction of other leukocytes. Chemoattraction by LTB_4 is one of the intended targets in current development of LTB_4 antagonists in treatment of COPD and asthma. LTB_4 antagonists have been shown to inhibit allergen-induced neutropenia in allergic asthmatics [60].

The cysteinyl leukotrienes (LTC_4 and D_4) stimulate vasodilation, increased vascular permeability, bronchoconstriction and mucous secretion. These actions undoubtedly provide targets for the cysteinyl leukotriene receptor antagonists currently marketed for treatment of asthma. PAF also mediates vasodilation, increased vascular permeability and bronchoconstriction.

Therefore, in addition to the priming role of macrophages in initiation of immune responses through release of cytokines including TNFα and IL-1, macrophages can also contribute to the generation of acute inflammation. In this context the interstitial as opposed to alveolar (lumenal) macrophages could be of greater significance due to their proximity to respiratory vasculature and diapedesing cells.

COX-2 is induced by inflammatory stimuli including LPS, PAF, IL-1 and mitogens and downregulated by the immunosuppressive cytokines IL-4 and IL-10. Macrophages thus produce significant amounts of PGE_2 on activation, which provides an inhibitory autocrine signal for macrophages and paracrine signal for inhibition of lymphocyte proliferation.

Enzymes

Macrophages release neutral proteinases (e.g. elastase, collagenase, plasminogen activator) although neutrophil elastase associated with macrophages could be present as a result of uptake from neutrophils. They also release alpha1-antiproteinase, which is targeted for inhibition by bacteria and plays a role in defending the lungs against catabolism.

Reactive oxygen intermediates

Macrophages produce several reactive intermediates including the following: hydrogen peroxide (H_2O_2), singlet oxygen (O:), hydroxyl radicals (OH^-) and super oxide (SO^-). Oxygen intermediates in reaction with nitric oxide (NO) from inflamed airway epithelium can form peroxynitrites, which are more reactive. Although rodent macrophages demonstrate upregulation of inducible NO synthase (iNOS), iNOS induction in human macrophages is difficult to obtain compared to macrophages from rodents and iNOS production in airway inflammation is far more obvious in the epithelium than in the alveolar macrophages.

There are other groups of macrophage activators in addition to inflammatory/immune cytokines. The plasma proteins include Hageman-Factor-related systems including kinins, clotting, fibrinolysis and complement [61].

Phagocytosis

Ligation of macrophage Fc receptors is involved in immunoglobulin-signalled phagocytosis. Macrophages express Fc receptors for IgA [62], the low affinity IgE receptor (CD23) [63] and IgG classes I, II and III [64]. Thus binding sites involved in phagocytosis include the following: FcR (IgG, IgE), CR3, C1qr, mannose receptors. Macrophage mannose receptors together with CD36 and vitronectin receptors are also involved in uptake of apoptotic cells [65].

A major question hangs over the concept of inhibiting macrophage function in general. This could result in reduced uptake of apoptotic cells. A consequence of diminution of this valuable macrophage function could be the promotion of necrotic focii where accumulated apoptotic cells are left to advance into necrosis. Endocytosis could be susceptible to interference from agents interacting with certain G-protein coupled processes, since the recycling of membrane material between intracellular and plasma membrane involves G-protein activity [66].

Macrophage influence over T-cell development

Macrophage products can direct T-cell development in either Th1 or -2 type directions. Thus Th1 promoters include IL-12 [67], TGFβ [68], IL-1β [68]. Th1 supressors include IL-10, PGE_2 [69], TGFβ [70]. TGFβ appears to be able to promote Th1 or Th2 responses depending upon conditions. When AMs encounter a foreign antigen a Th1 response is normally elicited. In asthma however, there appears to be a predominance of Th2 activity. Whether this is influenced by macrophage-derived mediators or those of other cells at the point of initial antigen detection such as the DC or epithelium is not established. Alternatively, the DC could be a major director of T-cell differentiation independently of the macrophage within the lymph node and therefore in the absence of cells at the mucosal surface. Activated T cells already present at the mucosal surface may be further stimulated by MHC II-bearing cells not expressing the required co-stimulatory molecules for activation of naive cells in lymph nodes by DC. Thus macrophages and epithelial cells could be involved in sustaining either Th-1 or -2 type responses at the mucosal surface in secondary immune responses [71].

Macrophage inhibition of antigen presentation by dendritic cells

Depletion of AM by intratracheal administration of liposomes containing diphosphonate toxic for macrophages results in marked upregulation of antibody production in regional lymph nodes following intrapulmonary administration of antigen [72]. Macrophage inhibition of T-cell activation could be mediated by a range of inhibitory factors including IL-1 receptor antagonist [73], soluble TNFα receptor [74], H_2O_2, PGE_2, IL-10 [75] and reduced IL-1 and B7 co-stimulatory molecule expression [76]. IL-1 receptor antagonist, while exhibiting anti-inflammatory activity has not demonstrated inhibition of APC-mediated T-cell activation [73]. Similarly the concentrations of TNFα receptor required to inhibit APC-mediated T-cell activation are several orders of magnitude higher than those required to inhibit TNFα induced inflammatory reactions, which are of the order of five times the active TNFα concentrations.

The concept of macrophages as modulators of antigen presentation raises the possibility that certain macrophage activities may be of some benefit under conditions of excessive inflammation.

Effects of drugs

Corticosteroids

Corticosteroids reduce the transcription of the early response gene JE, expression of TNFα [77], MCP-1 [32], MIP-1α [78], production of IL-8 [79] and metalloproteinases [80]. Pretreatment of AM with corticosteroids also inhibits AA release and consequent production of leukotrienes and prostaglandins [81]. Corticosteroids also inhibit RANTES production from the epithelium, which reflects the capacity of corticosteroids to indirectly influence macrophage recruitment and activity.

The damping of excessive macrophage immune/inflammatory product release by corticosteroids may also impinge upon the macrophage capacity for endocytosis of apoptotic cells. This could conceivably promote accumulation of necrotic cells as described above. This concept has not been adequately explored.

Elevation of cyclic AMP

Macrophages possess beta-adrenoceptors that function in terms of stimulation of production of cyclic adenosine monophosphate (cyclic AMP), but beta-adrenoceptor stimulation with the full agonist isoprenaline has not been found to inhibit alveolar macrophage superoxide production or release of thromboxane B2 [82]. Forskolin, a direct activator of adenylate cyclase and cyclic AMP production did in the same study inhibit macrophage activation. In addition AM β-receptor stimulation had no effect on oxidative metabolism or phagocytic activity [83]. The disparity in actions of forskolin and β-adrenoceptor agonists could be attributable to their relative efficacy in elevation of cyclic AMP; forskolin being far more efficacious than β-agonists. There is also the possibility that differential cell responsiveness to forskolin and β-receptor-stimulated cyclic AMP levels could involve differences in capacity of macrophage PDEs to remove cyclic AMP generated in response to these agents.

Phosphodiesterase inhibition

The potential for elevation of cyclic AMP to provide a means of inhibition of inflammatory cell activity or immunomodulation has lead to an extensive search for compounds that will inhibit the predominant PDE type 4 present in inflammatory cells responsible for hydrolysis of cyclic AMP. PDE4 is the predominant cell type present in monocytes and its inhibition results in marked inhibition of LPS-stimulated monocyte TNFα production. The relevance of this observation to macrophage activity and the enormous amount of data generated in finding a PDE4 inhibitor for treatment of inflammatory diseases may be reduced by our observation and others [84] that PDE4 inhibition alone does not influence LPS-stimulated macrophage TNFα production (Fig. 1) or stimulated macrophage TXB2 or LTB_4 production. The explanation for the disparity between the response of monocytes and macrophages to PDE4 inhibition is probably due to the large amount of PDE1 present in monocyte-derived macrophages and alveolar macrophages in addition to many of the other PDE types [85]. The large PDE1 type activity is far in excess of that of PDE4 in macrophages and will possibly provide sufficient cyclic AMP hydrolysis in the presence of full PDE4 inhibition. Combined PDE3 and 4 inhibition, however, has inhibited macrophage TNFα production [84], suggesting that PDE3 in addition to PDE1 and 4 is important.

Dendritic cells

The requirement for contact interaction between DCs and lymphocytes in initiation of primary responses underscores the significance of cell surface adhesion molecule and co-stimulatory molecules expression in these cells. This assists identity and staging in maturation of DCs and there is far more information concerning this aspect of DC behaviour than the production and release of cytokines.

DCs *in vitro* and *in vivo* display dendriform "veil"-like projections (lamellipodia). *In vivo*, DCs interdigitate with the airway epithelia at a density of 500–800 cells/mm^2 in the larger human bronchioles [86]. The dendritic network at the base of the airway epithelium provides an essentially continuous barrier, more so in the upper airways, ensuring detection of foreign material traversing the epithelium.

Antigen processing

Primary responses to antigen involve uptake and processing of antigen prior to presentation of antigen peptide fragments to T lymphocytes in lymphoid tissue *via* MHC II (Fig. 2). The morphology and activity in the immature DC indicate considerable energy expenditure in sampling and processing foreign material for presentation. Coupled with the potency of DCs in antigen presentation leading to lymphocyte activation, the DC exhibits the characteristics of a professional antigen presenting cell. Antigen uptake is mediated by relatively specific and nonspecific routes. A nonspecific route involves macropinocytosis using the lamellipodia to form vesicles and recycle extracellular fluid at a rate of one cell volume per hour [87]. Specific uptake of antigen is mediated by two identified multilectin-type receptors found on DCs with 8 or 10 carbohydrate recognition domains. The macrophage mannose receptor with 8 lectin binding domains recognises mannosylated proteins. The second receptor carrying 10 lectin domains (DEC-105) has not been associated with any particular ligand so far.

Therefore, while macrophages are phagocytic for removal of pathogens and debris, DCs are not phagocytic, but internalise antigen for the purpose of processing involving coupling to MHC II molecules for presentation to T cells at the cell surface upon maturation.

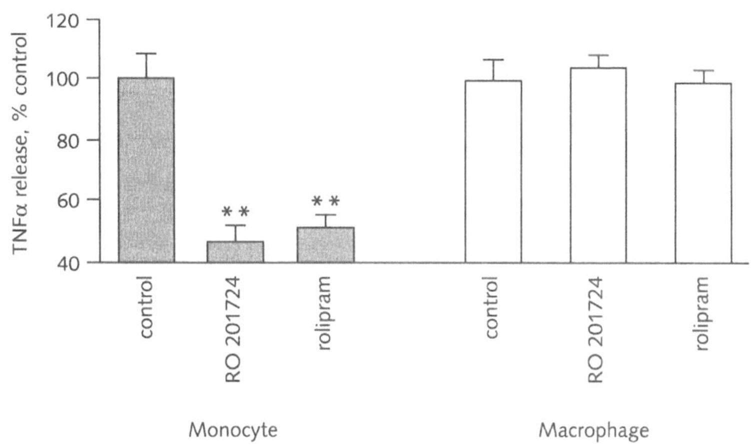

Figure 1
Effect of PDE4 inhibition on monocyte and macrophage TNFα production. Human peripheral blood monocytes and macrophages matured from the same monocyte population were exposed to LPS (100 ng/ml) in the presence and absence of PDE4 inhibitors rolipram (1 μM) and RO 201724 (1 μM). TNFα accumulation was measured after 18 h by ELISA.

Isolated DCs lacking the maturity for antigen presentation possess adequate antigen processing capacity [88]. The processing capacity diminishes as DCs mature in readiness for antigen presentation. This process is visible through changes in cell surface marker expression including upregulation of adhesion and co-stimulatory molecules [89, 90].

Cell surface markers and accessory molecules

The emergence of the DC as the professional antigen presenting cell raises the importance of the nature of cell surface protein interactions that are possible between the DC and lymphocyte. Many of these cell surface markers which vary depending upon the maturational status of the DC are involved in co-stimulation as accessory molecules (Fig. 2). The restrictive markers currently recognised are DEC-205 (murine), 0X62 (rat) and CD83 and p55 (human).

In primary immune responses GM-CSF and IL-4 induced DC maturation upregulate the expression of the primary accessory molecule-derived stimulation through B7-1 (CD80) or B7-2 (CD86) and CD-28. Blocking studies have shown that CD28 and CD86 are equally necessary in promoting the Th2 bias observed in allergic

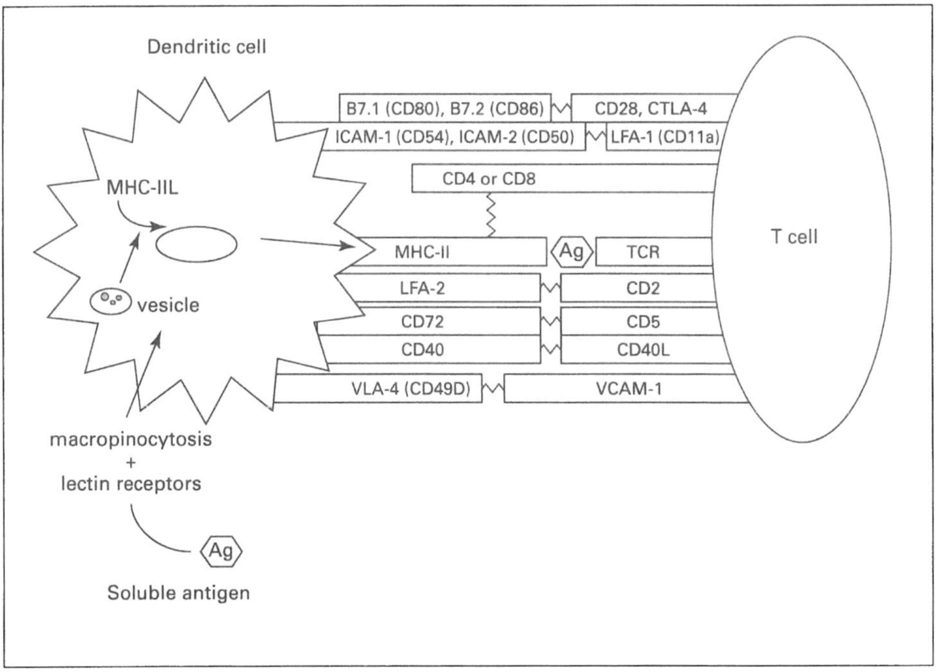

Figure 2
Antigen processing by dendritic cells and presentation to T lymphocytes.

immune states. In secondary immune responses, however, activated T cells (IL-2 producing) can be further activated by interaction with other MHC II expressing cells in conjunction with minimal co-stimulation; through ICAM-1 for example. This has relevance not only to secondary immune responses, but the maintenance of immune abnormalities in chronic diseases such as asthma.

Cytokine influence

The difficulty in isolating DCs contributes to the relatively small amount of information concerning DC release products compared with macrophages. The mechanisms utilised by DCs to transmit signals concerning antigen presentation that directs lymphocyte development toward either Th1 or Th2 pathways are now being explored. IL-12 , PGE_2 and IL-10 appear to play significant roles. IL-12 is released from DCs and facilitates T-cell IFNγ production [91]. Thus, IL-12, as observed in other tissues, promotes a Th1 bias, while PGE_2 and IL-10 promote Th2 bias. PGE_2 can also promote antigen presentation and lymphocyte responses, while IL-10 is inhibitory against presentation and lymphocyte response.

IL-1 in conjunction with GM-CSF enhances DC immunostimulatory capacity [92]. IL-2 and IFNγ are strong stimuli for increasing DC content in the airways. The actions of IL-2 and IFNγ suggest that Th1 responses facilitate recruitment of DC.

GM-CSF, TNFα and IL-4 appear to be the most effective promoters of DC differentiation from immature cells leading to a DC population exhibiting potent lymphocyte activation [93]. Blockade of TNFα activity markedly reduces antigen presentation-induced T-cell activation mediated by DCs or exposure to anti-CD3 antibodies [94]. TNFα enhances maturation of DCs and facilitates their antigen presenting activity. It is conceivable that activation of mast cells and consequent release of TNFα is involved in the priming of DC antigen presenting activity.

Macrophage depletion upregulates DC antigen presenting activity. Macrophages appear therefore to provide both autocrine and paracrine inhibition of macrophage and DC activation. IL-10 is a possible candidate for involvement in inhibition of DC activity by macrophages. IL-10 inhibits the expression of surface antigens on APCs including B7 and MHC II [95] and the release of TNFα [75], IL-10 may also reduce DC densities by facilitating apoptosis [96].

Immunoglobulins

Immunoglobulin receptors on DCs mediate enhancement of their antigen presenting activity by IgE and IgG. In this context the facilitiation of antigen presenting activity by IL-4 can occur through two routes. Firstly, IL-4 and GM-CSF are the primary stimuli for dendritic cell maturation [93]. Secondly, IL-4 promotes B-cell IgE production, an action that would sustain the atopic reactions through IgE facilitation of DC antigen presentation.

Chemoattraction

DCs are also stimulated to migrate by C5a, N-formyl-met-leu-phe (FMLP) and the CC chemokines monocyte chemoattractant protein (MCP-3), MIP-1α/LD78 and RANTES. IL-8 is not chemoattractant for DC and together these findings suggest a distinct pattern of chemoattractant stimuli for DCs and neutrophils. The migration of DCs, in other tissues (intestine, heart and kidneys) or analogous dermal "Langerhans cell" (LC) is promoted by TNFα; a process that is sensitive to blockade by MoAb to TNFα [97].

DC maturation

The contribution of groups engaged in airway immunology has been considerable in the context of knowledge gained concerning DC antigen presentation, but there is at present a relative deficit in the knowledge concerning the functional relationship between the DC and others in the airway, with the exception of the T cell.

Antigen challenge can induce a rapid (within hours) increase in the airway DC population. This implies that there is a resident population of dendritic precursors in readiness to mobilise immune responses. This is also implied by experiments involving irradiation [98]. Following local irradiation, the antigen-induced increase in monocytic cells within the airway is delayed to approximately 3 days, implying that a local source of cells contributes to the turnover. $CD14^+$ circulating monocytes can differentiate to DC, but it is not yet established that these cells provide the sole source of DC within the airway, or whether a bone marrow derived precursor is an alternative source.

DCs exist in a range of maturational states leading toward DC cell types with the capacity for antigen presentation at lymph nodes. The level of DC maturity is influenced by a range of local environmental factors including antigen exposure, cell-cell contact and local cytokine mileu. There are DCs within the airway that do not express MHC II and are possibly restricted from doing so by local factors until the DCs migrate from the epithelial region toward lymph node areas where maturation is completed in a lymphocytic environment. Mature dendritic cells express in the region of 10^6 MHC II molecules [99]. Although GM-CSF is an effective vector in driving DCs toward maturation for antigen presentation, exposure to GM-CSF alone is insufficient and the condition of precursor cells and local tissue environment are also important [100]. The conditioning of airway DCs is further complicated in the presence of chronic inflammation. Under such conditions GM-CSF, normally encountered at BALT and lymphocyte-derived, can be supplied by other cells in the mucosa including epithelia. Thus DC maturation for antigen presentation can be attained in the region of antigen entry under conditions of established inflammation and suggests the role of DCs in secondary immune responses at the epithelia. Under these circumstances activated interstitial macrophages could facilitate DC-mediated presentation. Furthermore, activated lymphocytes, particularly those in activation states, producing IL-2, have a reduced requirement for specific co-stimulatory molecule interaction. Under such conditions, many cells expressing MHC-II can facilitate antigen presentation provided they have certain surface molecules that have co-stimulatory function. This may include epithelial cells [71].

Effect of topical exposure to bacteria, virus and allergen on expansion of MHC II bearing DCs

McWilliams and colleagues [101] have investigated the effects of topical administration of bacteria, virus and allergen on airway MHC II bearing DC populations. Inhalation of bacteria (dead or live *Moxarella catarrhalis*) results in rapid upregulation of the MHC II bearing DCs and is maximal within 1 h of acute exposure (30–60 min). The morphology of the cells suggested an influx of immature Ia^+ DCs that underwent maturation over the following hours. Exposure to allergen in sensitised animals results in an increase in MHC II bearing DCs with a similar time-course to that following exposure to bacteria. Exposure to virus, however, while evoking an expansion of MHCII expressing DCs, exhibits a time course incorporating a lag phase of several days consistent with other immune/inflammatory responses to viral exposure.

Allergy and sensitised states

The DC population expands under conditions of sensitisation to allergen [102], allergic rhinitis [103] and asthma [104]. The sustained higher level of DCs in the airway of asthmatics may not represent a reduction of migration of cells to the lymph nodes, but a functional higher steady-state of equilibrium between recruitment and migration to lymph nodes. Thus elevated signalling for recruitment could ensure an accelerated supply of antigen, while the increased capacity for detection at the mucusoal surface is matched by increased volume of trafficking for signalling at the afferent lymphoid tissue.

The significant influence of GM-CSF in driving the differentiation toward DC has important implications in the maintenance of antigen presentation and its amplification in conditions such as asthma. GM-CSF is released from a range of cells in the airway, some of which are present in high concentration such the epithelium, mast cell and lymphocytes expressing predominantly Th2 in allergic states. The generation and enhancement of antigen presenting cell (APC) activity by GM-CSF is facilitated by interleukin-4 (IL-4), another cytokine released by the Th2-type phenotype and other cells in the airway including mast cells. These cytokines could therefore be involved in promoting DC activity in sensitised states under conditions of epithelial, mast cell and Th2 cell activation and elevated release of these cytokines from these cells.

Effects of drugs

Corticosteroids

Nelson and colleagues have demonstrated that inhaled commercially available corticosteroids including fluticasone, beclomethasone and budesonide significantly reduce rat airway DC density [105]. Systemic administration of high doses of dexamethasone were also accompanied by loss of DCs. The kinetics of the corticosteroid-mediated dendritic loss indicated that most of the effect is established within 24 h through either route of administration and recovery is achieved on removal of corticosteroid within 2 days. The recovery probably reflects the rapid turnover of DC in the airways, which appears to be more rapid than in the periphery.

The reduction in proportion of Ia^+ cells by corticosteroids was greater than the reduction in total DC density, but nevertheless demonstrates ablation of the APC section of the DC population. This group also demonstrated the inhibition by corticosteroids of increasing Ia^+ expression among DCs during weaning and DC expansion following irradiation and subsequent bone marrow administration. The latter finding indicates an interruption of the entry of DC to the airways, although whether this involves an inhibition of adhesion or subsequent diapedesis has not been established.

Nelson and colleagues also demonstrated the capacity of inhaled corticosteroids to undermine the bacteria-induced upregulation of MHC II cells [105]. Again it is not certain to what extent this inhibition measured at 24 h following exposure to bacteria involves interruption of upregulation of MHC II expression or the shift to a steady-state of cell concentration involving a greater DC content through cell influx in conjunction with upregulation of MHC II expression.

Moller and colleagues demonstrated elevated density in atopic asthmatics treated with bronchodilators alone compared with those treated with corticosteroids [106]. The level of DCs present in those treated with corticosteroid approached levels observed in nonasthmatic subjects.

Neuropeptides

DCs residing in the airway epithelium are in close proximity to neuronal cells. Interaction with neurotransmitters is therefore unavoidable. In this context substance P, a nonadrenergic noncholinergic (NANC) neuropeptide rerleased at this site promotes DC motility *in vitro* and DC accumulation *in vivo* can be blocked by capsaicin, which depletes substance P [107]. Calcitonin gene related peptide (CGRP) is a major neuropeptide and produced by airway epithelial cells [108] and suppresses B7-2 expression by DCs and peritoneal macrophages and antigen presentation by Langerhans cells [109]. This is interesting in the context of cyclic AMP, which usually provides a route for the damping of immune inflammatory responses. CGRP elevates cyclic AMP levels and this action in DC coupled with a reduction in B7-2 expression could be an indication that DCs respond to cyclic AMP in a manner consistent with other mononuclear cells. This does not, however, appear to be a universal finding of agents that stimulate cyclic AMP production as discussed below.

Modulation of Th1 and Th2 bias in lymphocytes by cyclic AMP

PGE_2 works in opposition to IL-12 in regulation of T-cell differentation. Thus, PGE_2, which is a stimulus of cyclic AMP production directs T-cell development toward Th2 type and assists in maturation [110]. IL-12 is a consistent promoter of the Th1 type and the direction of Th development appears to be under the influence of PGE_2:IL-12 ratio. Despite the significant effects of PGE_2 on T-cell responses to DC presentation, the range of possible effects of cyclic AMP elevating agents on DC function in terms of T-cell differentiation has not been fully explored.

Conclusions

A system of airway immunity is emerging in which macrophages and dendritic cells provide distinct roles. Macrophages provide efficient phagocytic activity, while dendritic cells are the professional antigen presenting cell. The activity of macrophages and dendritic cells is influenced by cytokines through paracrine and autocrine pathways. It is prudent to consider the influence of other cell types in close proximity in the execution of the roles of these cell types. For dendritic cells in the airway the influence of the epithelium appears to be unavoidable. The effects of application of exogenous agents on these cell types in the context of pharmacology have received relatively little attention compared to their roles in maintenance of immune and inflammatory activity.

References

1 Poulter LW, Janossy G (1985) The involvement of dendritic cells in chronic inflammatory disease. *Scand J Immunol* 21: 401–407

2 Burke C, Power CK, Norris A, Condez A, Schmekel B, Poulter LW (1992) Lung-function and immunopathological changes after inhaled corticosteroid-therapy in asthma. *Eur Respir J* 5: 73–79

3 Burke CM, Sreenan S, Pathmakanthan S, Patterson J, Schmekel B, Poulter LW (1996) Relative effects of inhaled corticosteroids on immunopathology and physiology in asthma: A controlled study. *Thorax* 51: 993–999

4 Reid CDL, Fryer PR, Clifford C, Kirk A, Tikerpae J, Knight SC (1990) Identification of hematopoietic progenitors of macrophages and dendritic Langerhans cells (Dl-cfu). In human bone-marrow and peripheral-blood. *Blood* 76: 1139–1149

5 Stein M, Keshav S (1992) The versatility of macrophages. *Clin Exp Allergy* 22: 19–27

6 Knight SC, Stagg A, Hill S, Fryer P, Griffiths S (1992) Development and function of dendritic cells in health and disease. *J Invest Dermatol* 99: S33–S38

7 Vanhaarst JMW, Dewit HJ, Drexhage HA, Hoogsteden HC (1994) Distribution and immunophenotype of mononuclear phagocytes and dendritic cells in the human lung. *Am J Respir Cell Mol Biol* 10: 487–492

8 Vanoudalblas AB, Vanfurth R (1982) The origin of pulmonary macrophages. *Immunobiology* 161: 186–192

9 Tarling JD, Lin H, Hsu S (1987) Self-renewal of pulmonary alveolar macrophages – evidence from radiation chimera studies. *J Leuk Biol* 42: 443–446

10 Chandler DB, Fuller WC, Jackson RM, Fulmer JD (1986) Studies of membrane-receptors and phagocytosis in subpopulations of rat alveolar macrophages. *Am Rev Respir Dis* 133: 461–467

11 Mcinnes A, Rennick DM (1988) Interleukin-4 induces cultured monocytes macrophages to form giant multinucleated cells. *J Exp Med*167: 598–611

12 Weinberg JB, Hobbs MM, Misukonis MA (1984) Recombinant human gamma-interferon induces human monocyte polykaryon formation. *Proc Natl Acad Sci USA* 81: 4554–4557
13 Parwaresch MR, Wacker HH (1984) Origin and kinetics of resident tissue macrophages – parabiosis studies with radiolabeled leukocytes. *Cell Tissue Kinet* 17: 25–39
14 Holt PG, Haining S, Nelson DJ, Sedgwick JD (1994) Origin and steady-state turnover of class-ii mhc-bearing dendritic cells in the epithelium of the conducting airways. *J Immunol* 153: 256–261
15 Rosen H, Gordon S (1990) Adoptive transfer of fluorescence-labeled cells shows that resident peritoneal-macrophages are able to migrate into specialized lymphoid organs and inflammatory sites in the mouse. *Eur J Immunol* 20: 1251–1258
16 Shellito J, Kaltreider HB (1985) Heterogeneity of immunological function among subfractions of normal rat alveolar macrophages. 2. Activation as a determinant of functional-activity. *Am Rev Respir Dis* 131: 678–683
17 Dethloff LA, Lehnert BE (1988) Pulmonary interstitial macrophages – isolation and flow cytometric comparisons with alveolar macrophages and blood monocytes. *J Leuk Biol* 43: 80–90
18 Thet LA, Wrobel DJ, Crapo JD, Shelburne JD (1983) Morphologic aspects of the protection by endotoxin against acute and chronic oxygen-induced lung injury in adult-rats. *Lab Invest* 48: 448–457
19 Doherty TM (1995) T-cell regulation of macrophage function. *Current Op Immunol* 7: 400–404
20 Nacy CA, Meltzer MS (1991) T-cell-mediated activation of macrophages. *Current Op Immunol* 3: 330–335
21 Paulnock DM (1992) Macrophage activation by T-cells. *Current Op Immunol* 4: 344–349
22 Strieter RM, Koch AE, Antony VB, Fick RB, Standiford TJ, Kunkel SL (1994) The immunopathology of chemotactic cytokines – the role of interleukin-8 and monocyte chemoattractant protein-1. *J Lab Clin Med* 123: 183–197
23 Xing Z, Jordana M, Kirpalani H, Driscoll KE, Schall TJ, Gauldie J (1994) Cytokine expression by neutrophils and macrophages *in vivo* – endotoxin induces tumor-necrosis-factor-alpha, macrophage inflammatory protein-2, interleukin-1-beta, and interleukin-6 but not rantes or transforming growth factor-beta(1). Messenger-RNA expression in acute lung inflammation. *Am J Respir Cell Mol Biol* 10: 148–153
24 Chavis C, Godard P, Michel FB, Depaulet AC, Damon M (1991) Sulfidopeptide leukotrienes contribute to human alveolar macrophage activation in asthma. *Prostagland Leukotrienes Essential Fatty Acids* 42: 95–100
25 Moqbel R (1994) Eosinophils, cytokines, and allergic inflammation. *Ann NY Acad Sci* 725: 223–233
26 Spessotto P, Dri P, Bulla R, Zabucchi G, Patriarca P (1995) Human eosinophil peroxidase enhances tumor-necrosis-factor and hydrogen-peroxide release by human monocyte-derived macrophages. *Eur J Immunol* 25: 1366–1373

27 Dackiw APB, Nathens AB, Ribeiro MB, Cheung PYC, Marshall JC, Rotstein OD (1995) Mast-cell modulation of macrophage procoagulant activity and tnf production. *J Surg Res* 59: 1–5
28 Standiford TJ, Kunkel SL, Kasahara K, Milia MJ, Rolfe MW, Strieter RM (1991) Interleukin-8 gene-expression from human alveolar macrophages – the role of adherence. *Am J Respir Cell Mol Biol* 5: 579–585
29 Murphy JF, Mcgregor JL, Leung LLK (1998) Senescent human neutrophil binding to thrombospondin (TSP) – evidence for a TSP-independent pathway of phagocytosis by macrophages. *Br J Haematology* 102: 957–964
30 Muller JM, Zieglerheitbrock HWL, Baeuerle PA (1993) Nuclear factor kappa-b, a mediator of lipopolysaccharide effects. *Immunobiology* 187: 233–256
31 Feng L, Xia YY, Garcia GE, Hwang D, Wilson CB (1995) Involvement of reactive oxygen intermediates in cyclooxygenase-2 expression induced by interleukin-1, tumor-necrosis-factor-alpha, and lipopolysaccharide. *J Clin Invest* 95: 1669–1675
32 Kawahara RS, Deng ZW, Deuel TF (1991) Glucocorticoids inhibit the transcriptional induction of je, a platelet-derived growth factor-inducible gene. *J Biol Chem* 266: 13261–13266
33 Beutler B (1990) The tumor necrosis factors – cachectin and lymphotoxin. *Hospital Practice* 25: 45–56
34 Dinarello CA (1988) Interleukin-1. *Ann NY Acad Sci* 546: 122–132
35 Waage A, Halstensen A, Espevik T (1987) Association between tumor-necrosis-factor in serum and fatal outcome in patients with meningococcal disease. *Lancet* 1: 355–357
36 Tracey KJ, Fong Y, Hesse DG, Manogue KR, Lee AT, Kuo GC, Lowry SF, Cerami A (1987) Anti-cachectin tnf monoclonal-antibodies prevent septic shock during lethal bacteremia. *Nature* 330: 662–664
37 Michie HR, Manogue KR, Spriggs DR, Revhaug A, Odwyer S, Dinarello CA, Cerami A, Wolff SM, Wilmore DW (1988) Detection of circulating tumor necrosis factor after endotoxin administration. *N Engl J Med* 318: 1481–1486
38 Sherry B, Cerami A (1988) Cachectin tumor necrosis factor exerts endocrine, paracrine, and autocrine control of inflammatory responses. *J Cell Biol* 107: 1269–1277
39 Dalton DK, Pittsmeek S, Keshav S, Figari IS, Bradley A, Stewart TA (1993) Multiple defects of immune cell-function in mice with disrupted interferon-gamma genes. *Science* 259: 1739–1742
40 Pace JL (1981) Activation of mouse macrophages for tumor-cell killing 1 Quantitative-analysis of interactions between lymphokine and lipopolysaccharide. *J Immunol* 126: 1863–1867
41 Bogdan C, Nathan C (1993) Modulation of macrophage function by transforming growth-factor-beta, interleukin-4, and interleukin-10. *Ann NY Acad Sci* 685: 713–739
42 Mulligan MS, Jones ML, Vaporciyan AA, Howard MC, Ward PA (1993) Protective effects of IL-4 and IL-10 against immune complex-induced lung injury. *J Immunol* 151: 5666–5674

43 Gordon S, Clarke S, Greaves D, Doyle A (1995) Molecular immunobiology of macrophages – recent progress. *Current Op Immunol* 7: 24–33

44 Chen GH, Curtis JL, Mody CH, Christensen PJ, Armstrong LR, Toews GB (1994) Effect of granulocyte-macrophage colony-stimulating factor on rat alveolar macrophage anticryptococcal activity *in vitro*. *J Immunol* 152: 724–734

45 Laskin DL, Pendino KJ (1995) Macrophages and inflammatory mediators in tissue-injury. *Ann Rev Pharmacol Toxicol* 35: 655–677

46 Kips JC, Tavernier J, Pauwels RA (1992) Tumor-necrosis-factor causes bronchial hyper-responsiveness in rats. *Am Rev Respir Dis* 145: 332–336

47 Strieter RM, Chensue SW, Basha MA, Standiford TJ, Lynch JP, Baggiolini M, Kunkel SL (1990) Human alveolar macrophage gene-expression of interleukin-8 by tumor necrosis factor-alpha, lipopolysaccharide, and interleukin-1-beta. *Am J Respir Cell Mol Biol* 2: 321–326

48 Martin TR, Pistorese BP, Chi EY, Goodman RB, Matthay MA (1989) Effects of leukotriene-b4 in the human-lung – recruitment of neutrophils into the alveolar spaces without a change in protein permeability. *J Clin Invest* 84: 1609–1619

49 Terashima T, Kanazawa M, Sayama K, Urano T, Sakamaki F, Nakamura H, Waki Y, Soejima K, Tasaka S, Ishizaka A (1995) Neutrophil-induced lung protection and injury are dependent on the amount of pseudomonas-aeruginosa administered *via* airways in guinea-pigs. *Am J Respir Crit Care Med* 152: 2150–2156

50 Khalil N, Greenberg AH (1991) The role of tgf-beta in pulmonary fibrosis. *Ciba Foundation Symposia* 157: 194–211

51 Reynolds HY (1988) Immunoglobulin-g and its function in the human respiratory-tract. *Mayo Clinic Proceedings* 63: 161–174

52 Bergamaschini L, Santangelo T, Faricciotti A, Ciavarella N, Mannucci PM, Agostoni A (1996) Study of complement-mediated anaphylaxis in humans – The role of IgG subclasses (IgG1 and/or IgG4) in the complement-activating capacity of immune complexes. *J Immunol* 156: 1256–1261

53 Burton DR (1985) Immunoglobulin-γ – functional sites. *Mol Immunol* 22: 161–206

54 Kerr MA (1990) The structure and function of human-IgA. *Biochem J* 271: 285–296

55 Mazanec MB, Nedrud JG, Kaetzel CS, Lamm ME (1993) A 3-tiered view of the role of iga in mucosal defense. *Immunol Today* 14: 430–435

56 Debecker G, Sornasse T, Nabavi N, Bazin H, Tielemans F, Urbain J, Leo O, Moser M (1994) Immunoglobulin isotype regulation by antigen-presenting cells *in vivo*. *Eur J Immunol* 24: 1523–1528

57 Petersgolden M, Mcnish RW, Hyzy R, Shelly C, Toews GB (1990) Alterations in the pattern of arachidonate metabolism accompany rat macrophage differentiation in the lung. *J Immunol* 144: 263–270

58 Coffey MJ, Wilcoxen SE, Petersgolden M (1994) Increases in 5-lipoxygenase activating protein expression account for enhanced capacity for 5-lipoxygenase metabolism that accompanies differentiation of peripheral-blood monocytes into alveolar macrophages. *Am J Respir Cell Mol Biol* 11: 153–158

59 Grimminger F, Sibelius U, Seeger W (1991) Amplification of LTB4 generation in ampmn cocultures – transcellular 5-lipoxygenase metabolism. *Am J Physiol* 261: L195–L203

60 Evans DJ, Barnes PJ, Spaethe SM, Vanalstyne EL, Mitchell MI, OConnor BJ (1996) Effect of a leukotriene B-4 receptor antagonist, LY293111, on allergen induced responses in asthma. *Thorax* 51: 1178–1184

61 Wachtfogel YT, Delacadena RA, Colman RW (1993) Structural biology, cellular interactions and pathophysiology of the contact system. *Thrombosis Res* 72: 1–21

62 Gauldie J, Richards C, Lamontagne L (1983) Fc-receptors for IgA and other immunoglobulins on resident and activated alveolar macrophages. *Mol Immunol* 20: 1029–1037

63 Williams J, Johnson S, Mascali JJ, Smith H, Rosenwasser LJ, Borish L (1992) Regulation of low affinity IgE receptor (Cd23) Expression on mononuclear phagocytes in normal and asthmatic subjects. *J Immunol* 149: 2823–2829

64 Kindt GC, Vandewinkel JGJ, Moore SA, Anderson CL (1991) Identification and structural characterization of fc-gamma-receptors on pulmonary alveolar macrophages. *Am J Physiol* 260: L403–L411

65 Ren Y, Silverstein RL, Allen J, Savill J (1995) Cd36 gene-transfer confers capacity for phagocytosis of cells undergoing apoptosis. *J Exp Med* 181: 1857–1862

66 Beron W, Alvarezdominguez C, Mayorga L, Stahl PD (1995) Membrane trafficking along the phagocytic pathway. *Trends Cell Biol* 5: 100–104

67 Hall SS (1995) Il-12 at the crossroads. *Science* 268: 1432–1434

68 Romagnani S (1994) Lymphokine production by human T-cells in disease states. *Ann Rev Immunol* 12: 227–257

69 Abe N, Katamura K, Shintaku N, Fukui T, Kiyomasu T, Iio J, Ueno H, Tai GX, Mayumi M, Furusho K (1997) Prostaglandin E-2 and IL-4 provide naive CD4(+) T cells with distinct inhibitory signals for the priming of IFN-gamma production. *Cell Immunol* 181: 86–92

70 Maeda H, Shiraishi A (1996) TGF-beta contributes to the shift toward Th2-type responses through direct and IL-10-mediated pathways in tumor-bearing mice. *J Immunol* 156: 73–78

71 Cunningham AC, Zhang JG, Moy JV, Ali S, Kirby JA (1997) A comparison of the antigen-presenting capabilities of class II MHC- expressing human lung epithelial and endothelial cells. *Immunology* 91: 458–463

72 Holt PG, Oliver J, Bilyk N, Mcmenamin C, Mcmenamin PG, Kraal G, Thepen T (1993) Down-regulation of the antigen presenting cell function(s). Of pulmonary dendritic cells *in vivo* by resident alveolar macrophages. *J Exp Med*177: 397–407

73 Nicod LP, Elhabre F, Dayer JM (1992) Natural and recombinant interleukin-1 receptor antagonist does not inhibit human T-cell proliferation induced by mitogens, soluble-antigens or allogeneic determinants. *Cytokine* 4: 29–35

74 Nicod LP, Galvederochemonteix B, Dayer JM (1994) Modulation of IL-1 receptor

antagonist and TNF-soluble receptors produced by alveolar macrophages and blood monocytes. *Ann NY Acad Sci* 725: 323–330
75 Nicod LP, Elhabre F, Dayer JM, Boehringer N (1995) Interleukin-10 decreases tumor-necrosis-factor-alpha and tumor- necrosis-factor-beta in alloreactions induced by human lung dendritic cells and macrophages. *Am J Respir Cell Mol Biol* 13: 83–90
76 Chelen CJ, Fang Y, Freeman GJ, Secrist H, Marshall JD, Hwang PT, Frankel LR, Dekruyff RH, Umetsu DT (1995) Human alveolar macrophages present antigen ineffectively due to defective expression of B7 costimulatory cell-surface molecules. *J Clin Invest* 95: 1415–1421
77 Ralph P, Jeong G, Welte K, Mertelsmann R, Rabin H, Henderson LE, Souza LM, Boone TC, Robb RJ (1984) Stimulation of immunoglobulin secretion in human lymphocytes-b as a direct effect of high-concentrations of IL-2. *J Immunol* 133: 2442–2445
78 Berkman N, Jose PJ, Williams TJ, Schall TJ, Barnes PJ, Chung KF (1995) Corticosteroid inhibition of macrophage inflammatory protein-1-alpha in human monocytes and alveolar macrophages. *Am J Physiol-Lung Cell Mol Physiol* 13: L443–L452
79 Standiford TJ, Kunkel SL, Kasahara K, Milia MJ, Rolfe MW, Strieter RM (1991) Interleukin-8 gene-expression from human alveolar macrophages – the role of adherence. *Am J Respir Cell Mol Biol* 5: 579-585
80 Shapiro SD, Campbell EJ, Kobayashi DK, Welgus HG (1991) Dexamethasone selectively modulates basal and lipopolysaccharide-induced metalloproteinase and tissue inhibitor of metalloproteinase production by human alveolar macrophages. *J Immunol* 146: 2724–2729
81 Petersgolden M, Thebert P (1986) Inhibition by methylprednisolone of zymosan-induced leukotriene synthesis in alveolar macrophages. *Am Rev Respir Dis* 133: A169
82 Baker AJ, Fuller RW (1990) Loss of beta-receptor function during maturation of monocytes to macrophages. *Eur J Pharmacol* 183: 876–877
83 Henricks PAJ, Vanesch B, Vanoosterhout AJM, Nijkamp FP (1988) Specific and non-specific effects of beta-adrenoceptor agonists on guinea-pig alveolar macrophage function. *Eur J Pharmacol* 152: 321–330
84 Gantner F, Kupferschmidt R, Schudt C, Wendel A, Hatzelmann A (1997) *In vitro* differentiation of human monocytes to macrophages: Change of PDE profile and its relationship to suppression of tumour necrosis factor-alpha release by PDE inhibitors. *Brit J Pharmacol* 121: 221–231
85 Tenor H, Hatzelmann A, Kupferschmidt R, Stanciu L, Djukanovic R, Schudt C, Wendel A, Church MK, Shute JK (1995) Cyclic-nucleotide phosphodiesterase isoenzyme activities in human alveolar macrophages. *Clin Exp Allergy* 25: 625–633
86 Holt PG, Schonhegrad MA, Oliver J, Holt BJ, Mcmenamin PG (1990) A contiguous network of dendritic antigen-presenting cells within the respiratory epithelium. *Internat Arch Allergy Applied Immunol* 91: 155–159
87 Lambrecht BN, Pauwels RA, Bullock GR (1996) The dendritic cell: Its potent role in the respiratory immune response. *Cell Biol Internat* 20: 111–120
88 Steinman RM (1998) Dendritic cells and the control of immunity. *Exp Hematol* 26: 4

89 Witmerpack MD, Swiggard WJ, Mirza A, Inaba K, Steinman RM (1995) Tissue distribution of the dec-205 protein that is detected by the monoclonal-antibody nldc-145. 2. Expression *in situ* in lymphoid and nonlymphoid tissues. *Cell Immunol* 163: 157–162
90 Sallusto F, Cella M, Danieli C, Lanzavecchia A (1995) Dendritic cells use macropinocytosis and the mannose receptor to concentrate macromolecules in the major histocompatibility complex class-II compartment – down-regulation by cytokines and bacterial products. *J Exp Med* 182: 389–400
91 Macatonia SE, Hosken NA, Litton M, Vieira P, Hsieh CS, Culpepper JA, Wysocka M, Trinchieri G, Murphy KM, Ogarra A (1995) Dendritic cells produce IL-12 and direct the development of th1 cells from naive CD4(+) T-cells. *J Immunol* 154: 5071–5079
92 Christensen PJ, Armstrong LR, Fak JJ, Chen GH, Mcdonald RA, Toews GB, Paine R (1995) Regulation of rat pulmonary dendritic cell immunostimulatory activity by alveolar epithelial cell-derived granulocyte-macrophage colony- stimulating factor. *Am J Respir Cell Mol Biol* 13: 426–433
93 Sallusto F, Lanzavecchia A (1994) Efficient presentation of soluble-antigen by cultured human dendritic cells is maintained by granulocyte-macrophage colony-stimulating factor plus interleukin-4 and down-regulated by tumor-necrosis-factor-alpha. *J Exp Med* 179: 1109–1118
94 Nicod LP, Isler P, Chicheportiche R, Songeon F, Dayer JM (1996) Production of prostaglandin E(2) and collagenase is inhibited by the recombinant soluble tumour necrosis factor receptor p55-human gamma 3 fusion protein at concentrations a hundred-fold lower than those decreasing T cell activation. *Eur Cytokine Network* 7: 757–763
95 Galvederochemonteix B, Nicod LP, Dayer JM (1996) Tumor necrosis factor soluble receptor 75: The principal receptor form released by human alveolar macrophages and monocytes in the presence of interferon gamma. *Am J Respir Cell Mol Biol* 14: 279–287
96 Ludewig B, Graf D, Gelderblom HR, Becker Y, Kroczek RA, Pauli G (1995) Spontaneous apoptosis of dendritic cells is efficiently inhibited by trap (CD40-ligand) and TNF-alpha, but strongly enhanced by interleukin-10. *Eur J Immunol* 25: 1943–1950
97 Cumberbatch M, Fielding I, Kimber I (1994) Modulation of epidermal langerhans cell frequency by tumor-necrosis- factor-alpha. *Immunology* 81: 395–401
98 Holt PG, Haining S, Nelson DJ, Sedgwick JD (1994) Origin and steady-state turnover of class-II MHC-bearing dendritic cells in the epithelium of the conducting airways. *J Immunol* 153: 256–261
99 Schuler G, Steinman RM (1985) Murine epidermal langerhans cells mature into potent immunostimulatory dendritic cells *in vitro*. *J Exp Med*161: 526–546
100 Nelson DJ, Holt PG (1995) Defective regional immunity in the respiratory-tract of neonates is attributable to hyporesponsiveness of local dendritic cells to activation signals. *J Immunol* 155: 3517–3524
101 Mcwilliam AS, Nelson D, Thomas JA, Holt PG (1994) Rapid dendritic cell recruitment is a hallmark of the acute inflammatory response at mucosal surfaces. *J Exp Med* 179: 1331–1336

102 Ohkawara Y, Yamauchi K, Tanno Y, Tamura G, Ohtani H, Nagura H, Ohkuda K, Takishima T (1992) Human lung mast-cells and pulmonary macrophages produce tumor-necrosis-factor-alpha in sensitized lung-tissue after ige receptor triggering. *Am J Respir Cell Mol Biol* 7: 385–392
103 Bellini A, Vittori E, Marini M, Ackerman V, Mattoli S (1993) Intraepithelial dendritic cells and selective activation of Th2-like lymphocytes in patients with atopic asthma. *Chest* 103: 997–1005
104 Fokkens WJ, Vroom TM, Rijntjes E, Mulder PGH (1989) Cd-1 (T6), HLA-DR-expressing cells, presumably langerhans cells, in nasal mucosa. *Allergy* 44: 167–172
105 Nelson DJ, Mcwilliam AS, Haining S, Holt PG (1995) Modulation of airway intraepithelial dendritic cells following exposure to steroids. *Am J Respir Crit Care Med* 151: 475–481
106 Moller GM, Overbeek SE, VanHeldenMeeuwsen CG, Vanhaarst JMW, Prens EP, Mulder PG, Postma DS, Hoogsteden HC (1996) Increased numbers of dendritic cells in the bronchial mucosa of atopic asthmatic patients: Downregulation by inhaled corticosteroids. *Clin Exp Allergy* 26: 517–524
107 Holzer P (1991) Capsaicin – cellular targets, mechanisms of action, and selectivity for thin sensory neurons. *Pharmacol Rev* 43: 143–201
108 Tazi A, Bouchonnet F, Grandsaigne M, Boumsell L, Hance AJ, Soler P (1993) Evidence that granulocyte macrophage colony-stimulating factor regulates the distribution and differentiated state of dendritic cells Langerhans cells in human lung and lung cancers. *J Clin Invest* 91: 566–576
109 Hosoi J, Murphy GF, Egan CL, Lerner EA, Grabbe S, Asahina A, Granstein RD (1993) Regulation of Langerhans cell-function by nerves containing calcitonin gene-related peptide. *Nature* 363: 159–163
110 Kalinski P, Schuitemaker JHN, Hilkens CMU, Kapsenberg ML (1998) Prostaglandin E-2 induces the final maturation of IL-12-deficient CD1a(+)CD83(+) dendritic cells: The levels of IL-12 are determined during the final dendritic cell maturation and are resistant to further modulation. *J Immunol* 161: 2804–2809

Contribution of endothelial cells to airway inflammation

Anne Burke-Gaffney[1] *and Paul G. Hellewell*[2]

[1]Unit of Critical Care, Imperial College School of Medicine at the National Heart and Lung Institute, Dovehouse St., London SW3 6LY, UK; [2]Cardiovascular Research Group, University of Sheffield, Clinical Sciences Centre, Northern General Hospital, Herries Rd, Sheffield S5 7AU, UK

Introduction

The single layer of endothelial cells that lines the microvessels of the bronchial circulation plays a key role in orchestrating airway inflammation. As a result of their strategic position at the blood-tissue interface, endothelial cells can interact with inflammatory cells and mediators at their luminal and abluminal surface. The response of endothelial cells to an inflammatory stimuli can be broadly divided into vascular and cellular events and this is summarized in Figure 1. The vascular changes include an increase in endothelial permeability of post-capillary venules and vasodilation of arterioles, as a result of the release of, amongst others, endothelial-derived vasodilators. Increased expression of endothelial adhesion molecules and the production of leukocyte chemoattractants from endothelial cells triggers the cellular changes. Together, the vascular and cellular changes culminate in an increase in plasma leakage and leukocyte emigration through the endothelium into the underlying tissue at the site of inflammation.

This chapter aims to (i) outline the generalized structure of endothelial cells, highlighting specialized features of endothelium in the bronchial circulation; (ii) provide an overview of endothelial cell activation, relevant to airway inflammation; (iii) describe the contribution of endothelial adhesion molecules, release of chemoattractants, increase in endothelial permeability and release of endothelial-derived vasodilators to the inflammatory response in the airways; and finally (iv) describe how modulating these endothelial functions may provide useful therapeutic tools for reducing airways inflammation.

Cellular structure

Endothelial cells from different organs display remarkable heterogeneity in structure and function and even within the same organ, large and small vessels may vary significantly [1]. Despite this heterogeneity there are characteristics common to all

Cellular Mechanisms in Airways Inflammation, edited by Clive P. Page, Katharine H. Banner and Domenico Spina

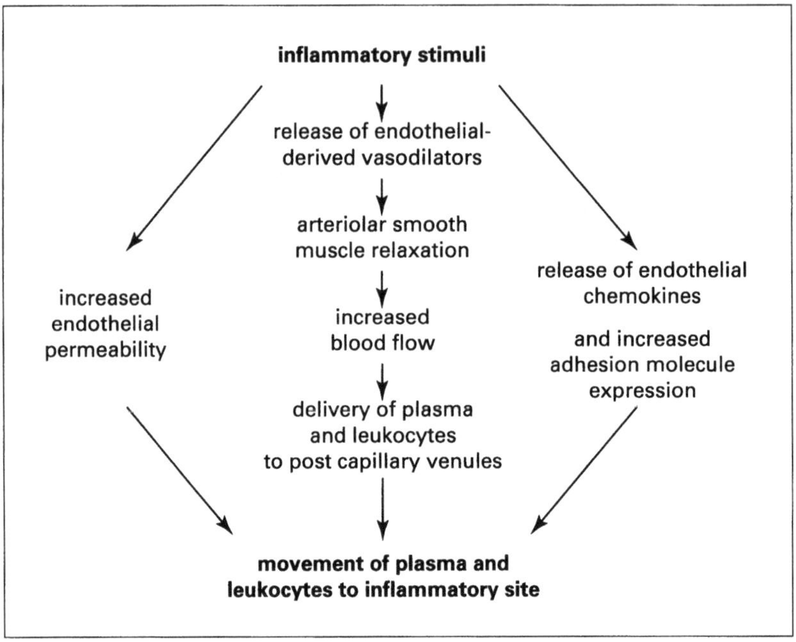

Figure 1
Vascular and cellular events associated with airway inflammation.

endothelial cells and those that, in particular, contribute to the role of endothelial cells in airway inflammation will be discussed.

Each endothelial cell is between 25 to 50 μm long and 10 to 15 μm wide. The thickness varies from less than 0.1 μm at the edges of vein or capillary endothelial cells, up to 3–5 μm at the nucleus. Endothelial cells lie with their long axis in the direction of blood flow [2]. The luminal surface is in direct contact with the blood and the abluminal surface next to the basal lamina. In arterioles of the upper and lower airways, the basal lamina separates endothelial cells from one or two layers of smooth muscle cells that lie in a radial position underneath the endothelium [3]. This spatial arrangement allows an endothelial cell to contact many smooth muscle cells and this facilitates the rapid transfer of information between these cells resulting in, for example, smooth muscle relaxation in response to endothelial-derived vasodilators. In contrast, the basal lamina of capillaries that are situated under the epithelium and near submucosal glands separates the endothelial layer from only a few pericytes, rather than a smooth muscle layer [3]. In post capillary venules that arise from the subepithelial capillary network, the basal lamina separates the endothelium from a discontinuous layer of pericytes, in small vessels, or a continuous layer, in vessels of a diameter of 30–50 μm [3].

The luminal and abluminal surfaces of endothelial cells have a carbohydrate-rich glycocalyx [4] which is thought to play a role in controlling plasma movement across the endothelium. Endothelial surfaces also have a negative charge [2] which, in the case of the luminal surface, may act to repel circulating blood cells with a similar negative charge. Another feature of endothelial cells is the presence of plasmalemmal vesicles [2]. These are numerous, small, vesicular invaginations about 500–700 Å in diameter which are more abundant in capillary than in arteriolar endothelial cells [3]. These vesicles may fuse to form transendothelial channels and are thought to be one way in which fluid and plasma proteins can pass through the capillary wall.

Endothelial cells in microvessels of the airways form either a continuous endothelial layer, as seen in post-capillary venules [5], or a fenestrated endothelial layer usually found in the subepithelial capillaries of the nose, or upper airways [3]. Fenestrae are circular structures of 50–60 nm that appear as gaps or openings in the endothelium [6]. Fenestrated and continuous endothelium have a similar permeability to plasma proteins but fenestrated endothelium show considerably higher permeability to water, ions and small molecules [6]. In the lower airways of most species, including healthy humans, fenestrations are only seen near the glands, neuro-epithelial bodies and bronchus-associated lymphoid tissue. In contrast, in asthmatic patients fenestrations have been shown to develop in the tracheobronchial subepithelial capillaries [7]. It is unclear whether these fenestrations develop as a marker of injury or whether they provide a functional advantage.

The inter-endothelial junctions also vary in different microvessels. Arterioles have a well developed network of tight junctions whereas capillaries have a less well organised system [3]. Endothelial cells of the post-capillary venules have the appearance of being loosely connected and their inter-cellular junctions are the least well organised, which may aid the separation of endothelial cells during inflammation [3, 5]. Many inflammatory mediators act at the endothelial junction allowing plasma and plasma proteins to pass, *via* a paracellular pathway, from the blood to the underlying tissue [3]. Emigration of leukocytes from the blood is also thought to occur at the endothelial junctions [3]. Disruption of endothelial junctions and increased permeability may be secondary to changes in the endothelial cytoskeleton as actin-binding proteins provide a direct link between junctional proteins and actin microfilaments.

Finally, an organelle characteristic of endothelial cells, which also contributes to the inflammatory role of the endothelium, is the Weibel-Palade body. In response to inflammatory stimuli, such as histamine, thrombin or C5a, Weibel-Palade bodies rapidly fuse with the plasma membrane and release von Willebrand factor (vWF, also known as Factor VIII) and express P-selectin on the endothelial surface [4, 8]. P-selectin plays a key role in the initial phase of leukocyte rolling on the endothelium [8] and will be described in detail in the section on biological activity. Factor VIII has always been regarded as a marker for endothelial cells because it is present only in endothelial cells, megakaryocytes and platelets [1]. It is now clear, however, that Factor VIII is not uniformly expressed by all endothelial cells and is absent in a variety of microvascular endothelium. In contrast, platelet endothelial cell adhesion molecule-1 (PECAM-1 or CD31), expressed at endothelial junctions, is expressed by all endothelial cells and is often used as an endothelial marker [1].

Mechanisms of activation

Early studies of endothelial cells identified certain proinflammatory substances, such as cytokines and bacterial products, as important stimuli of many endothelial functions [9]. Endothelial cells are also constantly exposed to a range of hemodynamic forces generated by pulsatile blood flow. There is increasing evidence that these biomechanical stimuli can directly influence endothelial function [10]. Also, it has recently become apparent that leukocyte binding to endothelial cells, *via* adhesion molecules, may directly trigger changes in endothelial cell function independent of soluble mediator release [11]. Figure 2 summarizes these mechanisms of endothelial activation.

In this section we will (i) give details of endothelial-activating cytokines which are increased in airway inflammatory diseases, to illustrate soluble mediator activation. We will also describe activation by bacterial products; other soluble activators of endothelial function will be referred to in the biological activity section of this chapter. Finally, we will describe (ii) biomechanical activation and (iii) adhesion-dependent activation of endothelial function relevant to airway inflammation.

Cytokine activation

Many cytokines have been implicated in the pathophysiology of airway inflammation. Those that may, in part, contribute to an inflammatory response by altering endothelial function include tumor necrosis factor α (TNFα), interleukin (IL)-1, -4, -13 and -6. The actual cytokine profile depends on the inflammatory disease; for example, increased expression of all the above are detected in asthmatic airways [12, 13], whereas in chronic bronchitis only TNFα and IL-4 are increased [14].

IL-1 is secreted predominantly from monocytes and macrophages but may also be produced by other cell types including endothelial cells [9, 15]. The two forms of IL-1, IL-1α and IL-1β, are two distinct gene products. Despite limited amino acid sequence homology, IL-1α and β have similar effects on endothelial cells [9, 15]. There are also two known forms of the IL-1 receptor and IL-1 is thought to activate endothelial cells *via* the type I receptor as the type II, or decoy, receptor is not expressed on endothelial cells [15]. IL-1 activation of endothelial cells increases adhesion molecule expression and the release of chemoattractant and vasoactive

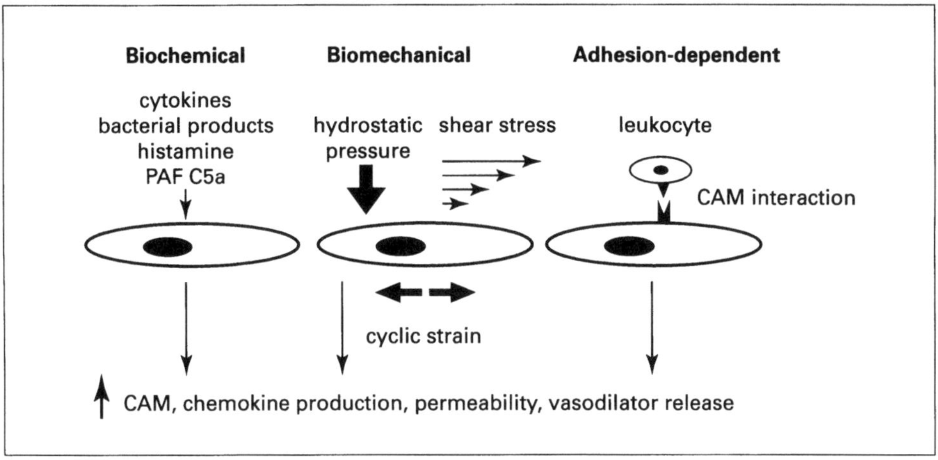

Figure 2
Mechanisms of endothelial activation
CAM, cell adhesion molecule.

mediators. TNFα, produced by many cells including macrophages, mast cells and epithelial cells, mimics every known action of IL-1 on cultured endothelial cells [9, 15]. The effects of TNFα and IL-1 are often additive. There are also two known forms of the TNF receptor, p55 and p75, expressed on endothelial cells [15]. TNFα activates endothelial cells predominantly *via* p55 which is expressed, overall, at higher levels than p75. At the cell membrane, however, p75 is expressed at higher levels and is thought to present TNFα to p55. This effect is seen at low ligand concentrations and is known as "ligand passing" [15].

IL-4, a 20 kDa glycoprotein secreted by activated T lymphocytes and mast cells [16] induces vascular cell adhesion molecule-1 (VCAM-1) expression on endothelial cells derived from several vascular sites including human lung microvascular endothelial cells (HLMVEC) [17]. Unlike IL-1 or TNFα, IL-4 does not increase intercellular adhesion molecule-1 (ICAM-1) or E-selectin expression [17] although it may decrease expression of these adhesion molecules induced by other cytokines [18]. In contrast, IL-4 enhances LPS, IL-1 or TNFα-induced VCAM-1 expression [17, 18]. The presence of IL-4 may thus result in selective VCAM-1 expression. The leukocyte ligand for VCAM-1, VLA-4, is expressed on eosinophils or monocytes, but not neutrophils. Raised levels of IL-4 may therefore trigger the recruitment to the airways of eosinophils and mononuclear cells seen in certain airway inflammatory diseases such as asthma.

Effects of IL-4 on chemokine production may further fine-tune the leukocyte subtype recruited in the airways. RANTES is a CC chemokine that activates eosinophils and mononuclear cells and IL-4 can inhibit TNFα/IFNγ-induced production of

RANTES from endothelial cells [19]. In contrast, IL-4 increases the production, from fibroblasts, of eotaxin [20] a CC chemokine active on eosinophils but not mononuclear cells. IL-13 has similar activities to IL-4 on endothelial cells because both cytokines bind to the IL-4 receptor α chain (IL-4Rα) expressed on endothelial cells [21]. We have shown that HLMVEC express IL-4Rα and that TNFα increases its expression [17]. Endothelial IL-4Rα expression is also significantly increased in bronchial mucosa biopsies from asthmatics compared with normal controls [22], although the mediators responsible for this have not been identified.

IL-6 is produced in copious amounts by endothelial cells but until recently this cytokine was not thought to affect inflammatory endothelial functions. This is because endothelial cells do not express the cytokine-binding alpha subunit of the IL-6 receptor (IL-6Rα) although they do express the signal-transducing gp130 chain known to be associated with IL-6Rα in leukocytes [23]. Soluble IL-6Rα together with constitutively produced endothelial IL-6 is sufficient to induce expression of ICAM-1, VCAM-1 and E-selectin and also production of IL-8 [24]. Activated neutrophils are known to shed significant amounts of IL-6Rα which could be utilized by endothelial cells to further increase leukocyte recruitment [24]. IL-6 may therefore play a previously unsuspected role in amplifying leukocyte recruitment.

Gram-negative and gram-positive bacterial products also activate endothelial cells and these may play a role in exacerbating airway inflammation. Lipopolysaccharide (LPS), a major component of the cell wall of gram-negative bacteria, triggers a profile of endothelial activation, for example adhesion molecule expression, similar to that seen with TNFα and IL-1 [17]. Levels of LPS binding protein and soluble CD14, molecules involved in LPS activation of endothelial cells, are increased in post antigen challenge BALF of asthmatics [25]. Moreover, asthma severity in patients exposed to house dust mite has been shown to be related to LPS, rather than allergen, concentration in house dust [26]. Gram-positive bacteria are more heterogenous than gram-negative bacteria and it is more difficult to pin-point one agent (such as lipopolysaccharide for gram-negative bacteria) that might exacerbate airway inflammation. Cell wall products, peptidoglycans and teichoic acid and/ or exotoxins released from gram-positive bacteria, may be involved. We have shown that lipotechoic acid from *Staphylococcal aureus* (*S. aureus*) increases ICAM-1 and E-selectin expression on HLMVEC [27]. Exotoxin from *S. aureus* also increases P-selectin expression [28]. *S. aureus* is found in the early stages of airway inflammation associated with cystic fibrosis and exotoxin and/or lipotechoic acid activation of endothelial cells may contribute to this inflammation [29].

Biomechanical activation

There is increasing evidence that hemodynamic forces generated by blood flow in vessels can directly influence endothelial function and may thus constitute a novel paradigm of endothelial activation [10]. Flow-dependent changes in endothelial function have been described for large vessel endothelial cells and implicated in the development of atherosclerotic lesions [10]. In contrast, although it is known that inflamed microvessels are subjected to acute increases in blood flow, little is known about the direct consequences of these changes on endothelial function.

The hemodynamic forces generated in the blood vessel include (i) hydrostatic pressure that acts at right angles to the vessel wall and causes compressive stress within the cells; (ii) cyclic strain or stretch that results from the elongation to which cells are subjected following blood vessel distention; (iii) shear stress, which is the frictional force that acts parallel to the endothelial cell as blood flows across it (Fig. 2) [10]. Of these, the effects of shear stress on endothelial function have been best characaterised. Considerable progress has been made in defining positive and negative shear stress responsive elements (SSRE) in the promoters of biomechanically active genes and also the transcription factors that regulate their activation [30]. A positive SSRE has been identified in the promoter of the ICAM-1, but not E-selectin or VCAM-1, gene. This may account for why subjecting cultured endothelial cells to laminar shear stress (LSS; 2.5–46 dyn/cm^2) induces a time-dependent increase in ICAM-1, but not VCAM-1 or E-selectin expression [30]. Biomechanical stimuli may therefore act as differential regulators of adhesion molecule expression and may also enhance or inhibit effects of soluble mediators.

The release of endothelial-derived vasodilators, nitric oxide (NO) and prostacyclin (PGI_2), is also increased when endothelial cells are subjected to biomechanical stimuli [30]. LSS induces expression of endothelial NO synthase (eNOS) and cyclooxygenase-2 (COX-2), the enzymes involved in the synthesis of NO and PGI_2, respectively [30]. NO and PGI_2 cause smooth muscle relaxation and arteriolar vasodilation characteristic of inflammation. MCP-1, a CC-chemokine that increases endothelial transmigration of mononuclear cells, is also induced by LSS [30]. To date, it is unknown whether changes in blood flow alter production of other chemokines.

Adhesion-dependent activation

Leukocyte adhesion, *via* interactions of CD11/CD18 integrins with endothelial ICAM-1, also activates endothelial cells [11]. Adhesion molecule interactions were thought to simply facilitate close contact between endothelial cells and leukocytes and to allow the release of toxic leukocyte products into a microenviroment close to the endothelium. Recent evidence suggests, however, that adhesion molecule activation directly trigger changes in endothelial function. For example, ICAM-1-CD11/CD18 interactions in endothelial-monocyte co-cultures trigger E-selectin induction and chemokine generation, independent of soluble mediators [11, 31]. The mechanisms by which direct changes in endothelial function are triggered have yet to be determined, but may involve the cytoskeleton transducing signals from adhesion molecules into functional responses in endothelial cells. Another endothelial adhesion molecule that also provides a signalling function is PECAM-1. Engagement of endothelial PECAM-1 with anti-PECAM-1 monoclonal mAb induces a slow but sustained release in intracellular calcium and a time-dependent increase in PGI_2 release [32]. These changes may facilitate leukocyte migration and enhance the vasodilator response of the blood vessel during inflammation.

Biological activity

The principle endothelial functions that contribute to the pathophysiology associated with airway inflammation are (i) adhesion molecule expression; (ii) chemokine production; (iii) alteration of endothelial permeability; (iv) production of vasoactive mediators. These are summarized in Figures 3–5. In this section we will consider each of these and give specific examples of their involvement in airway inflammation. Increases in adhesion molecule expression and chemokine production are thought to represent cellular changes of inflammation and increased permeability and release of vasoactive mediators, the vascular changes. Vascular and cellular changes are not, however, mutually exclusive; for example, leukocyte adhesion is known to increase endothelial permeability [33] and the endothelial-derived vasoactive mediator, NO, alters adhesion molecule expression [34].

Adhesion molecule expression

Endothelial adhesion molecules play a key role in the three distinct phases of leukocyte recruitment described as rolling/ tethering, firm adhesion and transmigration (Fig. 3) [8, 35]. We will briefly describe each phase with specific emphasis on the role, in each, of endothelial adhesion molecules.

Leukocyte rolling only occurs under flow conditions and is normally associated with post capillary venules rather than arterioles [35]. Small changes in blood flow, and/or release of inflammatory mediators, induce expression of endothelial P- and E-selectin and this triggers rolling. The selectins are a family of three closely related cell surface molecules: E-selectin, expressed exclusively on endothelial cells; P-selectin, on endothelial cells and platelets; and L-selectin, expressed on most leukocytes but not endothelial cells [36]. The selectins have a unique and characteristic extracellular region made up of an amino-terminal calcium-dependent lectin domain, an epidermal growth factor (EGF)-like domain and a varying number of short consensus repeats (SCR) similar to those found in complement regulatory proteins [36]. Although these domains are found in numerous other proteins, the selectins are the only known example in which the three domains are found in

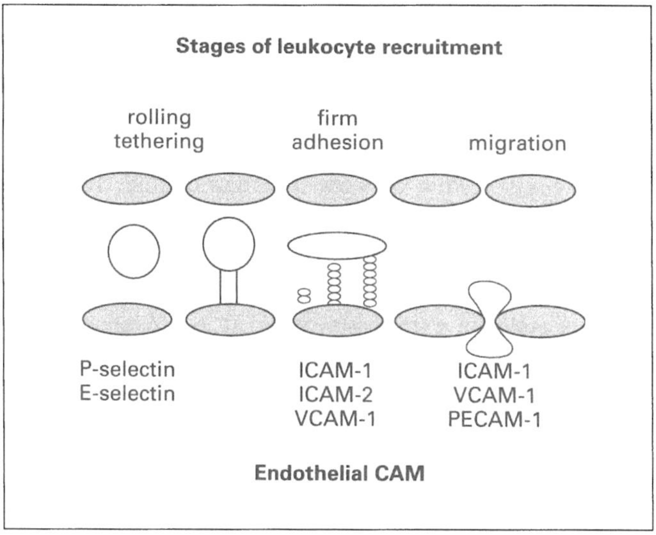

Figure 3
Involvement of endothelial adhesion molecules in the three stages of leukocyte recruitment; rolling/tethering, firm adhesion and migration.

immediate juxtaposition. This suggests that the spatial arrangement is important for receptor function [36].

The lectin domain plays an essential role in selectin-mediated adhesion because it binds to specific carbohydrate sugar residues, such as sialic acid and fucose, known to be essential components of selectin ligands [36]. The EGF-like domain is thought to contribute structural information required for the correct presentation of the lectin domain [36]. The SCR domain extends the ligand binding domain away from the cell surface and thus may facilitate contact with selectin ligands presented on moving leukocytes [36]. As suggested above the selectin ligands are, at least in part, carbohydrate. The prototype ligand for selectins is sialyl Lewis X, a tetrasaccharide containing a fucose and sialic acid residue [36]. Selectin adhesion is uniformly dependent on sialic acid and there is strong evidence that all three selectins require fucose. It is now also apparent that L- and P-selectin, but not E-selectin, requires a sulphate group, expressed on one of the sugar residues, for adhesion [36]. Several glycoprotein ligands for E-selectin have been identified including E-selectin ligand-1 (ESL-1). P-selectin glycoprotein-1 (PSGL-1) is a counter receptor for P-selectin and also for E-selectin which it binds with a lower affinity [36].

P-selectin is thought to mediate the very earliest leukocyte rolling since this stage is absent in P-selectin knock-out mice [36]. This early rolling is probably triggered following the release of histamine from tissue mast cells because histamine is known to rapidly mobilize P-selectin from the Weibel-Palade bodies to the cell surface [8].

Thrombin, complement fragments, free radicals and cytokines can also cause a rapid (peaks at 10 min), but transient (return to basal levels at 20–30 min), increase in P-selectin [8]. In addition to the rapid expression of P-selectin at the cell surface, LPS and cytokines increased in airway inflammation, such as TNFα, can up-regulate P-selectin at a transcriptional level [8].

E-selectin also supports leukocyte rolling at sites of inflammation, however, because of the requirement of *de novo* gene transcription for E-selectin expression, it does not contribute to rolling at the earliest phase of leukocyte recruitment. E-selectin is detected following stimulation with inflammatory cytokines or bacterial products (see previous section). E-selectin expression peaks at 4–6 h on cultured endothelial cells, for example HLMVEC, and returns to basal levels within about 24 h [17]. E-selectin expression is also increased in bronchial biopsy tissue from patients with rhinitis compared with control patients which may indicate a role for E-selectin in this airway inflammatory disease [37]. Also, monoclonal antibodies against E-selectin block neutrophil influx and late phase bronchoconstriction, after a single inhalation challenge, in a primate model of asthma [37].

When selectin-mediated rolling has slowed down the leukocytes sufficiently, firm adhesion can occur. Firm adhesion requires the interaction of endothelial immunoglobulin (Ig)-like adhesion molecules, ICAM-1, ICAM-2 and VCAM-1, with their respective leukocyte integrin counter-ligands [8, 38]. ICAM-1 binds the leukocyte β_2-integrin ligand $\alpha_L\beta_2$ (CD11a/CD18) and $\alpha_M\beta_2$ (CD11b/CD18) [8]. In contrast, ICAM-2 which has 2 Ig domains partly homologous with the first two domains of ICAM-1, binds only CD11a/CD18 [8]. VCAM-1, binds the β_1-integrin, $\alpha_4\beta_1$ (VLA-4), and this will be discussed below. Unlike E-selectin, ICAM-1 is expressed under non-inflammatory basal conditions and on leukocytes, epithelial cells and smooth muscle cells, in addition to endothelial cells. It is possible that the selective basal expression of ICAM-1 may result from the LSS effects of blood flow through a vessel, described in the previous section. TNFα, IL-1, LPS, thrombin and exposure to oxygen radicals, upregulate ICAM-1 expression [8]. In general, expression is detectable at 2–4 h, maximal at 24 h and may be sustained up to 72 h; this has also been demonstrated for HLMVEC [17]. In contrast to ICAM-1, inflammatory stimuli do not up-regulate expression of ICAM-2. Compelling evidence showing that ICAM-1 is up-regulated, 5–6 h post antigen challenge in human asthma [37] and that ICAM-1 mAb inhibits airway eosinophilia and hyperresponsiveness in a primate model of asthma [39], suggests an involvement of ICAM-1 in airway inflammation.

A third member of the Ig family, expressed on endothelial cells, involved in firm adhesion is VCAM-1 [8]. There are two known forms of VCAM-1; one, with six Ig domains, is an alternatively spliced variant of the predominant seven domain form [8]. VCAM-1, like ICAM-1, is expressed on other cell types in addition to endothelial cells but like E-selectin, VCAM-1 is not normally constitutively expressed. The cytokines that induce VCAM-1 expression include, IL-1, 4, 13 and TNFα [17, 40].

LPS also induces VCAM-1 expression [17]. Increased expression can usually be detected within 2 h of stimulation and this upregulation may last for 72 h, although this is dependent on the induction stimulus. For example, LPS induces maximal expression on HLMVEC at 6 h and TNFα at 24 h, whereas no effect is detected with IL-4 alone until 72 h [17]. Evidence for the involvement of VCAM-1 in airway inflammation comes from studies showing that VCAM-1 expression is increased in nasal biopsies from patients with rhinitis [37]. Also increased VCAM-1 expression and subsequent eosinophil and T lymphocyte accumulation are found after bronchial allergen challenge in asthmatics [37].

Finally, following firm adhesion of leukocytes to the endothelium, leukocytes undergo dramatic shape change that allows them to pass through the inter-endothelial junction of the vessel wall and migrate into the surrounding tissue. For transmigration to occur a chemotactic gradient is usually essential but this does not negate the need for adhesion molecules. In addition to facilitating firm adhesion, ICAM-1 and VCAM-1 are also thought to aid transmigration. Another member of the Ig family that is not involved in firm adhesion but plays a key role in transmigration is PECAM-1 [8]. PECAM-1 has six Ig-like domains and homotypically binds PECAM-1 expressed on leukocytes [8], and the integrin $\alpha_v\beta_3$. PECAM-1 is expressed in large amounts on resting endothelium, but is specifically located at the endothelial junctions. This localization is thought to facilitate its role in migration and it may act to guide leukocytes through the inter-endothelial junction. It has recently been shown that TNFα/IFNγ decreases PECAM-1 expression [41], although the significance of this is unclear.

Chemokine production

A second aspect of endothelial function, namely the ability of endothelial cells to produce leukocyte chemoattractants, also contributes towards the cellular changes associated with airway inflammation. Endothelial cells are a rich source of PAF and they may also metabolize LTB_4, from neutrophil-derived LTA_4 [42]. Endothelial cells can also produce, given the appropriate stimulus, several members of a recently described family of chemoattractant proteins called chemokines [43, 44]. Unlike classical chemoattractants, chemokines are specific, to a varying degree, for leukocyte subsets and may therefore contribute to the recruitment of different leukocyte subsets during airway inflammation [44]. In this section we will describe the role in leukocyte recruitment of IL-8, RANTES, and eotaxin which can be produced by endothelial cells and are increased during airways inflammation [44].

Chemokines are 8–10 kd proteins with 20 to 70 % homology in amino acid sequences that have been subdivided into families on the basis of the relative position of their cysteine residues [43, 44]. There are two main chemokine families, CXC (α) and CC (β) [43, 44]. In the CXC chemokine family, one amino acid separates the first two cysteine residues, whereas in the CC family the first two cysteine residues are adjacent to each other [43, 44]. The CXC chemokines can be further subdivided functionally into those that are chemotactic for neutrophils for example IL-8, and those that act on lymphocytes, such as IP-10 [44]. The CC chemokines, in general, do not act on neutrophils but attract monocytes, eosinophils, basophils and lymphocytes, with variable selectivity [44].

IL-8 is the most prominent neutrophil chemoattractant of the CXC chemokines. The involvement of IL-8 in neutrophil recruitment is three-fold (Fig. 4). First, IL-8 causes L-selectin shedding and upregulates CD11b/CD18 expression and affinity for its ICAM-1 ligand [43]. Together these actions disengage leukocyte rolling and trigger firm adhesion. Second, IL-8 provides a chemotactic gradient to facilitate neutrophil emigration into thc tissuc [43]. Third, IL-8 activates neutrophil function, for example release of degradative enzymes and respiratory burst [43]. Uncontrolled neutrophil activation may contribute to the tissue damage associated with airway inflammation. Cultured endothelial cells, activated with TNFα, IL-1 or LPS, release soluble IL-8 (first detected at 4 h), but also present IL-8 on the endothelial surface [45]. Presentation of IL-8, in this way, may facilitate L-selectin shedding and CD11b/CD18 up-regulation on leukocytes, because blood flow is less likely to remove or dilute it. The kinetics of IL-8 production are similar to E-selectin expression and it is thought that simultaneous expression of an adhesion molecule involved in leukocyte rolling and a chemokine that activates leukocyte integrins, is instrumental in converting rolling to firm adhesion [35]. Increased levels of IL-8 are detected in BALF fluid of cystic fibrosis patients [46] and asthmatics [12] and may correlate with the influx of neutrophils into the airways in these diseases.

Many CC chemokines have been detected in the airways of patients with asthma, including RANTES and this chemokine is thought to contribute to the accumulation of and/ or activation of eosinophils, T cells, monocytes and basophils [44]. Modulation of RANTES production from endothelial cells by cytokines was discussed in the previous section. In addition, the amount of RANTES released from TNFα/IFNγ-stimulated human nasal mucosal microvascular endothelial cell obtained from patients with nasal allergy is higher than from patients without allergy [47]. As described for IL-8, there is evidence for the involvement of RANTES at most steps of leukocyte recruitment. *In vitro* studies have shown effects on chemoattraction, transendothelial migration, release of eosinophil cationic protein (ECP) and induction of production of reactive oxygen species; there is some disagreement however, as to whether RANTES increase the expression of CD11b/CD18 [43]. In contrast to RANTES, eotaxin is thought to activate eosinophils but not mononuclear cells because the CCR3 receptor, the only known eotaxin receptor, is not expressed on mononuclear cells [44]. Murine endothelial cells produce eotaxin following cytokine stimulation [48]. Eotaxin can increase CD11b/CD18 expression on eosinophils, increase eosinophil adhesion and chemotaxis and also trigger eosinophil oxidative burst [49–51].

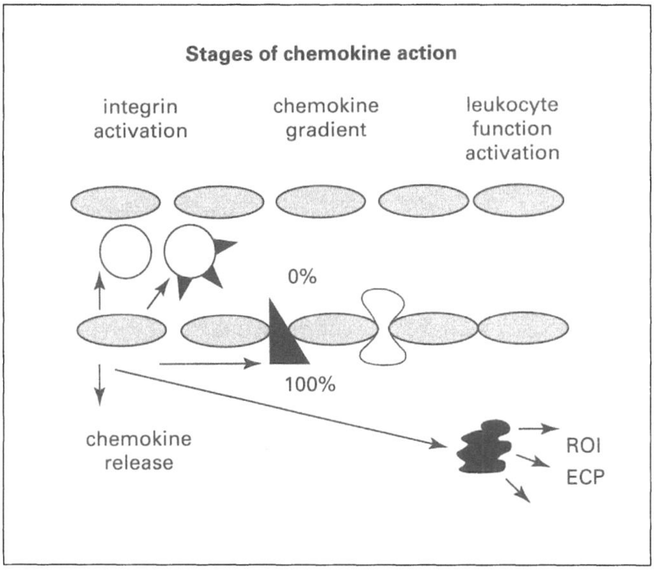

Figure 4
Involvement of endothelial-derived chemokines in leukocyte activation and migration. ROI, reactive oxygen intermediates; ECP, eosinophil actionic protein.

Finally, a recently identified chemokine that does not fit into the CC or CXC chemokine families is fracktalkine [44]. To date, this is the only known member of the CXXXC chemokine family and is a membrane-bound glycoprotein in which the first two cysteine residues are separated by three amino acids and the chemokine domain sits on a mucin-like stalk. Fractalkine is induced on cultured human endothelial cells and promotes adhesion of monocytes and activated T cells *in vitro* [44]. The presentation of a chemokine on the cell surface puts it in an ideal position to stimulate circulating leukocytes without being removed by blood flow or cleared by DARC, a promiscuous chemokine receptor on the surface of erythrocytes. To date, it is not clear whether the unique structure of fractalkine allows this chemokine to directly mediate adhesion in addition to activating adhesion molecules.

Permeability

One of the most prominent homeostatic activities of the endothelium is the regulation of exchanges between the blood and the underlying tissue. Changes in endothelial permeability of bronchial post-capillary venules lead to plasma exudation and tissue oedema characteristic of airway inflammation. Oedema formation causes

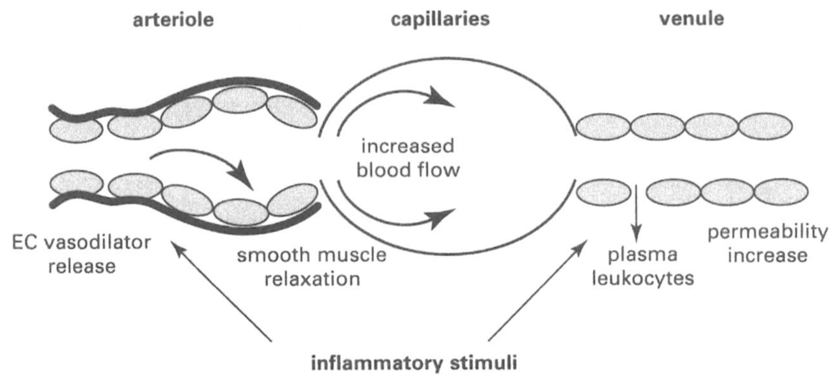

Figure 5
Involvement of increased endothelial permeability and release of endothelial-derived vasodilators in plasma and leukocyte leakage from the circulation.

mucosal thickening which may contribute to the bronchoconstriction associated with airway inflammatory diseases such as asthma. Whether or not the venular endothelial junctions of these microvessels are abnormally leaky in patients with such diseases is unknown. What is known, however, is that many of the inflammatory mediators implicated in the pathogenesis of airway inflammation increase endothelial permeability (Fig. 5). In this section, we will give examples of two mediators, histamine and PAF, that are thought to directly alter endothelial permeability.

Histamine, a biogenic amine stored in cytoplasmic granules of mast cells, is one of the first inflammatory mediators released in response to an inflammatory trigger during airway inflammation. When mast cells degranulate the released histamine activates local target cells including the endothelium [52]. Histamine increases transendothelial permeability of cultured endothelial cells to albumin [52]. This is associated with reorganisation of the F-actin fibres of the cytoskeleton and increases in $[Ca^{2+}]_i$ and phosphoinositide turnover [52]. Local installation of histamine onto human nasal mucosa leads to increased recovery of albumin in the nasal lavage fluid, suggesting transient increases in epithelial and endothelial permeabilities [53].

PAF is a lipid mediator which is newly synthesised and released during airway inflammation, mainly from mucosal mast cells but smaller quantities are also produced by endothelial cells. PAF like histamine, causes the contraction of human endothelial cells and increase permeability of endothelial cells in culture [52]. PAF is also known to be one of the most potent inducers of microvascular leakage throughout the guinea-pig airway, when administered intravenously [53]. It is approximately 10,000-fold more potent than histamine, although its duration of action is shorter. It has been suggested that oedema resulting from increased airway microvascular permeability may be responsible for airway narrowing in human subjects after the inhalation of PAF since PAF does not contract airway smooth muscle *in vitro* [53].

In response to inflammatory stimuli, macromolecules and plasma move from the blood to the surrounding tissue either *via* paracellular pathways, at the intercellular junctions, or transcellular pathways across the cell membrane [6]. It is thought that many inflammatory mediators, including PAF and histamine act directly at the endothelial junctions [52]. It has been known for some time that actin filament reorganization is involved in endothelial permeability changes [52]. In general, stabilization of actin cytoskeleton reduces endothelial permeability and inhibition of actin microfilament assembly increases it. Until recently, however, little was known about the molecular targets at the cell junctions [54]; whether permeability increasing agents can alter the distribution or function of these molecules remains to be seen.

Production of vasoactive mediators

Endothelial cells are a rich source of vasodilators including NO, prostaglandins (PG) E_2 and PGI_2 and also vasoconstrictors such as endothelin and angiotensin II [9]. These mediators have direct effects on vascular smooth muscle (Fig. 5), but may also have more wide-reaching effects on airway smooth muscle. These "long distance" effects may occur because of the close anatomic relationship between microvascular endothelial cells and airway tissue. In this section, however we will only discuss the effects of vasodilators on vascular smooth muscle relaxation.

NO, a highly reactive gas with a half-life of seconds in biological systems, is formed when NO synthase (NOS) enzymes convert L-arginine to L-citrulline [55]. It has now become clear that there are at least three different NOS isoforms: (i) neuronal (nNOS), (ii) macrophage or inducible (iNOS) and (iii) endothelial (eNOS) [56]. Despite the terminology, NOS expression is not restricted to these cells. NO plays a key role in the regulation of cellular processes in the cardiovascular, nervous and immune systems but the complexity of its role in the airways and its involvement in airway inflammation is still being unravelled. Increased levels of NO are detected in the BALF of asthmatics and it is thought that this may be an important marker of inflammation in the airway [57]. There is controversy, however, as to the main cell source of NO in airways disease but certainly endothelial cells in the nasal mucosa of rhinitic patients stain strongly for eNOS and to a lesser extent, iNOS [58].

NO increases blood flow in the bronchial circulation and this may contribute, in part, to the increase in plasma exudation and oedema formation associated with airway inflammation [57]. NOS inhibitors, applied to the surface of guinea-pig airways, have however, also been shown to increase plasma exudation into the airway lumen [57]. It is possible that the latter effect of NOS inhibitors may be at the level of the epithelium. In support of this we have shown that NOS inhibitors increase cytokine-induced damage of lung epithelial cells in culture [59]. These results suggest that NO may have pro and anti-inflammatory effects in airway inflammation. The site of NO production, the target cells on which it acts and/ or the amount of NO produced may combine to determine the predominant effect.

There are also two isoforms to the COX enzyme involved in the synthesis of prostaglandins. These are COX-1, thought to be responsible for the production of prostaglandins during acute inflammation and COX-2 which is thought to be the predominant isoform present during chronic inflammation [60]. PGI_2 and PGE_2 are the vasodilators produced by most arteries and high yields of PGI_2 are especially characteristic of endothelial cells. Microvascular endothelial cells, however, produce predominantly PGE_2 and $PGF_{2\alpha}$ although the profile of prostaglandins produced by endothelial cells from the bronchial microcirculation circulation, has not been specifically addressed. As described for NO, PGs will act directly on the vascular smooth muscle of arterioles to cause vasodilation which contributes to the associated plasma exudation. PGE_2 and PGI_2 have been shown to synergise with mediators such as histamine that act directly on the endothelium of the post capillary venules, to increase permeability and greatly potentiate oedema formation [60]. This synergism is probably the result of increased blood flow through the capillary bed with the delivery of more plasma to venules downstream. The resulting increase in hydrostatic pressure in the venules also contribute to enhanced plasma protein leakage.

Pharmacological modulation *in vitro*

In this last section, we will describe ways in which endothelial function can be modulated *in vitro*. In particular, we will emphasise the endothelial modulatory effects of anti-inflammatory agents that are routinely used in the treatment of airway inflammation, such as glucocorticoids and β-agonists. Other ways in which endothelial function may be inhibited *in vitro* will not be covered in detail but include tyrosine kinase inhibition and antisense. Tyrosine kinase inhibitors suppress endothelial functions, including adhesion molecule expression [61] and the induction of COX-2 [60]. Identification of specific tyrosine kinases involved with individual endothelial functions might lead to the development of specific inhibitors of these functions. Another approach that might result in selective inhibition of the inflammatory response is the use of anti-sense oligonucleotides to inhibit the expression of mRNA for adhesion molecules [62]. These targeted approaches may provide useful therapeutic tools for reducing airway inflammation, in the future.

Glucocorticoids, used in the treatment of asthma and rhinitis, have potent and wide ranging anti-inflammatory effects including inhibition of leukocyte influx into the airways, inhibiton of inflammatory mediator release and reduction of microvascular leakage. The relative contribution to these effects of endothelial function inhibition is hard to assess *in vivo*. *In vitro* studies, however, provide strong evidence that glucocorticoids inhibit, to a varying degree, the endothelial functions discussed in the biological activity section of this chapter. Glucocorticoids, such as dexamethasone, inhibit, in part, ICAM-1 and E-selectin expression on human endothelial cells, in culture [63, 64], and also abolish cytokine-induced increases in endothelial monolayer permeability [65]. Glucocorticoids also block chemokine release from endothelial cells [66]. Finally, inhibition of induction of the inducible isoenzymes iNOS and COX-2 may also contribute significantly to the anti-inflammatory effects of glucocorticoids [60, 67].

Steroids have, however, many harmful side-effects when used chronically and thus the development of drugs with an effective anti-inflammatory profile but with fewer side-effects would be highly desirable. A strategy that has received much attention recently, especially in the context of asthma, concerns increasing intracellular cAMP levels in cells involved in the inflammatory process [68]. Activation of adenylate cyclase or inhibition of phosphodiesterases, the enzymes involved in the synthesis and breakdown of cAMP respectively, elevate intracellular cAMP. Inhaled β-agonists, used to treat bronchoconstriction associated with airway disease, cause relaxation of the airway smooth muscle as a result of adenylate cyclase activation and subsequent cAMP elevation in these cells. Elevation of intracellular cAMP in endothelial cells may also contribute, in part, to the anti-inflammatory potential of cAMP elevating agents used to treat airway inflammation.

Endothelial cells express PDE3 and 4 as the major cAMP hydrolysing enzymes. We have shown that inhibition of PDE4, with appropriate activation of adenylate cyclase, is sufficient to inhibit TNFα-induced E-selectin expression and neutrophil adhesion, whereas combined inhibition of PDE3 and 4 is required for inhibition of VCAM-1 and eosinophil adhesion [69]. In contrast, neither condition inhibited ICAM-1 expression. Selective inhibition of adhesion molecule expression may have therapeutic implications for the treatment of leukocyte recruitment associated with airway inflammation. Activation of adenylate cyclase with simultaneous PDE3 and 4 inhibition, also blocks thrombin-induced endothelial permeability increases [70]. These studies provide clear evidence that increasing intracellular cAMP within endothelial cells may have important anti-inflammatory effects.

In summary, we have outlined the generalized structure of endothelial cells highlighting specialized features of endothelium of the bronchial circulation; provided an overview of endothelial cell activation relevant to airway inflammation; described the role of endothelial adhesion molecules and chemokines in orchestrating leukocyte recruitment and the implications for airway inflammation of increased endothelial permeability and release of endothelial-derived vasodilators. Finally, we have described how these endothelial functions may be modulated *in vitro*. In conclusion, the single layer of endothelial cells that line the microvessels of the bronchial circulation play a pivotal role in orchestrating airway inflammation. Inhibition of endothelial function may therefore provide a useful therapeutic strategy for reducing airways inflammation.

Acknowledgements
Work in the authors laboratories is funded by the National Asthma Campaign, British Heart Foundation, British Lung Foundation and the Wellcome Trust.

References

1 Garlanda C, Dejana E (1997) Heterogeneity of endothelial cells. Specific markers. *Arterioscler Thromb Vasc Biol* 17: 1193–1202
2 Wehrmacher WH (1988) Endothelium: from whence to whither. *Semin Thromb Hemost* 14: 1–11
3 Widdicome, JG (1995) Microvascular anatomy of the airways. In: WW Busse, ST Holgate (eds): *Rhinitis and asthma*. Blackwell Scientific Publications, Boston, 722–732
4 Borsum T (1991) Biochemical properties of vascular endothelial cells. *Virchows Arch B Cell Pathol Incl Mol Pathol* 60: 279–286
5 McDonald DM (1990) The ultrastructure and permeability of tracheobronchial blood vessels in health and disease. *Eur Respir J* 12 (Suppl): 572S–585S
6 Renkin EM (1992) Cellular and intercellular transport pathways in exchange vessels. *Am Rev Respir Dis* 146: S28–S31
7 Laitinen A, Laitinen LA (1990) Vascular beds in the airways of normal subjects and asthmatics. *Eur Respir J* 12 (Suppl): 658S–661S
8 Carlos TM, Harlan JM (1994) Leukocyte-endothelial adhesion molecules. *Blood* 84: 2068–2101
9 Pober JS, Cotran, RS (1990) Cytokines and endothelial biology. *Physiol Rev* 70: 427–44
10 Gimbrone MA Jr, Nagel T, Topper JN (1997) Biomechanical activation: an emerging paradigm in endothelial adhesion biology. *J Clin Invest* 100: S61–S65
11 Noble KE, Panayiotidis P, Collins PW, Hoffbrand AV, Yong KL (1996) Monocytes induce E-selectin gene expression in endothelial cells: role of CD11/CD18 and extracellular matrix proteins. *Eur J Immunol* 26: 2944–2951
12 Barnes PJ (1994) Cytokines as mediators of chronic asthma. *Am J Respir Crit Care Med* 150: S42–S49
13 Humbert M, Durham SR, Kimmitt P, Powell N, Assoufi B, Pfister R, Menz G, Kay AB, Corrigan CJ (1997) Elevated expression of messenger ribonucleic acid encoding IL-13 in the bronchial mucosa of atopic and nonatopic subjects with asthma. *J Allergy Clin Immunol* 99: 657–665

14 Mueller R, Chanez P, Campbell AM, Bousquet J, Heusser C, Bullock GR (1996) Different cytokine patterns in bronchial biopsies in asthma and chronic bronchitis. *Respir Med* 90: 79–85
15 Mantovani A, Bussolino F, Introna M (1997) Cytokine regulation of endothelial cell function: from molecular level to the bedside. *Immunol Today* 18: 231–240
16 Bradding P, Feather IH, Howarth PH, Mueller R, Roberts JA, Britten K, Bews JP, Hunt TC, Okayama Y, Heusser CH (1992) Interleukin 4 is localized to and released by human mast cells. *J Exp Med* 176: 1381–1386
17 Blease K Seybold J, Adcock IM, Hellewell PG Burke-Gaffney A (1998) Interleukin-4 and LPS synergise to induce vascular cell adhesion molecule-1 expression in human lung microvascular endothelial cells. *Am J Respir Cell Mol Biol* 18: 620–630
18 Thornhill MH, Haskard DO (1990) IL-4 regulates endothelial cell activation by IL-1, tumor necrosis factor, or IFN-gamma. *J Immunol* 145: 865–872
19 Marfaing-Koka A, Devergne O, Gorgone G, Portier A, Schall TJ, Galanaud P, Emilie D (1995) Regulation of the production of the RANTES chemokine by endothelial cells. Synergistic induction by IFN-gamma plus TNF-alpha and inhibition by IL-4 and IL-13. *J Immunol* 154: 1870–1878
20 Mochizuki M, Bartels J, Mallet AI, Christophers, E. Schroder, J-M (1998) IL-4 induces eotaxin: a possible mechanism of selective eosinophil recruitment in helminth infection and atopy. *J Immunol* 160: 60–68.
21 Synder B, Lugli S, Feng N, Etter R, Lutz A, Ryffel B, Sugamura K, Wunderli-Allenspach H, Moser R (1996) Interleukin-4 (IL-4) and IL-13 bind to a shared heterodimeric complex on endothelial cells mediating vascular cell adhesion molecule-1 induction in the absence of the common γ chain. *Blood* 87: 4286–4295
22 Kotsimbos ATC, Minshall E, Durham, S, Pfister R, Menz G, Thomas EK, Troutt T, Kay AB, Hamid Q (1997) Upregulation of alpha IL-4 receptor in asthma. *Am J Respir Crit Care Med* 155: A816
23 Romano M, Sironi M, Toniatti C, Polentarutti N, Fruscella P, Ghezzi P, Faggioni R, Luini W, van Hinsbergh V, Sozzani et al (1997) Role of IL-6 and its soluble receptor in induction of chemokines and leukocyte recruitment. *Immunity* 6: 315–325
24 Modur V, Li Y, Zimmerman GA, Prescott SM, McIntyre TMJ (1997) Retrograde inflammatory signalling from neutrophils to endothelial cells by soluble interleukin-6 receptor alpha. *J Clin Invest* 100: 2752–2756
25 Dubin W, Martin TR, Swoveland P, Leturcq DJ, Moriarty AR, Tobias PS, Bleecker, ER, Goldblum SE, Hasday JD (1996) Asthma and endotoxin: lipopolysaccharide-binding protein and soluble CD14 in bronchoalveolar compartment. *Am J Physiol* 270: L736–L744
26 Michel O, Kips J, Duchateau J, Vertongen F, Robert L, Collet H, Paulwels R, Sergysels R (1996) Severity of asthma is related to endotoxin in house dust. *Am J Respir Crit Care Med* 154: 1641–1646
27 Blease K, Burke-Gaffney A, Hellewell PG (1998) Lipoteichoic acid induces cell adhesion

molecule expression and IL-8 release from human lung microvascular endothelial cells. *FASEB J* 12: A576

28 Krull M, Dold C, Hippenstiel S, Rosseau S, Lohmeyer J, Suttorp N (1996) *Escherichia coli* hemolysin and *Staphylococcus aureas* alpha-toxin potently induce neutrophil adhesion to cultured human endothelial cells. *J Immunol* 157: 4133–4140

29 Branger C, Gardye C, Lambert-Zechovsky N (1996) Persistence of *Staphylococcus aureus* strains among cystic fibrosis patients over extended periods of time. *J Med Microbiol* 45: 294–301

30 Resnick N, Gimbrone MA (1995) Hemodynamic forces are complex regulators of endothelial gene expression. *FASEB J* 9: 874–882

31 Lukacs NW, Strieter RM, Elner V, Evanoff HL, Burdick MD, Kunkel SL (1995) Production of chemokines, interleukin-8 and monocyte chemoattractant protein-1, during monocyte: endothelial cell interactions. *Blood* 86: 2767–2773

32 Gurubhagavatula I, Amrani Y, Practico D, Ruberg, FL, Albelda, SM (1998) Engagement of human PECAM-1 (CD31) on human endothelial cells increases intracellular calcium ion concentration and stimulates prostacyclin release. *J Clin Invest* 101: 212–222

33 Wedmore CV, Williams TJ (1981) Control of vascular permeability by polymorphonuclear leukocytes in inflammation. *Nature* 19 289: 646–650

34 De Caterina R, Libby P, Peng HB, Thannickal VJ, Rajavashisth TB, Gimbrone MA Jr, Shin WS, Liao JK (1995) Nitric oxide decreases cytokine-induced endothelial activation. Nitric oxide selectively reduces endothelial expression of adhesion molecules and proinflammatory cytokines. *J Clin Invest* 96: 60–68

35 Albelda SM, Smith CW, Ward PA (1994) Adhesion molecules and inflammatory injury. *FASEB J* 8: 504–512

36 Kansas GS (1996) Selectins and their ligands: current concepts and controversies. *Blood* 88: 3259–3287

37 Montefort S, Holgate ST, Howarth PH (1993) Leucocyte-endothelial adhesion molecules and their role in bronchial asthma and allergic rhinitis. *Eur Respir J* 6: 1044–1054

38 Malik AB, Lo SK (1996) Vascular endothelial adhesion molecules and tissue inflammation. *Pharmacol Rev* 48: 213–229

39 Wegner CD, Gundel RH, Reilly P, Haynes N, Letts LG, Rothlein R (1990) Intercellular adhesion molecule-1 (ICAM-1) in the pathogenesis of asthma. *Science* 247: 456–459

40 Bochner BS, Klunk DA, Sterbinsky SA, Coffman RL, Schleimer RP (1995) IL-13 selectively induces vascular cell adhesion molecule-1 expression in human endothelial cells. *J Immunol* 154: 799–803

41 Rival Y, Del Maschio A, Rabiet MJ, Dejana E, Duperray A (1996) Inhibition of platelet endothelial cell adhesion molecule-1 synthesis and leukocyte transmigration in endothelial cells by the combined action of TNF-alpha and IFN-gamma. *J Immunol* 157: 1233–1241

42 Feinmark SJ (1992) The role of the endothelial cell in leukotriene biosynthesis. *Am Rev Respir Dis* 146 S51–S55

43 Teran LM, Davies DE (1996) The chemokines: their potential role in allergic inflammation. *Clin Exp Allergy* 26: 1005–1019
44 Luster AD (1998) Chemokines – chemotactic cytokines that mediate inflammation. *N Engl J Med* 338: 436–445
45 Rot A (1992) Endothelial cell binding of NAP-1/IL-8: role in neutrophil emigration. *Immunol Today* 13: 291–294
46 Bonfield TL, Panuska JR, Konstan MW, Hilliard KA, Hilliard JB, Ghnaim H, Berger M (1995) Inflammatory cytokines in cystic fibrosis lungs. *Am J Respir Crit Care Med* 152: 2111–2118
47 Terada N, Maesako K, Hamano N, Ikeda T, Sai M, Yamashita T, Fukuda S, Konno A (1996) RANTES production in nasal epithelial cells and endothelial cells. *J Allergy Clin Immunol* 98: S230–S237
48 Rothenberg ME, Luster AD, Leder P (1995) Murine eotaxin: an eosinophil chemoattractant inducible in endothelial cells and in interleukin 4-induced tumor suppression. *Proc Natl Acad Sci USA* 92: 8960–8964
49 Burke-Gaffney A, Hellewell PG (1996) Eotaxin stimulates eosinophil adhesion to human lung microvascular endothelial cells. *Biochem Biophys Res Commun* 227: 35–40
50 Elsner J, Hochstetter R, Kimmig D, Kapp A (1996) Human eotaxin represents a potent activator of the respiratory burst of human eosinophils. *Eur J Immunol* 26: 1919–1925
51 Tenscher K, Metzner B, Schopf E, Norgauer J, Czech W (1996) Recombinant human eotaxin induces oxygen radical production, Ca(2+)-mobilization, actin reorganization, and CD11b upregulation in human eosinophils *via* a pertussis toxin-sensitive heterotrimeric guanine nucleotide-binding protein. *Blood* 88: 3195–3199
52 Lum H, Malik AB (1994) Regulation of vascular endothelial barrier function. *Am J Physiol* 267: L223–L241
53 Chung KF, Rogers DF, Barnes PJ Evans TW (1990) The role of increased airway microvascular permeability and plasma exudation. *Eur Respir J* 3: 329–337
54 Dejana E, Corada M, Lampugnani, MG (1995) Endothelial cell-to-cell junctions. *FASEB J* 9: 910–918
55 Palmer RMJ, Moncada S (1989) A novel citrulline-forming enzyme implicated in the formation of nitric oxide by vascular endothelial cells. *Biochem Biophys Res Commun* 158: 348–352
56 Snyder J (1995) Nitric oxide. No endothelial NO. Nature 377: 196–197
57 Curran AD (1996) The role of nitric oxide in the development of asthma. *Int Arch Allergy Immunol* 111: 1–4
58 Furukawa K, Harrison DG, Saleh D, Shennib H, Chagnon FP, Giad, A (1996) Expression of nitric oxide synthase in the nasal mucosa. *Am J Respir Crit Care Med* 153: 847–850
59 Burke-Gaffney A, Hellewell, PG (1997) Endogenous nitric oxide limits cytokine-induced damage of murine lung epithelial cells. *Am J Physiol* 272: L707–L713.
60 Mitchell JA, Larkin S, Williams TJ (1995) Cyclooxygenase-2: regulation and relevance in inflammation. *Biochem Pharmacol* 50: 1535–1542

61 Burke-Gaffney A, Hellewell PG (1996) Tumour necrosis factor-alpha-induced ICAM-1 expression in human vascular endothelial and lung epithelial cells: modulation by tyrosine kinase inhibitors. *Br J Pharmacol* 119: 1149–1158

62 Bennett CF, Condon TP, Grimm S, Chan H, Chiang MY (1994) Inhibition of endothelial cell adhesion molecule expression with antisense oligonucleotides. *J Immunol* 152: 3530–3540

63 Cronstein BN, Kimmel SC, Levin RI, Martiniuk F, Weissmann G (1992) A mechanism for the antiinflammatory effects of corticosteroids: the glucocorticoid receptor regulates leukocyte adhesion to endothelial cells and expression of endothelial-leukocyte adhesion molecule 1 and intercellular adhesion molecule 1. *Proc Natl Acad Sci USA* 89: 9991–9995

64 Burke-Gaffney A, Hellewell PG (1996) Regulation of ICAM-1 by dexamethasone in a human vascular endothelial cell line EAhy926. *Am J Physiol* 270: C552–C561

65 Burke-Gaffney A, Keenan AK (1993) Does TNF-alpha directly increase endothelial cell monolayer permeability? *Agents Actions* 38: C83–C85

66 Deleuran B, Kristensen M, Paludan K, Zachariae C, Larsen CG, Zachariae E, Thestrup-Pedersen K (1992) The effect of second-line antirheumatic drugs on interleukin-8 mRNA synthesis and protein secretion in human endothelial cells. *Cytokine* 4: 403–409

67 Palmer RMJ, Bridge L, Foxwell NA, Moncada S (1992) The role of nitric oxide in endothelial cell damage and its inhibition by glucocorticoids. *Br J Pharmacol* 105: 11–12

68 Teixeira MM, Gristwood RW, Cooper N, Hellewell PG (1997) Phosphodiesterase (PDE)4 inhibitors: anti-inflammatory drugs of the future? *Trends Pharmacol Sci* 18: 164–171

69 Blease K, Burke-Gaffney A, Hellewell, PG (1998) Modulation of cell adhesion molecule expression and function on human lung microvascular endothelial cells by inhibition of phosphodiesterases 3 and 4. *Brit J Pharmacol* 124: 229–237

70 Suttorp N, Ehreiser P, Hippenstiel S, Fuhrmann M, Krull M, Tenor H, Schudt C (1996) Hyperpermeability of pulmonary endothelial monolayer: protective role of phosphodiesterase isoenzymes 3 and 4. *Lung* 174: 181–194

Airway epithelial cells

Jagdish Laxman Devalia, Jia Hua Wang and Robert James Davies

Academic Department of Respiratory Medicine, St. Bartholomew's and The Royal London School of Medicine and Dentistry, The London Chest Hospital, London E2 9JX, UK

Introduction

The epithelial lining of the airways forms the first line of defence against toxic and infectious agents in the inspired air. Although airway epithelial cells have traditionally been seen to play a vital role in providing an impermeable barrier and clearing the airways of noxious inhaled agents, through efficient mucociliary clearance, there is now increasing evidence to suggest that airway epithelial cells play a more important physico-chemical role. Several studies have demonstrated that epithelial cells are capable of synthesising and releasing several biologically active mediators which directly or indirectly influence the activity of inflammatory cells important in allergic airway diseases, including allergic rhinitis and asthma [1].

The airway epithelium as a physical barrier

The airway epithelium is a membrane-like barrier, comprised of several epithelial cell types (Fig. 1), and provides an interface between the respiratory system and the external environment. Whilst the anterior third of the nasal cavity is covered by a squamous epithelium, the posterior two-thirds is covered by a pseudo-stratified ciliated columnar epithelium. Although the distribution and characteristics of the cells in the upper epithelial lining are consistent with those of the lower airways [2, 3], the basal cells gradually decrease in number distally in the lower airways, until there are none in the terminal and respiratory bronchioles, and the pseudo stratified columnar epithelium is replaced by a single cuboidal epithelium.

Basal cells

The basal cells, which appear polygonal to ovoid in section, form a single cell layer along the airway basement membrane and are thought to play a major role in both

Cellular Mechanisms in Airways Inflammation, edited by Clive P. Page, Katharine H. Banner and Domenico Spina

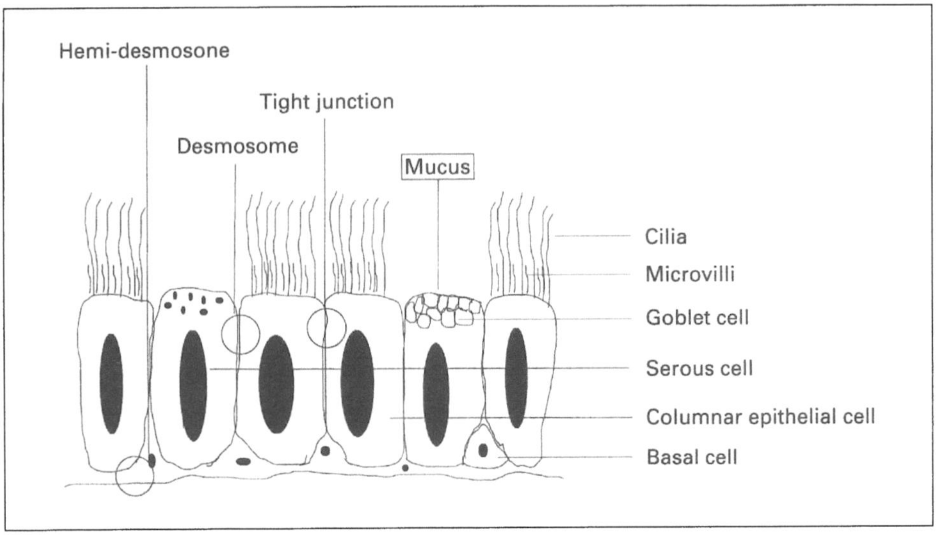

Figure 1
Schematic diagram of the major epithelial cell types in the airway epithelium.

the generation of columnar and goblet cells [4] and the attachment of columnar cells to airway basement membrane [5].

Ciliated columnar epithelial cells

The columnar cells constitute the superficial luminal borders of the epithelium and are composed of both ciliated and non-ciliated cells. The terminally differentiated ciliated cells form an upper cell layer at the apical surface of the airway epithelium and play a central role in mucociliary clearance, which is an integral component of defence against infectious agents and inhaled toxic materials in the respiratory system [2]. Electron microscopic studies of the airways have demonstrated that the ciliated cells are each covered with 50-100 hair-like mobile structures (cilia), each 4–6 µm in length and 0.33 µm in diameter in thickness, and are joined to each other at the luminal surface by tight junctions, which serve in maintaining a permeability barrier [2, 6] and preserving the integrity of the epithelium [7]. The cilia beat in synchrony to transport mucus efficiently and it has been suggested that the ciliary activity of the epithelial cells may be under the influence of the autonomic nervous system, since both adrenergic and cholinergic agents can stimulate the ciliary beat frequency of these cells [8].

In addition to cilia, the columnar cells are also covered by 300–400 microvilli, which are small finger-like projections from the cell surface: these are up to a maximum of 2 μm in length, approximately 0.1 μm in diameter, and unlike the cilia are immobile [9]. The microvilli prevent drying of the surface of the nasal mucosa and may also help in the transport of fluid and electrolytes between the cells and nasal fluid. The microvilli are not thought to be the precursors for cilia.

Non-ciliated columnar epithelial cells

The non-ciliated cells (also referred to as mucus cells) comprise goblet, serous, Clara and pre-secretory cell types, and are involved primarily in the production of airway secretions. These cells are also thought to be progenitor cells for terminally differentiated ciliated cells [10]. Goblet cells are unicellular mucous glands, with basally situated nuclei, and produce abundant droplets of mucus in the more superficial part of the cells before releasing them directly onto the surface of the ciliated epithelium [11]. Goblet cells are widely distributed throughout the surface of the respiratory epithelium and thought to be under the control of capsaicin-sensitive sensory nerves, since they can be induced to secrete mucus by neuropeptides released from capsaicin-sensitive sensory nerve endings [11].

The airway epithelium as a biochemically active barrier

Airway epithelium and hyperresponsiveness

Although increased airway responsiveness is a cardinal feature of bronchial asthma, this phenomenon is also associated with several other disease states, where airway inflammation and damage to the airway mucosa is well established. Consequently, it has been suggested that airway hyperresponsiveness may be related to the disruption of airway epithelium and airway inflammation. It is, however, not clear whether the loss of epithelial integrity in bronchial asthma contributes to the increased bronchial responsiveness or whether it is itself a result of airway inflammation and the consequential hyperreactivity. Nevertheless, there are several possible mechanisms through which epithelial abnormalities could lead to increased airway reactivity, including (i) increased permeability to allergen [12, 13]; (ii) changes in osmolarity of the airway surface lining fluid [13]; (iii) exposure of sensory nerve fibres to irritants and potentiation of local axon reflexes [12]; (iv) increased production of inflammatory mediators [1] and reduction of putative "protective" (both anti-inflammatory and relaxing) mediators [14, 15]; and (v) modulation of the immune system [16]. Of these mechanisms, the latter two have been the most widely studied and suggest that airway epithelial cells may play an important role in the modulation of airway function (under both normal and abnormal conditions) by influencing the expression, synthesis, release and degradation of substances such as nitric oxide, endothelin, metabolites of arachidonic acid, specific pro-inflammatory cytokines, "protective" substances, cell adhesion molecules and major histocompatibility complex (MHC) class II antigens. For the purpose of this chapter, some of these studies will be discussed in greater detail.

Culture of human airway epithelial cells *in vitro*

In spite of the increasing evidence for an important physico-chemical role of airway epithelium *in vivo*, it has, however, not proved easy to assign a specific pathogenic role to the airway epithelium, due to the presence of other cell types and underlying tissues. Consequently, a large number of mechanistic studies have employed human airway epithelial cell cultures as an ideal *in vitro* model system for investigating the association between airway epithelial cells, inflammation and hyperresponsiveness in airway disease. Although nasal and bronchial epithelial cells have been cultured *in vitro* by several groups, a major difficulty experienced by many of workers in the field has been to consistently grow these cells to confluence and to the terminally differentiated ciliated cell type. We have addressed these difficulties and have demonstrated that both nasal and bronchial ciliated epithelial cells can indeed grow to confluence to the fully differentiated ciliated cell types [17], and can be used in further investigations.

Airway epithelial cell-derived mediators

Nitric oxide

Studies have demonstrated that nitric oxide (NO) is a highly reactive multi-functional chemical produced by many diverse cell types, including epithelial cells, from L-arginine by the action of the enzyme nitric oxide synthase (NOS) [18, 19]. NOS is present as three isoforms, of which two are expressed constitutively and one is inducible. The constitutive isoforms (cNOS) are activated by calcium influx in response to physiological stimuli, to synthesise endogenous NO at picomolar concentrations required for the maintenance of physiological homeostasis [18–21]. In contrast, the inducible isoform (iNOS) is calcium-independent and transcribed in response to endotoxin and cytokines such as interferon γ (IFNγ), interleukin (IL)-1β and tumour necrosis factor α (TNFα) [18, 19, 22]. It is thought that the nanomolar concentrations of NO synthesised by the action of iNOS may lead to generation of peroxynitrites and hydroxyl radicals, which subsequently damage tissue [21].

Indeed, Guo and colleagues have demonstrated that in normal human airways iNOS mRNA is expressed abundantly and predominantly in airway epithelial cells, and that NO synthesis was due to continuous expression of the iNOS isoform in airway epithelial cells [23]. Other studies have suggested that bronchial epithelial cells of asthmatics may express increased levels of iNOS, compared with cells of non-asthmatic individuals, and consequently may contribute to increased epithelial damage and shedding observed in these individuals [21, 24].

Endothelin

The endothelins (ETs) are a family of three isopeptides, ET-1, ET-2 and ET-3 synthesised and released from both bronchial and nasal epithelial cells [25, 26] and mediating a number of effects including vasoconstriction, a slow but prolonged bronchocontraction and mucus secretion. Wu and colleagues have shown that ET-1 can also stimulate the synthesis of the eicosanoids, prostaglandin (PG) E_2, $PGF_{2\alpha}$, PGD_2, thromboxane B_2, and 15-hydroxyeicosatetraenoic acid (15-HETE) in human nasal explant cultures [27].

Several studies have demonstrated that bronchial epithelial cells express ETs and that mediators such as IL-1, TNFα, histamine and endotoxin can upregulate the expression of epithelial ET [28, 29]. These studies suggest that epithelial-derived ET play a role in the aetiology and pathogenesis of airway disease, particularly asthma. Indeed, several studies have demonstrated that the concentration of ET is raised in airways of asthmatics.

Studies investigating bronchoalveolar lavage (BAL) samples collected from asthmatics have demonstrated that ET-1 and ET-3 are raised in symptomatic individuals [30, 31]. Similarly, bronchial biopsy studies have also demonstrated that ET-immunoreactive material is present in increased concentration in airway epithelium of asthmatic individuals [32, 33]. Vittori and colleagues have investigated bronchial epithelial cells isolated from bronchial biopsies of patients with symptomatic asthma, patients with chronic obstructive pulmonary disease (COPD) and healthy non-smoking volunteers, and demonstrated that epithelial cells of asthmatics and COPD patients, but not cells of healthy non-smokers, expressed and released increased amounts of immunoreactive ET-1, *in vitro* [34].

Arachidonic acid metabolites

We and others have shown that cultured human tracheal and bronchial epithelial cells can metabolise arachidonic acid to PGE_2, $PGF_{2\alpha}$, leukotriene (LT) B_4, LTC_4 and additionally 12-HETE and 15-HETE [35–38]. Although there is evidence that many arachidonic acid metabolites may act as potent bronchial constrictors as well as cell activators and chemoattractants, the generation of these mediators and their relevance in airway inflammation and the initiation of hyperreactivity in asthma remains unclear. However, LTC_4 and its metabolites LTD_4 and LTE_4- have significant bronchoconstrictor activities. LTC_4 and LTD_4 can also increase membrane permeability and cause microvascular leakage and/or airway oedema. LTB_4 and LTE_4 have been shown to be potent chemoattractants for eosinophils and may further activate either eosinophils or the vascular endothelium to increase the migration of these cells [39, 40]. Similarly, PGD_2 and $PGF_{2\alpha}$ have potent "bronchoconstrictive" effects [41].

Inflammatory cytokines

Recent studies have demonstrated that human airway epithelial cells can generate a wide variety of cytokines, which either directly or in conjunction with one another influence the growth, differentiation, activation, migration, and survival of other inflammatory cells and therefore feature prominently in the allergic inflammatory response [42–45]. The epithelial cytokines can be divided into four groups according to their functions: (1) chemotactic factors, (2) colony stimulating factors, (3) growth factors and (4) pro-inflammatory multifunctional cytokines; and include IL-1β, IL-3, IL-6, IL-8, granulocyte macrophage colony stimulating factor (GM-CSF), granulocyte colony stimulating factor (G-CSF), TNFα and regulated on activation, normal T cell expressed and secreted (RANTES) and monocyte chemotactic protein-1 (MCP-1).

However, recent studies have demonstrated that there are differences in the ability of epithelial cells of atopic and non-atopic individuals to synthesise different amounts and/or profiles of pro-inflammatory cytokines, and suggest that genetic predisposition and manifestation of the symptoms of allergic airway disease in the atopic individuals may, at least in part, account for these differences.

Studies of epithelial cells cultured from nasal tissue of non-atopic non-rhinitic subjects, patients with allergic rhinitis and patients with nasal polyps have demonstrated that epithelial cells from rhinitics and individuals with nasal polyps synthesise significantly greater quantities of GM-CSF and IL-8, than cells of healthy non-atopic non-rhinitic individuals [46, 47]. Studies from our laboratory have demonstrated that epithelial cells cultured from nasal biopsies of atopic non-rhinitic and atopic rhinitic patients, release significantly greater amounts of IL-8, GM-CSF and TNFα, than non-atopic non-rhinitic healthy volunteers [48]. Additionally, our studies have demonstrated that epithelial cells from atopic rhinitics release significantly greater amounts of IL-1, TNFα, GM-CSF and RANTES during the pollen season [48]. Furthermore, epithelial cells of atopic rhinitics are more sensitive to stimulants, and exposure to ambient concentrations of ozone (O_3 10 ppb) exacerbates the release of RANTES only from the cells of atopic rhinitics during the pollen season (Fig. 2).

Similarly, studies of bronchial epithelial cells have demonstrated that asthmatics synthesise greater quantities of IL-1β, IL-16, GM-CSF and MCP-1 than non-asthmatic subjects *in vivo* [49–51] and the expression of IL-16 correlates well with the numbers of $CD4^+$ cells [51]. Preliminary studies of epithelial cells cultured from bronchial biopsies of well characterised groups of asthmatic and non-asthmatic subjects in our laboratory have also demonstrated that bronchial epithelial cells of

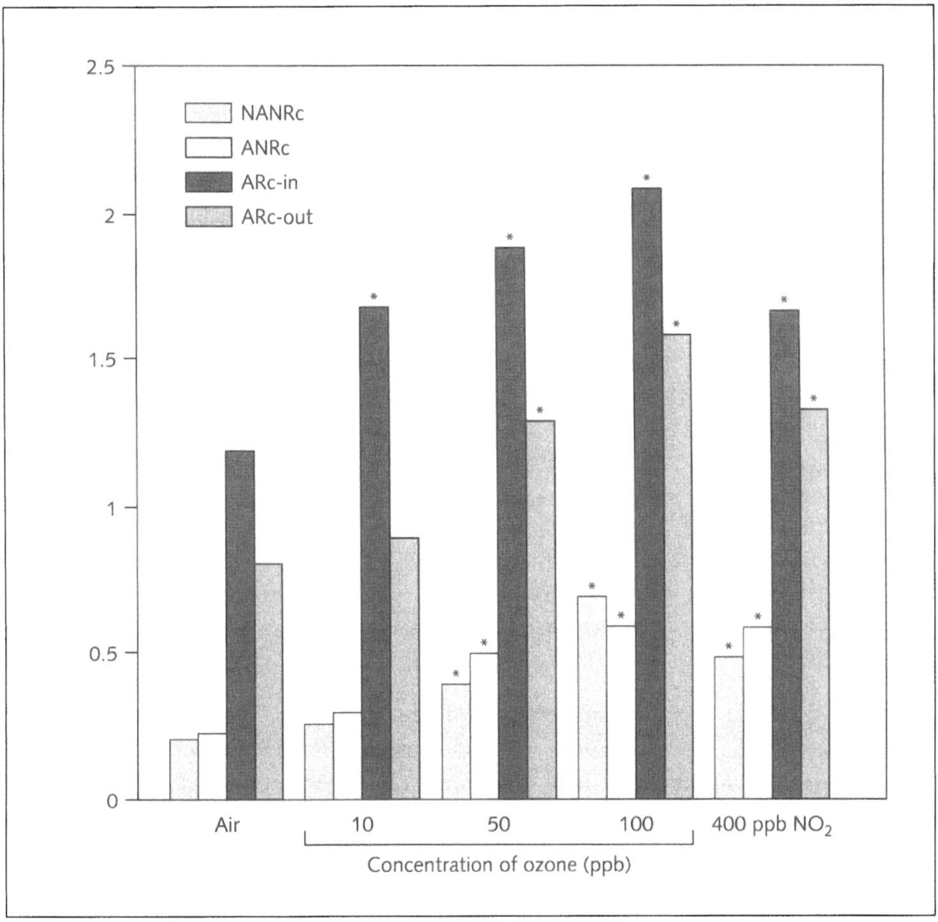

Figure 2
*Effect of exposure to ozone (O_3)/nitrogen dioxide (NO_2) on the release of RANTES from nasal epithelial cells of non-atopic non-rhinitic subjects (NANRc), atopic non-rhinitic subjects (ANRc) and atopic rhinitic patients outside of the pollen season (ARc-out) and during the pollen season (ARc-in). Results are expressed as median (n = 9 for each set of experiments; *$p < 0.05$ vs air).*

atopic asthmatics release significantly greater amounts of constitutive IL-8, GM-CSF, RANTES and soluble intercellular adhesion molecule-1 (sICAM-1) than non-atopic non-asthmatics [52] (Fig. 3). Similar to our findings for nasal epithelial cells of atopic rhinitic and non-atopic non-rhinitic individuals, epithelial cells of atopic asthmatics are also more susceptible after exposure to pollutants such as NO_2 and O_3 (Fig. 4), compared with non-atopic/non-asthmatics.

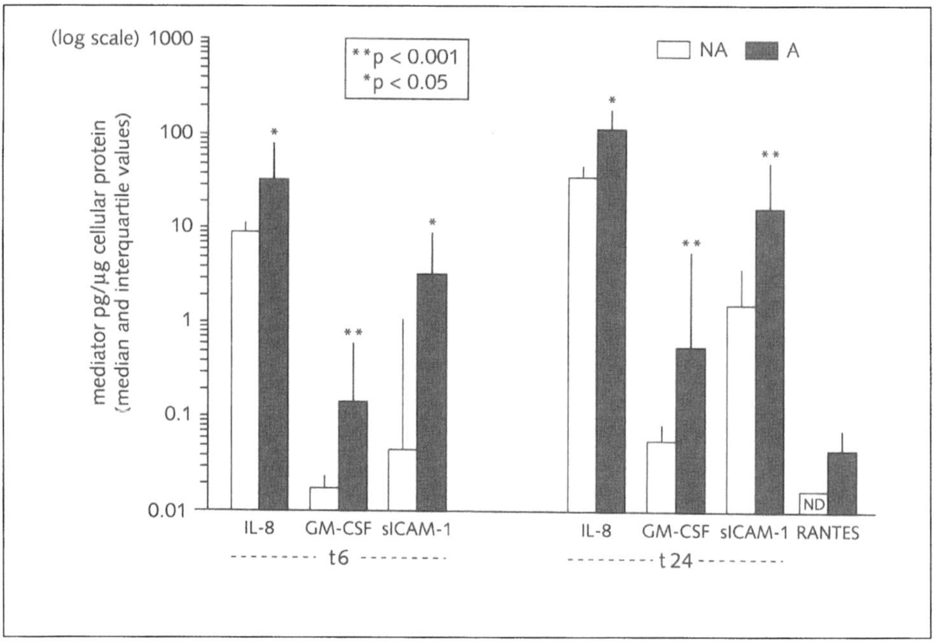

Figure 3
*Constitutive release of pro-inflammatory mediators by bronchial epithelial cells cultured from non-atopic non-asthmatic subjects (NA) and atopic asthmatic patients (A). Results are expressed as median and interquartile values (n = 8 for each set of experiments; *p < 0.05 and **p < 0.001 for NA vs A; ND, not detected).*

Collectively, these studies suggest that genetic pre-disposition and manifestation of symptoms of allergic airway disease in atopic individuals may, at least in part, be a consequence of increased expression, synthesis and release of specific pro-inflammatory mediators from airway epithelial cells, both constitutively and following exposure to external factors such as allergens and pollutants.

"Protective" mediators

In contrast to the bronchoconstrictive and inflammatory mediators expressed and synthesised by human airway epithelial cells, several studies have demonstrated that these cells are also capable of expressing naturally occurring protective mediators. PGE_2 is synthesised by human airway epithelium and is a potent inhibitor of both early and late phase asthmatic responses when given prior to allergen [53]. Other studies have shown that PGE_2 also has inhibitory effects on a variety of cytokines, leukotrienes and histamine [54, 55].

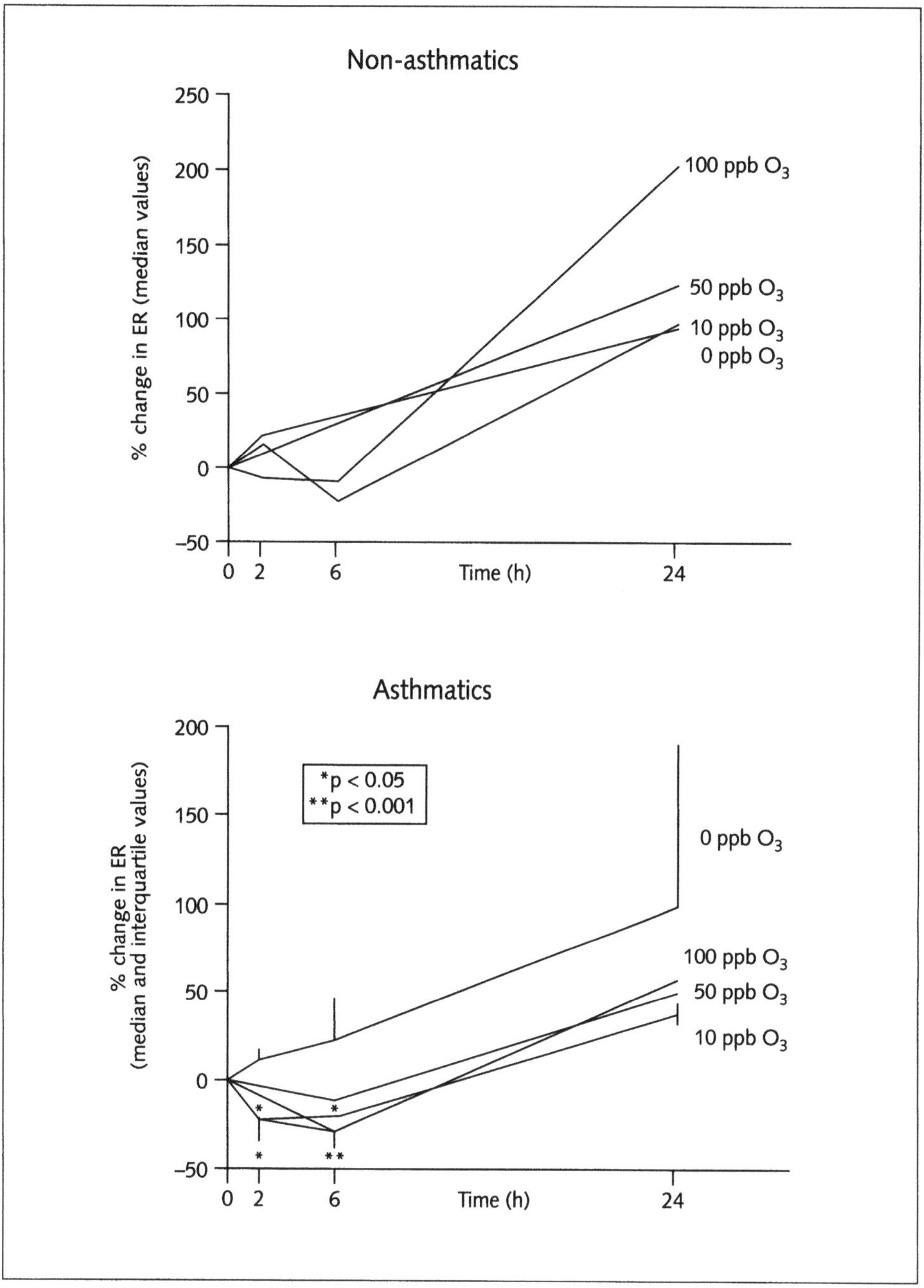

Figure 4

*Effect of exposure to ozone (O_3) on the electrical resistance of confluent bronchial epithelial cell cultures of non-atopic non-asthmatic subjects and atopic asthmatic patients (n = 8 for each set of experiments; *p < 0.05 vs air; **p < 0.001 vs air at each time-point).*

Some studies have suggested that airway epithelial cells may play a protective role against the adverse effects of neuropeptides such as substance P and bradykinin, by expressing and modulating the activity of a specific group of enzymes, including neutral endopeptidase (NEP), angiotensin-converting enzyme (ACE) and carboxypeptidase N (CPN) [56]. Ohkubo and co-workers have investigated the localization of these three enzymes in human nasal mucosa by immunohistochemical techniques and demonstrated that both NEP and ACE-immunoreactivity were strongly prominent in nasal epithelium [56, 57]. In contrast, immunoreactivity for CPN was most prominent in the superficial lamina propria [57]. More recently, in collaboration with others, we have investigated the distribution of NEP gene expression in human bronchial mucosa and also demonstrated that NEP-immunoreactive material and NEP mRNA were present in bronchial epithelium [58].

Similarly, animal studies have demonstrated that mechanical removal of airway epithelium leads to increased sensitivity of underlying airway smooth muscle to spasmogens, suggesting that this effect is a consequence of the removal or reduction of a naturally occurring epithelium derived smooth muscle relaxing factor [59, 60].

Consequently, it is possible that airway epithelial cell damage, as seen in asthma for example, could lead to changes in the concentrations of the naturally occurring "protective" substances, subsequently leading to airway inflammation and hyperresponsiveness.

Cell adhesion molecules

Cell adhesion molecules are specific cell surface receptors which mediate adhesion of cells to one another and to extracellular matrix [61, 62]. They play a crucial role in embryonic development, maintenance of tissue architecture, tumour metastasis, wound healing and inflammatory response [61–63]. The cell adhesion molecules are divided broadly into four main classes: (i) integrins, (ii) immunoglobulin superfamily, (iii) selectins and (iv) cadherins, of which members of the former two groups have been greatly studied.

Several studies have demonstrated that the α-integrin family, and more specifically members of the β_1 integrin subfamily, are expressed on human bronchial and nasal epithelial cells. The members of the β_1 integrin subfamily function as cell surface receptors which bind extracellular matrix components collagen, fibronectin, vitronectin and laminin [63–65], and influence (i) adherence of epithelial cells to basement membrane and underlying connective tissue, (ii) migration of leucocytes through endothelium and (iii) localisation of leucocytes at sites of inflammation in the epithelium. Our studies with cultured cells have shown that both nasal [66] and bronchial [67] epithelial cells are capable of expressing the $\beta_1\alpha_{2-6}$ integrins, *in vitro*. In contrast, marked expression of only $\beta_1\alpha_{2,\ 3\ \&\ 6}$ integrins is seen in the nasal and bronchial epithelium *in vivo*, with no difference in the expression between non-allergic subjects and patients with perennial rhinitis/seasonal allergic rhinitis/asthma [66–68].

Studies of the immunoglobulin superfamily have demonstrated that this is a large group of molecules with multiple immunoglobulin-like domains. This group includes the adhesion molecules ICAM-1, ICAM-2, ICAM-3 and VCAM-1, which play an important role in interactions involving leucocytes [69, 70]. ICAM-1 is perhaps the most widely studied of this group of molecules which is expressed constitutively at low levels by several cell types, including airway epithelial cells, and is markedly unregulated by inflammatory stimuli such as endotoxin, IL-1β, TNFα and IFNγ [66–73].

Functional studies have suggested that ICAM-1 may play a role in respiratory tract viral infections since this is thought to be the surface receptor for the major group of rhinoviruses which can cause airway epithelial cell damage [74]. More importantly, other studies have suggested that ICAM-1 influences the inter-tissue trafficking of neutrophils, eosinophils and lymphocytes [70, 75], and therefore may play a more ubiquitous role in the pathogenesis of airway disease.

Studies in animals have demonstrated that ICAM-1 expression is upregulated in inflammed airway epithelium *in vivo*, and may play an important role in airway eosinophilia and hyperresponsiveness, since antibodies against ICAM-1 can attenuate both the eosinophilia and hyperresponsiveness in these animals [76,77]. Similarly, studies in humans have demonstrated that the expression of airway epithelial cell adhesion molecules is enhanced in allergic conditions such as asthma and rhinitis. Manolitsas and co-workers have demonstrated that expression ICAM-1 is upregulated on bronchial tissue of patients with bronchial asthma [68]. Similarly, Montefort and colleagues have demonstrated that expression of ICAM-1 is significantly increased on nasal mucosa in perennial allergic rhinitis patients, compared to non-rhinitic individuals [78]. Furthermore, several studies have demonstrated that levels of serum sICAM-1 are also raised in stable atopic asthmatic patients, compared with healthy non-asthmatic subjects, and are elevated further during exacerbations of asthma [79–82].

HLA class II antigens

Several studies have demonstrated that type II alveolar epithelial cells and ciliated bronchial epithelial cells are capable of expressing class II major histocompatibility complex antigens (MHC II, HLA-DR) and that cytokines can increase the expression of these cell surface molecules [83–85]. The findings from these studies suggest that airway epithelial cells may additionally have a potentially important role in antigen processing/presentation and subsequent initiation and propagation of immune-mediated airway inflammation.

The putative mechanisms and consequences of the interaction between antigen presenting cells (APCs) and T lymphocytes have been reviewed recently [16]. It has been suggested that preferential binding of specific allergenic peptides to the HLA-class II antigens may lead to recognition by activation and proliferation of specific

T cell clones (either Th1 or Th2), which pre-dispose the individual to the development of certain diseases [86, 87].

Poston and colleagues have demonstrated that expression of HLA class II antigen is significantly upregulated in basal epithelial cells of asthmatic bronchial epithelium [88]. Similarly, Stoop and colleagues have investigated biopsy specimens of turbinates from both healthy subjects and patients with nasal polyps, by immunohistochemical staining, and demonstrated that there was a significant increase in the number of HLA-DR positive cells (including epithelial cells) in the nasal mucosa of patients with nasal polyps, compared to healthy subjects [89]. Further, these authors demonstrated that there was a concomitant increase in the number of $CD4^+$ and $CD8^+$ cells, suggesting a likely interaction between the HLA-DR positive cells and T lymphocytes. More recently, Nag and colleagues have demonstrated that complexes formed between soluble major histocompatibility (sMHC) class II molecules and antigenic peptides, which can be recognised by T cell receptors (TCRs) on $CD4^+$ T cell clones and render these cells non-responsive, also induces antigen-specific apoptosis in murine T cell clones, independently of non-responsiveness [90]. Thus, manipulation of T cell activity may offer novel therapeutic strategies for the management of T cell-associated diseases.

Summary

In view of the multi-functional role of the airway epithelium, and particularly the different types of epithelial cells which predominate in the epithelium, it is not difficult to envisage how perturbation of this barrier may bring about adverse changes in and around the surrounding tissues and possibly help to explain the pathogenesis of allergic airway diseases. It is tempting to hypothesise that in allergic airway diseases dysfunction of the airway epithelium, resulting from either acute exposure to airborne irritants such as air pollutants, allergen, viruses, bacteria, etc, or as a consequence of genetic pre-disposition to a specific allergen, itself results in the initiation, maintenance and potentiation of inflammation at the site/s of exposure. This may be expressed either in the form of generation of pro-inflammatory mediators, which interact with mediators derived from other inflammatory cells such as mast cells and T lymphocytes, and act as potent eosinophil and neutrophil chemoattractants and activators or up-regulate cell adhesion molecules involved in the inter-tissue trafficking of these and other "inflammatory" cell types. Alternatively, depletion of any naturally occurring anti-inflammatory mediators and smooth muscle relaxing agents, which help to maintain the integrity of the airways and the surrounding tissues, may ensue and also lead to adverse reactions in the airways.

Consequently, it is likely that agents which influence the generation, bioavailability and/or biological activity of both pro- and anti-inflammatory cytokines will play an important therapeutic role in the management of airway disease.

References

1 Devalia JL, Davies RJ (1993) Airway epithelial cells and mediators of inflammation. *Respir Med* 87: 405–408
2 Carson JL, Collier AM, Boucher RC (1987) Ultrastructure of the respiratory epithelium in the human nose. In: N Mygind, U Pipkorn (eds): *Allergic and vasomotor rhinitis: pathophysiological aspects*. Munksgaard, Copenhagen, 11–27
3 Mygind N, Bisgaard H (1990) Applied anatomy of the airways. In: N Mygind, U Pipkorn, R Dahl (eds): *Rhinitis and asthma: similarities and differences*. Munksgaard, Copenhagen, 21–37
4 Jacquot J, Hayem A, Galabert C (1992) Functions of proteins and lipids in airway secretions. *Eur Respir J* 5: 343–358
5 Evans MJ, Plopper CG (1988) The role of basal cells in adhesion of columnar epithelium to airway basement membrane. *Am Rev Respir Dis* 138: 481–483
6 Farquhar MG, Palade GE (1963) Junctional complexes in various epithelia. *J Cell Biol* 17: 375–412
7 Elia C, Bucca C, Rolla G, Scappaticci E, Cantino DA (1988) Freeze-fracture study of human bronchial epithelium in normal, bronchitic and asthmatic subjects. *J Submicrosc Cytol Pathol* 20: 509–517
8 Rusznak C, Devalia JL, Lozewicz S, Davies RJ (1994) The assessment of nasal mucociliary clearance and the effect of drugs. *Respir Med* 88: 89–101
9 Nils G. (1981) Structure and ultrastructure of the nose. In: N Mygind (ed): *Nasal allergy*. Blackwell Scientific Publications, Oxford, 3–38
10 Evans MJ, Shami SG, Cabral-Anderson LJ, Dekker NP (1986) Role of non-ciliated cells in renewal of the bronchial epithelium of rats exposed to NO_2. *Am J Pathol* 123: 126–133
11 Rogers DF (1994) Airway goblet cells: responsive and adaptable front-line defenders. *Eur Respir J* 7: 1690–1706
12 Hulsmann AR, De Jongste JC (1996) Modulation of airway responsiveness by airway epithelium in humans: putative mechanisms. *Clin Exp Allergy* 26: 1236–1242
13 Lozewicz S, Wells C, Gomez E, Ferguson H, Richman P, Devalia J, Davies RJ (1990) Morphological integrity of the bronchial epithelium in mild asthmatics. *Thorax* 45: 12–15
14 Vanhoute PM (1988) Epithelium-derived relaxing factor(s) and bronchial reactivity. *Am Rev Respir Dis* 138: 24S–30S
15 Wilkens JH, Wilkens H, Forstermann U, Frolich JC (1990) The effect of bronchial epithelium on bronchial contractility. *Pneumologie* 44: 373–374
16 Ricci M, Rossi O (1990) Dysregulation of IgE responses and airway allergic inflammation in atopic individuals. *Clin Exp Allergy* 20: 601–609
17 Devalia JL, Sapsford RJ, Wells C, Richman P, Davies RJ (1990) Culture and comparison of human bronchial and nasal epithelial cells *in vitro*. *Respir Med* 84: 303–312
18 Lyons CR (1996) The role of nitric oxide in inflammation. *Adv Immunol* 60: 323–370

19 Barnes PJ, Belvisi MG (1996) Exhaled nitric oxide: a new lung function test. *Thorax* 51: 233–237
20 Barnes PJ, Belvisi MG (1993) Nitric oxide and lung disease. *Thorax* 48: 1034–1043
21 Howarth PH, Redington AE, Sringall DR et al (1995) Epithelially derived endothelin and nitric oxide in asthma. *Int Arch Allergy Immunol* 107: 228–230
22 Robbins RA, Barnes PJ, Springall DR, Warren JB, Kwon OJ, Buttery LDK, Wilson AJ, Geller DA, Polak JM (1994) Expression of inducible nitric oxide in human lung epithelial cells. *Biochem Biophys Res Commun* 203: 209–218
23 Guo FH, DeRaeve HR, Rice TW et al (1995) Continuous nitric oxide synthesis by inducible nitric oxide synthase in normal airway epithelium *in vivo*. *Proc Natl Acad Sci USA* 92: 7809–7813
24 Hamid Q, Springall DR, Riveros-Moreno V et al (1993) Induction of nitric oxide synthase in asthma. *Lancet* 342: 1510–1513
25 Inoue A, Yanagisawa M, Kimura S, Kasuya Y, Miyauchi T, Goto K, Masaki T (1989) The human endothelin family: three structurally and pharmacologically distinct isopeptides predicted by three separate genes. *Proc Natl Acad Sci USA* 86: 2863–2867
26 Mullol J, Chowdhury BA, White MV, Ohkubo K, Rieves RD, Baraniuk J, Hausfeld JN, Shelhamer JH, KalinerMA (1993) Endothelin in human nasal mucosa. *Am J Respir Cell Mol Biol* 8: 393–402
27 Wu T, Mullol J, Rieves RD et al (1992) Endothelin-1 stimulates eicosanoid production in cultured human nasal mucosa. *Am J Respir Cell Mol Biol* 6: 168–174
28 Nakano J, Takizawa H, Ohtoshi T, Shoji S, Yamaguchi M, Ishii A, Yanagisawa M, Ito K (1994) Endotoxin and pro-inflammatory cytokines stimulate endothelin-1 expression and release by airway epithelial cells. *Clin Exp Allergy* 24: 330–336
29 Ackerman V, Carpi S, Bellini A, Vassalli G, Marini M, Mattoli S (1995) Constitutive expression of endothelin in bronchial epithelial cells of patients with symptomatic and asymptomatic asthma and modulation by histamine and interleukin-1. *J Allergy Clin Immunol* 96: 618–627
30 Nomoura A, Uchida Y, Kameyama M, Saotome M, Oki K, Hasegawa S (1989) Endothelin and bronchial asthma. *Lancet* 2: 747–748
31 Marini M, Fasoli A, Mattoli S (1991) Release of endothelin in the airways of patients with symptomatic asthma and reversible airflow obstruction. *Am Rev Respir Dis* 143 (Suppl): A158
32 Springall DR, Howarth PH, Counihan H et al (1991) Endothelin immunoreactivity of airway epithelium in asthmatic patients. *Lancet* 337: 697–701
33 Redington AE, Springall DR, Ghatei MA et al (1995) Endothelin in bronchoalveolar lavage fluid and its relationship to airflow obstruction in asthma. *Am J Respir Crit Care Med* 151: 1034–1039
34 Vittori E, Marini M, Fasoli A et al (1992) Increased expression of endothelin in bronchial epithelial cells of asthmatic patients and effect of corticosteroids. *Am Rev Respir Dis* 146: 1320–1325

35 Bradding P, Redington AE, Djukanovic R et al (1995) 15-Lipoxygenase immunoreactivity in normal and in asthmatic airways. *Am J Respir Crit Care Med* 151: 1201–1204
36 Hunter JA, Finkbeiner WE, Nadel JA, Goetzl EJ, Holtzman MJ (1985) Predominant generation of 15-lipoxygenase metabolites of arachidonic acid by epithelial cells from human trachea. *Proc Natl Acad Sci USA* 82: 4633–4637
37 Churchill L, Chilton FH, Resau JH, Bascom R, Hubbard WC, Proud D (1989) Cyclooxygenase metabolism of endogenous arachidonic acid by cultured human tracheal epithelial cells. *Am Rev Respir Dis* 140: 449–459
38 Devalia JL, Sapsford RJ, Cundell DR Campbell AM, Davies RJ (1993) Human bronchial epithelial cell dysfunction following exposure to nitrogen dioxide *in vitro*. *Eur Respir J* 6: 1308–1316
39 Henderson W (1987) Eicosanoids and lung inflammation. *Am Rev Respir Dis* 135: 1176–1185
40 Laitinen LA, Laitinen A, Haahtela T, Vilkka V, Spur BW, Lee TH (1993) Leukotriene E4 and granulocyte infiltration into asthmatic airways. *Lancet* 341: 989–900
41 Wenzel SE, Westocott JY, Smith HR, Larsen GL (1989) Spectrum of prostanoid release after bronchoalveolar allergen challenge in atopic asthmatics and in control group. *Am Rev Respir Dis* 139: 450–457
42 Denburg JA, Jordana M, Gibson P, Hargreave F, Gauldie J, Dolovich J (1990) Cellular and molecular basis of allergic airways inflammation. In: SGO Johanssen (ed): *Pharmacia allergy research foundation award book*. AW Grafiska, Uppsala, 15–22
43 Devalia JL, Campbell AM, Sapsford RJ, Rusnak C, Quint D, Godard P, Bousquet J, Davies RJ (1993) The effect of nitrogen dioxide on synthesis of inflammatory cytokines expressed by human bronchial epithelial cells *in vitro*. *Am J Respir Cell Mol Biol* 9: 271–278
44 Wang JH, Devalia JL, Xia C, Sapsford RJ, Davies RJ (1996) Expression of RANTES in human bronchial epithelial cells *in vitro* and *in vivo*, the effect of corticosteroids. *Am J Respir Cell Mol Biol* 9: 271–278
45 Levine SJ (1995) Bronchial epithelial cell-cytokine interactions in airway inflammation. *J Invest Med* 3: 241–249
46 Mullol J, Xaubet A, Gaya A et al (1995) Cytokine gene expression and release from epithelial cells. A comparison study between healthy nasal mucosa and nasal polyps. *Clin Exp Allergy* 25: 607–615
47 Ohtoshi T, Tsuda T, Vancheri C et al (1991) Human upper airway epithelial cell-derived granulocyte-macrophage colony-stimulating factor induces histamine-containing cell differentiation of human progenitor cells. *Int Arch Allergy Appl Immunol* 95: 376–384
48 Calderon MA, Devalia JL, Prior AJ, Sapsford RJ, Davies RJ (1997) A comparison of cytokine release from epithelial cells cultured from nasal biopsy specimens of atopic patients with and without rhinitis and nonatopic subjects without rhinitis. *J Allergy Clin Immunol* 99: 65–76
49 Sousa AR, Lane SJ, Nakhosteen JA, Yoshimura T, Lee TH, Poston RN (1994) Increased

expression of the monocyte chemoattractant protein-1 in bronchial tissue from asthmatic subjects. *Am J Respir Cell Mol Biol* 10: 142–147

50 Marini M, Vittori E, Hollomberg T, Mattoli S (1992) Expression of the potent inflammatory cytokines granulocyte macrophage-colony stimulating factor and interleukin-6 and interleukin-8 in bronchial epithelial cells of patients with asthma. *J Allergy Clin Immunol* 89: 1001–1009

51 Laberge S, Ernst P, Ghaffar O, Song YL, Cruikshank WW, Center DM, Hamid Q (1996) Increase in interleukin-16 (IL-16) expression in baseline asthma. *J Allergy Clin Immunol* 97: 1 (Part 3); 313 (abstract)

52 Bayram H, Devalia JL, Khair OA, Abdelaziz MM, Sapsford RJ, Ohtoshi T, Davies RJ (1997) Effect of diesel exhaust particles (DEP) on release of inflammatory mediators from bronchial epithelial cell cultures of non-atopic non-asthmatic and atopic asthmatic subjects *in vitro*. *Eur Respir J* 10 (Suppl 25): 414s

53 Pavord I, Wong C, Williams J, Tattersfield A (1993) Effect of inhaled prostaglandin E2 on allergen-induced asthma. *Am Rev Respir Dis* 148: 87–90

54 Marone G, Kagey-Sobotka, Lichtenstein L (1979) Effects of arachidonic acid and its metabolites on antigen-induced histamine release from human basophils *in vitro*. *J Immunol* 123: 1669–1677

55 Christman BW, Christman JW, Dworski R, Blair IA, Prakash C (1993) Prostaglandin E2 limits arachidonic acid availability and inhibits leukotriene B4 synthesis in rat alveolar macrophages by a non phospholipase A2 mechanism. *J Immunol* 151: 1096–1104

56 Ohkubo K, Baraniuk JN, Hohman RJ et al (1993) Human nasal mucosal neutral endopeptidase (NEP): location, quantitation and secretion. *Am J Respir Cell Mol Biol* 9: 557–567

57 Ohkubo K, Okuda M, Kaliner MA (1994) Immunological localization of neuropeptide-degrading enzymes in the nasal mucosa. *Rhinology* 31: 130–133

58 Baraniuk JN, Ohkubo K, Kwon OJ et al (1995) Localizatrion of neutral endopeptidase (NEP) mRNA in human bronchi. *Eur Respir J* 8: 1458–1464

59 Hay DWP, Farmer SC, Raeburn D, Robinson VA, Flemming WW, Feaden JS (1986) Airway epithelium modulates the reactivity of guinea pig respiratory smooth muscle. *Eur J Pharmacol* 129: 11–18

60 Vanhoute PM (1988) Epithelium-derived relaxing factor(s) and bronchial reactivity. *Am Rev Respir Dis* 138: 24S–30S

61 Macky CR, Imhof BA (1993) Cell adhesion in immune system. *Immunol Today* 14: 99–104

62 Frenete PS, Wagner DD (1996) Adhesion molecules. *N Eng J Med* 6: 1526–1529

63 Albelda SM, Buck CA (1990) Integrins and other cell adhesion molecules. *FASEB J* 4: 2868–2880

64 Hynes RO (1987) Interins, a family of cell surface receptors. *Cell* 48: 549–555

65 Hemler ME (1987) VLA proteins in the integrin family: structures, functions and their role on leucocytes. *Ann Rev Cell Biol* 3: 179–205

66 Devalia JL, Calderon M, Sapsford RJ, McAulay AE, d'Ardenne AJ, Davies RJ (1991)

Cell adhesion molecules expressed by human nasal epithelial cells. *Clin Exp Allergy* 22: 120 (abstract)
67 Devalia JL, Sapsford RJ, McAulay AE, d'Ardenne AJ, Davies RJ (1991) Comparison of cell adhesion molecules synthesised by human bronchial epithelial cells *in vitro* and *in vivo*. *Schweiz Med Wsch* 21 (Suppl 40/1): 48 (abstract)
68 Manolitsas ND, Trigg CJ, McAulay AE, Wang JH, Jordan SE, d'Ardenne AJ, DaviesRJ (1994) The expression of intercellular adhesion molecule-1 and the β_1-integrins in asthma. *Eur Respir J* 7: 1439–1444
69 Kishimoto TK, Anderson DC (1992) The role of integrins in inflammation. In: JI Gallin, IM Goldstein, R Snyderman (eds): *Inflammation: basic principles and clinical correlates*, 2nd ed. Raven Press, New York, 353–406
70 Wegner CD, Gundel RH, Rothlein R, Letts G (1992) Expression and probable roles of cell adhesion molecules in lung inflammation. *Chest* 101S: 34–39
71 Calderon E, Lockey RF (1992) A possible role of adhesion molecules in asthma. *J Allergy Clin Immunol* 90: 852–865
72 Tosi MF, Stark JM, Smith CW, Hamedani A, Gruenert DC, Infeld MD (1992) Induction of ICAM-1 expression on human airway epithelial cells by inflammatory cytokines: effects on neutrophil-epithelial cell adhesion. *Am J Respir Cell Mol Biol* 7: 214–221
73 Bloemen PGM, van den Tweel MC, Henricks PAJ, Engels F, Wagenaar SS, Rutten AAJJL, Nijkamp FP (1993) Expression and modulation of adhesion molecules on human bronchial epithelial cells. *Am J Respir Cell Mol Biol* 9: 586–593
74 Staunton DE, Merluzzi VJ, Rothlein R, Barton R, Martin SD, Springer TA (1989) A cell adhesion molecule, ICAM-1, is the major receptor for Rhinoviruses. *Cell* 56: 849–853
75 Dobrina A, Menegazzi R, Carlos TM, Nardon E, Cramer R, Zacchi T, Harlen JM, Patriarca P (1991) Mechanisms of eosinophils adherence to cultured vascular endothelial cells. *J Clin Invest* 88: 20–26
76 Wegner CD, Gundel RH, Reilly P, Haynes N, Letts G, Rothlein R (1990) Intercellular adhesion molecule-1 (ICAM-1) in the pathogenesis of asthma. *Science* 247: 456–459
77 Keelan E, Hashard D (1992) CAMS and anti-CAMs. *J Royal Coll Phys Lon* 149: 4021–4028
78 Monterfort S, Feather IH, Wilson SJ, Haskard DO, Lee TH, Holgate ST, Howarth PH (1992) The expression of leukocyte-endothelial adhesion molecules is increased in perennial allergic rhinitis. *Am J Respir Cell Mol Biol* 7: 393–398
79 Hashimoto S, Imai K, Kobayashi T, Amemiya E, Takahashi Y, Tomita Y, Iwata T, Suguro H, Yamaguchi M, Yachi A (1993). Elevated levels of soluble ICAM-1 in sera from patients with bronchial asthma. *Allergy* 48: 370–372
80 Kobayashi T, Hashimoto S, Imai K, Amemiya E, Yamaguchi M, Yachi A, Horie T (1994) Elevation of serum soluble intercellular adhesion molecule-1 (sICAM-1) and sE-selectin levels in bronchial asthma. *Clin Exp Immunol* 96: 110–115
81 Montefort S, Lai CKW, Kapahi P, Leung J, Lai KN, Chan HS, Haskard DO, Howarth PH, Holgate ST (1994) Circulating adhesion molecules in asthma. *Am J Respir Crit Care Med* 149: 1149–1152

82 Koizumi A, Hashimoto S, Kobayashi T, Imai K, Yachi A, Horie T (1995) Elevation of serum soluble vascular cell adhesion molecule-1 (sVCAM-1) levels in bronchial asthma. *Clin Exp Immunol* 101: 468–473

83 Komatsu T, Yamamoto M, Shimokata K, Nagura H (1989) Phenotypic characterisation of alveolar capillary endothelial cells, alveolar epithelial cells and alveolar macrophages in patients with pulmonary fibrosis, with special reference to MHC class II *antigens. Virchows Arch* 415: 79–90

84 Liversidge JM, Sewell HF, Forrester JV (1988) Human retinal pigment epithelial cells differentially express MHC class II (HLA, DP, DR and DQ) antigens in response to *in vitro* stimulation with lymphokine or purified IFNγ. *Clin Exp Immunol* 73: 489–494

85 Motojima K, Matsuo S, Mullen Y (1989) DR antigen expression on vascular endothelium and duct epithelium in fresh or cultured human fetal pancreata in the presence of gamma-interferon. *Transplantation* 48: 1022–1026

86 Mosmann TR, Coffman RL (1989) Heterogeneity of cytokine secretion patterns and function of helper T cells. *Adv Immunol* 46: 111–147

87 Maggi E, Macchia D, Parronchi P, Del Prete G, De Carli M, Piccinni MP, Simonelli C, Biswas P, Romagnani S, Ricci M (1991) The IgE response in atopy and infections. *Clin Exp Allergy* 21 (Suppl 1): 72–78

88 Poston RN, Chanez P, Lacoste JY, Litchfield T, Lee TH, Bousquet J (1992) Immunohistochemical characterization of the cellular infiltrate in asthmatic bronchi. *Am Rev Respir Dis* 145: 918–921

89 Stoop AE, Hameleers DMH, v Run PEM, Biewenga J, van der Baan S (1989) Lymphocytes and non lymphoid cells in the nasal mucosa of patients with nasal polyps and of healthy subjects. *J Allergy Clin Immunol* 84: 734–741

90 Nag B, Kendrick T, Arimilli S, Yu SC, Sriram S (1996) Soluble MHC II-peptide complexes induce antigen-specific apoptosis in T cells. *Cell Immunol* 170: 25–33

Airway smooth muscle cells

Alastair G. Stewart[1], *Darren J. Fernandes*[1], *Valentina Koutsoubos*[1], *Aurora Messina*[2], *Claire E. Ravenhall*[1], *Ross Vlahos*[1] *and Kai-Feng Xu*[3]

[1]Department of Pharmacology, University of Melbourne, Parkville, Victoria 3052, Australia; [2]Bernard O'Brien Institute of Microsurgery, St Vincent's Hospital, Fitzroy, Victoria 3065, Australia; [3]Peking Union Medical College Hospital, Beijing, China

Introduction

Airway smooth muscle (ASM) cell complexity is becoming increasingly apparent. Initially considered to be merely a contractile element, it is now known that smooth muscle cells actively regulate their function and microenvironment by producing a range of cytokines and low molecular weight products in addition to extracellular matrix. Growth and proliferation of smooth muscle cells within the airway is also recognised as a component of airway pathology, especially in asthma. This chapter is intended to provide an overview of smooth muscle function and to highlight recent advances in areas of active research.

Structural and functional characteristics

Ultrastructure

ASM cells are elongated and spindle shaped, and contain a thin elongated central oval nucleus with a prominent nucleolus and dense cytoplasm. They measure up to 600 μm in length and are oriented such that the thick middle portion of the cells lie against the thin tapered end of adjacent cells. In transverse section, light and dark cells can be identified which appear to correspond to differing contents of myofilaments (Fig. 1a). At the ultrastructural level, the perinuclear sarcoplasm is devoid of fibrils and contains the majority of organelles including rough endoplasmic reticulum, Golgi apparatus, mitochondria, dilated cisternae, ribosomes and vesicles (Fig. 1b). The sarcoplasmic membrane contains numerous invaginations known as caveoli. The remainder of the cell body is occupied predominantly by myofibrils (mostly actin) (Fig. 1c). Individual muscle fibres are surrounded by an extracellular matrix (ECM) comprising a continuous basement membrane of reticular fibres and collagenous bundles embedded in a protein polysaccharide ground substance (Fig. 1c).

Cellular Mechanisms in Airways Inflammation, edited by Clive P. Page, Katharine H. Banner and Domenico Spina

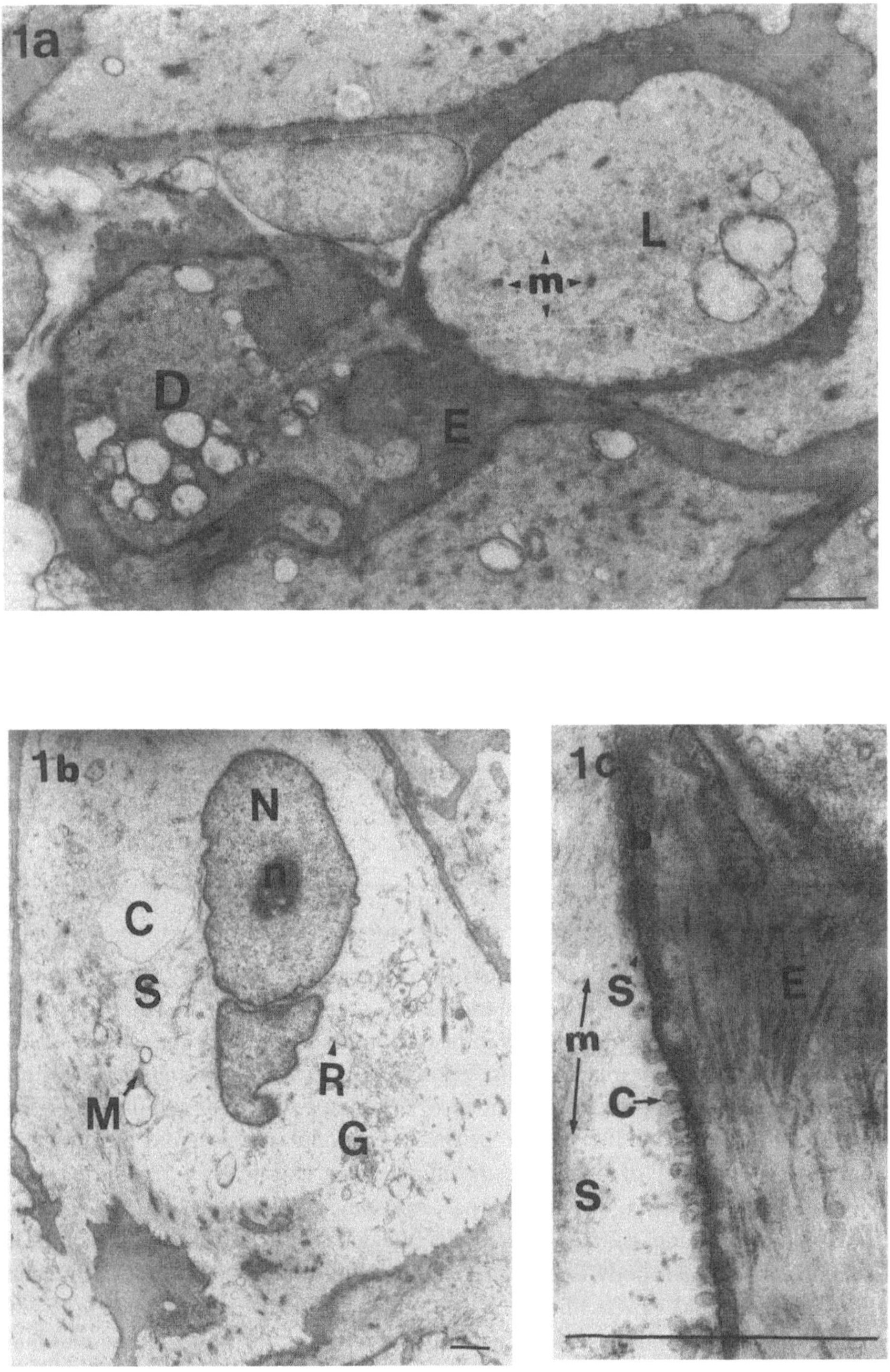
1a
L
m
D
E
1b
N
n
C
S
R
M
G
1c
n
S
E
m
C
S

Smooth muscle cells cultured from large airways become flattened and spindle shaped and contain a central oval shaped nucleus [1]. Two nuclear sizes, 9 μm and 15 μm across the shortest diameter, can be identified and these contain 2–7 or 1–2 prominent nucleoli, respectively. The smaller of the two cell types predominates. At the ultrastuctural level, the perinuclear sarcoplasm contains an abundance of synthetic organelles including rough endoplasmic reticulum, Golgi apparatus, mitochondria, dilated cisternae, ribosomes and vesicles (Fig. 2a). Unlike smooth muscle cells in the trachealis *in situ*, cultured smooth muscle cell processes also contain organelles consisting of mitochondria and free ribosomes as well as homogeneous scattered myofibrils. There is a dense band of longitudinally oriented myofibrils just below the sarcolemma which is continuous along the whole length of the cell (Fig. 2b).

Contractile mechanisms

The contractile apparatus of smooth muscle enables slow, sustained contractions which overcome resting loads to shorten. These loads comprise viscous and elastic structural elements in the airway wall and surrounding tissue, cartilage in large airways and transmural pressures [2]. The circumferential orientation of the shortening smooth muscle cells reduces the calibre of the airway, thereby increasing airway resistance [2]. The central airways control resistance and airflow distribution, while the peripheral airways contribute to the regulation of regional ventilation to perfusion ratio (V/Q) [3].

Smooth muscle contraction

Smooth muscle cells are connected *via* cell junctions, enabling co-ordinated contraction of the whole muscle sheet. Adherens junctions and their constitutive dense bands provide insertion points for the myofilaments of the contractile apparatus and the cytoskeleton. Activation of the contractile apparatus results in an inward pull on the sarcolemma through the attachments of the contractile elements to the basal lamina of the cell [4]. The contractile apparatus itself, shortens by the energy-depen-

Figure 1
Transmission electron micrographs (TEM) of normal human bronchial smooth muscle cells in situ; *sarcoplasm (S), sarcolemma (s), nucleus (N), and nucleolus (n); showing (1a) light (L) and dark (D) cells containing myofilaments (m) surrounded by dense extracellular matrix (E) (1b), organelles including rough endoplasmic reticulum (R), Golgi apparatus (G), mitochondria (M), and dilated cisternae (D) in the perinuclear sarcoplasm, and (1c) myofilaments (m) in the peripheral sarcoplasm, caveoli (c), basement membrane (b) and extracellular matrix (E). Bar = 1 μm*

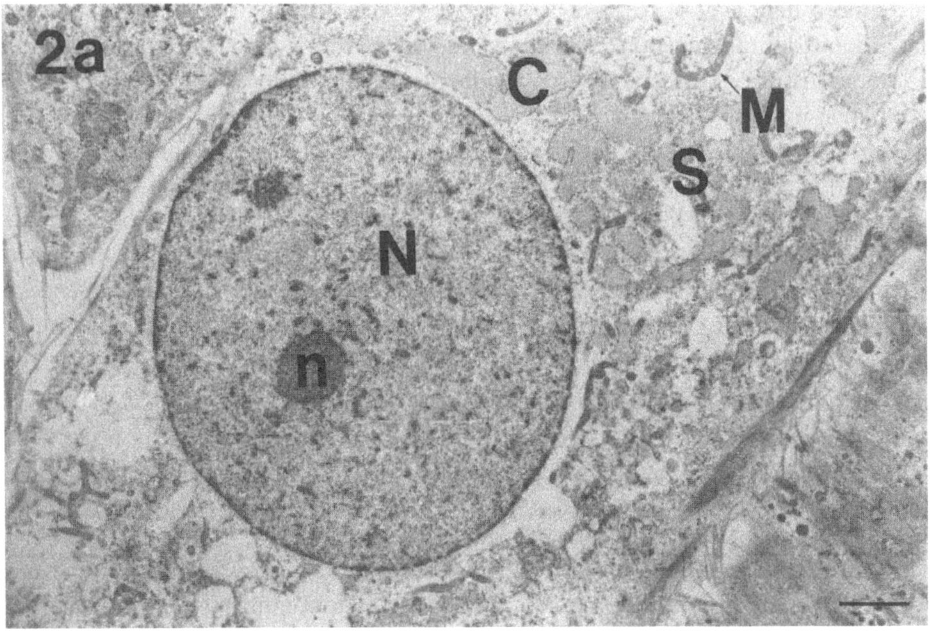
2a
C
M
S
N
n

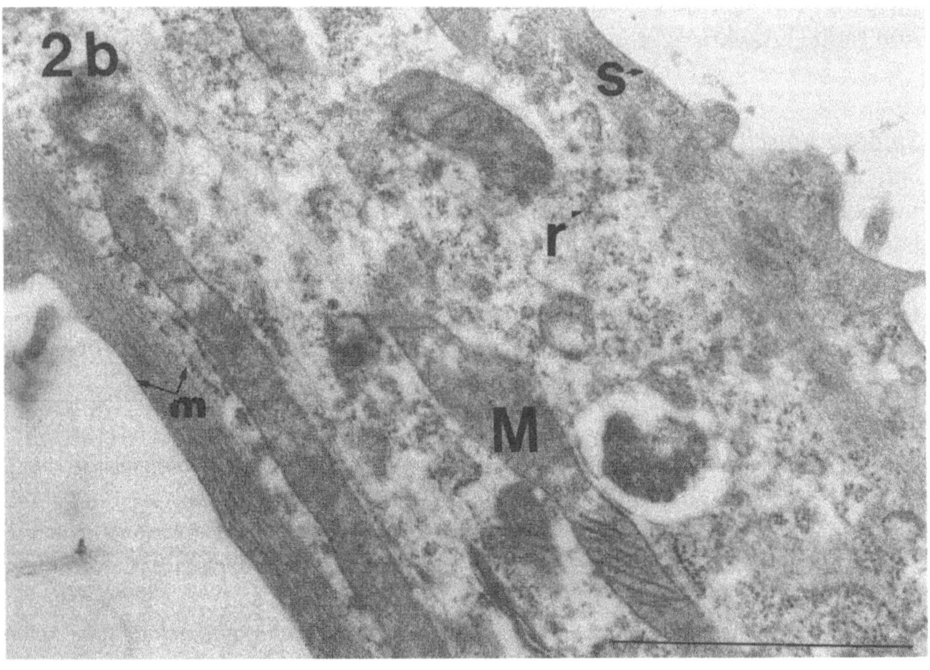
2b
s
r
m
M

dent sliding of actin and myosin filaments, whereas force maintenance occurs through complex and poorly understood mechanisms.

There remains considerable variation in the methods used to evaluate contractile processes *in vitro* [5, 6]. The commonly used methods involve measuring isometric force development, isotonic shortening and more recently pressure changes in perfused bronchial segments. In cultured ASM, cell stiffness has been measured magnetically [7] and contraction may be measured directly by microscopic determination of cell length. These methods simulate the behaviour of ASM *in situ* to a variable extent. The perfused bronchial segment appears to approximate the *in vivo* condition most closely, but lung volume-dependent parenchymal loading is not a feature of this method.

The mechanical properties of smooth muscle contraction have been analysed by generation of length-tension curves in canine ASM [8]. Length-tension curves of isolated ASM give an indication of the elasticity of the muscle (without the influence of resistance from surrounding tissue). The change in muscle tension, divided by cross-sectional area, over the corresponding change in muscle length (divided by optimal muscle length) is an index of the muscle stiffness. Measurement of stiffness is of particular use for the comparison of the mechanical properties of muscles [8]. However, stiffness and active tension curves represent equilibrium responses and do not provide information about the rate of shortening which may be more significant for smooth muscle regulation of airways resistance. Importantly, ASM shortening occurs in a dynamic environment with cyclically varying loads [9]. Shortening occurs at a velocity which is load-dependent: the greater the load, the slower the force activation.

Regulation of smooth muscle contraction

Smooth muscle contraction is regulated biochemically by phosphorylation and dephosphorylation of myosin and actin filaments in response to changes in the cytosolic calcium concentration [10]. Calcium bound to calmodulin (at μM intracellular calcium concentrations) activates myosin light-chain kinase (MLCK) and hence the activity of the actomyosin ATPase. MLCK phosphorylates the 20 kDa light chain subunit (LC_{20}) of myosin, facilitating the interaction between the myosin head and actin filaments, increasing actomyosin ATPase activity, thereby enabling cross-bridge cycling and contraction (Fig. 3). The calcium-calmodulin complex may

Figure 2
TEM of cultured normal human bronchial smooth muscle cells; sarcoplasm (S), sarcolemma (s), nucleus (N), nucleolus (n); showing perinuclear (2a) and peripheral (2b) sarcoplasm, rough endoplasmic reticulum (R), ribosomes (r), mitochondria (M), dilated cisternae (D) and myofilaments (m). Bar = 1 μm

also inactivate myosin light chain phosphatase thereby increasing the amount of phosphorylated LC_{20}.

Normal cycling cross-bridges are primarily active for the first 2–3 s of the contraction by which time 75% of the total smooth muscle shortening occurs, followed by slowing of cross-bridge cycling to about one-fourth of the initial rate [8]. The greater the load, the longer the contraction time. When the contraction time exceeds 3 s, there is a higher reliance on latch bridges than on cross bridge cycling for generation of force [8].

The calcium-calmodulin complex activates MLCK by binding to a sequence of the MLCK (pseudosubstrate inhibitory region, PSI) which, in the non-activated state, occludes the LC_{20} binding domain on the MLCK [11]. The PSI region shares sequence homology with the site of the LC_{20} that is dephosphorylated by LC_{20} phosphatase. The unfolded PSI region also indirectly inhibits LC_{20} phosphatase by providing a decoy binding site [10]. A reduction in the concentration of calcium to nM levels leads to the dissociation of the calcium-calmodulin complex from MLCK, a loss of kinase activity and smooth muscle relaxation as a result of the dephosphorylation of LC_{20} by myosin light chain phosphatases and the termination of ATP hydrolysis [10].

Sensitised canine tracheal and bronchial smooth muscle have an increased maximum shortening capacity, an elevated early maximum shortening velocity and the increased levels of actomyosin ATPase have been attributed to increased levels of MLCK activity and content [12].

Mechanisms sustaining contraction

During prolonged contraction there is a slowing of cross-bridge cycling concomitant with decreases in myosin phosphorylation, calcium concentration and energy consumption. A second regulatory mechanism has been invoked to explain the maintenance of force in carotid arterial smooth muscle, despite dephosphorylation of LC_{20}. This second contractile process occurs through the formation of attachments between dephosphorylated actomyosin cross-bridges [13] or possibly by the slowing of normally cycling cross-bridges [8]. The mechanisms responsible for maintaining the latch bridge state are not clearly defined. However, several proteins, including leiotonin, caldesmon and calponin may have a role in latch bridge formation [10].

Contractile regulatory proteins

Caldesmon and calponin are candidate molecules for the maintenance of force in the absence of an elevated calcium concentration or LC_{20} phosphorylation by tethering actin to myosin [14, 15]. Caldesmon, which inserts between the grooves between the actin double helix, inhibits actomyosin ATPase activity at resting calcium concentrations, but in the presence of calcium/calmodulin dissociates from actomyosin fila-

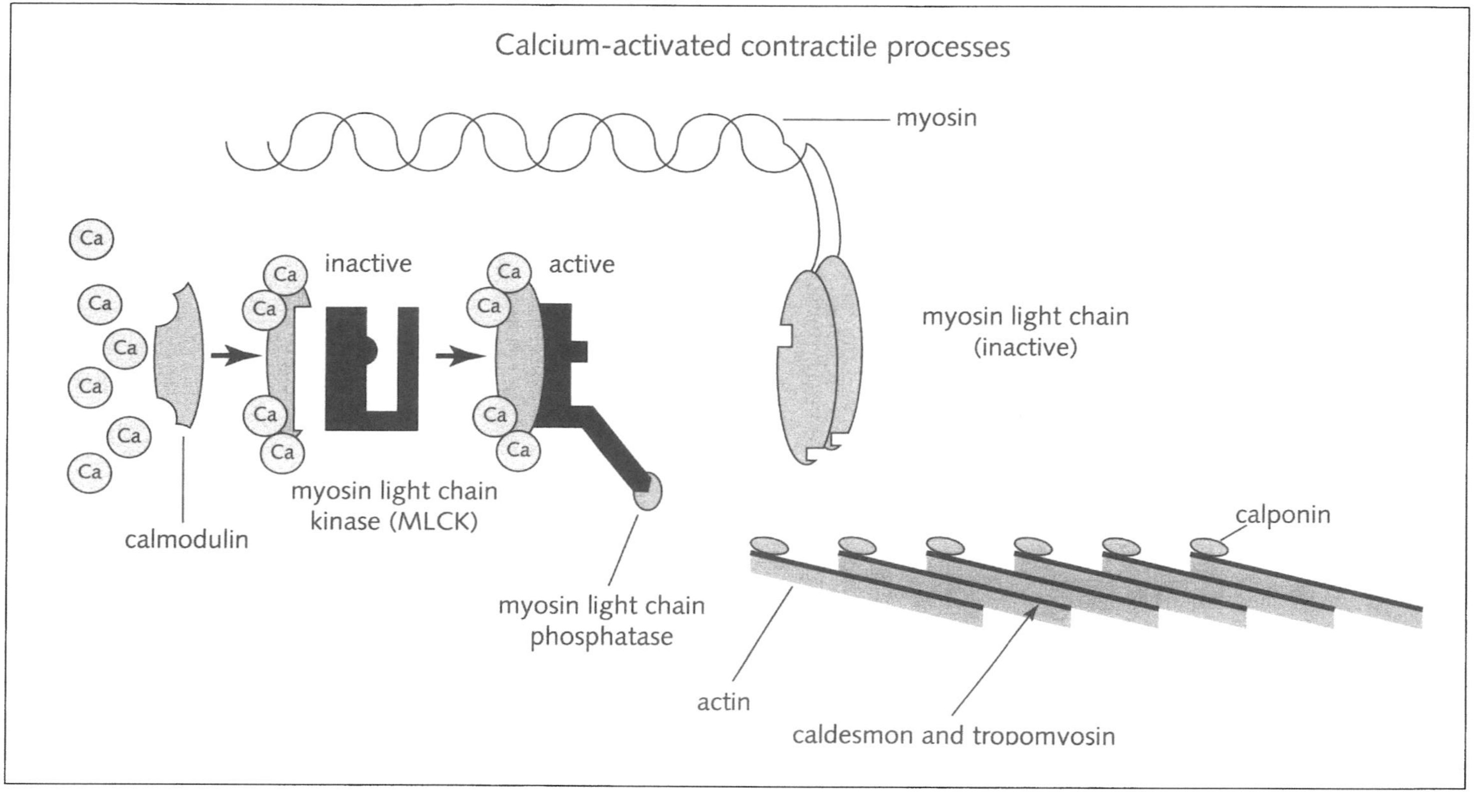

Figure 3
The contractile process involves calcium binding to calmodulin and activation of myosin light chain kinase (MLCK) to phosphorylate myosin light chain (LC20). The consequent increase in actomyosin ATPase activity provides energy for the sliding of the myosin and actin filaments to achieve contractile fibre shortening.

ments, activating actomyosin ATPase [16]. Calponin, a 33 kDa protein present in most forms of smooth muscle, also inhibits actomyosin ATPase activity. The inhibitory activity of calponin or caldesmon may be reversed by phosphorylation [17].

Heterogeneity

Smooth muscle cells in normal airway, blood vessels and in the viscera can exist in different phenotypes characterised by variable expression of contractile proteins. Studies of cultured vascular smooth muscle revealed modulation to a synthetic phenotype upon exposure to mitogens such as fetal calf serum which resembled the phenotype in the neointimal smooth muscle cells of atherosclerotic lesions [18]. More recently, phenotypic heterogeneity has been recognised in the absence of disease. Digestion of canine trachealis muscle and flow cytometric analyses of size and contractile protein expression indicate the existence of at least two phenotypes: a predominant (75%) population of smaller cells with reduced actin and myosin content and a minor population of larger cells with higher levels of contractile protein expression. These distinct phenotypes also show different contractile and calcium-handling properties [19–21]. There appears to be a bidirectional regulation between ECM and smooth muscle phenotype [22]: high levels of collagen type IV and fibronectin greatly enhance proliferative responses [23]; and synthetic state, proliferative smooth muscle makes large amounts of ECM.

Transpulmonary pressures are often increased in asthma in order to facilitate adequate ventilation. ASM cells are therefore subject to increased physical stress, which can increase the contractile enzyme activity of the muscle [24, 25]. In canine ASM cells subjected to strain there was increased calcium-dependent MLCK activity and myosin heavy chain levels accompanied by increases in LC_{20} phosphorylation and actomyosin ATPase activity, and decreased LC_{20} phosphatase activity [24]. Moreover, cyclic deformational strain increases amounts of total cellular protein, myosin and MLCK suggesting that strain is a stimulus for the contractile phenotype of ASM cells in culture [25].

The prevalence of contractile and synthetic phenotypes at different levels in the bronchial airways and their expression in different airways diseases has yet to be explored. Modulation of ASM to diminish the contractile phenotype represents a potential alternative therapeutic approach to treatment of bronchospasm in obstructive airways disease.

Signal transduction mechanisms

The signal transduction mechanisms controlling ASM function have received much attention as targetting these processes may lead to identification of novel agents to treat the bronchospastic component of obstructive airways diseases. Signalling mechanisms for contraction [26] and relaxation [27] have been reviewed in detail. The following section highlights important and well established regulatory mechanisms; signal transduction of ASM proliferation is covered in a later section.

Intracellular calcium

Intracellular free calcium concentrations ($Ca^{2+}{}_i$) are the primary determinant of the level of tone in ASM. There are four main regulatory mechanisms for $Ca^{2+}{}_i$: release from internal stores; influx through receptor- and voltage-operated membrane channels; and transmembrane transport, which is either directly or indirectly energy-dependent. Activation of the contractile process by agonists such as carbachol and histamine is associated with increases in production of inositol 1,4,5-trisphosphate (IP_3) as a consequence of phospholipase C activation [28]. Depolarization-induced activation of calcium influx into human ASM has also been described [29], but these voltage-operated channels are not considered to be important for responses to contractile agonists [30]. Thus, inhibitors of these channels such as verapamil have only modest inhibitory effects on agonist-induced contraction of ASM [31]. Receptor-operated calcium channel activity has been directly demonstrated in voltage-clamp experiments in histamine-stimulated human ASM [32]. These channels are believed to mediate the slow and persistent contractions associated with protein kinase C activation [33] and may play a role in the maintenance of the contractile response to histamine.

Cyclic nucleotides

Many ASM relaxants, including β_2-adrenoceptor agonists, vasoactive intestinal peptide (VIP) and prostaglandin E_2 (PGE_2) activate receptors coupled *via* Gs proteins to adenylate cyclase. Elevation of cyclic AMP and activation of protein kinase A leads to phosphorylation of several proteins which regulate $Ca^{2+}{}_i$. The net result of these phosphorylations is a decrease in $Ca^{2+}{}_i$ and thereby a relaxation of ASM tone [27]. Inhibition of phospholipase C activation, as evidenced by suppression of IP_3 formation is likely to be quantitatively important in cAMP-mediated relaxant responses [34]. Additional mechanisms include increased calcium re-uptake and extrusion *via* plasma membrane transport systems.

Nitric oxide relaxes ASM *via* activation of soluble guanylate cyclase. Cyclic GMP elevation decreases $Ca^{2+}{}_i$ elevated by either receptor-operated stimuli such as acetylcholine or by depolarisation [35].

Phosphodiesterases

Non-selective inhibitors of phosphodiesterase (PDE) relax both spontaneous and induced ASM tone. Identification of multiple subtypes of PDE with distinct cellular distribution has renewed interest in development of selective inhibitors as useful anti-inflammatory and smooth muscle relaxant agents [36]. The predominant types of PDE in human ASM are III and IV and the latter is also present in inflammatory cell types. PKA-dependent phosphorylation of PDE III activates this isoform resulting in a negative feedback on PKA activation, whereas expression of the type IV isoform is increased by cAMP. Dual inhibitors of types III and IV PDE in combination with β-agonists may produce a more efficacious treatment regimen for bronchospasm with additional anti-inflammatory effects to those of β-agonists alone.

Protein kinases

Protein kinase C represents a large family of related kinases exhibiting differences in activation properties. Isoforms detected in bovine and canine ASM include α, β1, β2, δ, ε, λ, μ and θ [37]. Activation of protein kinase C in ASM activates calcium influx, stimulates Na/K ATPase activity [38], increases the calcium sensitivity of LC_{20} phosphorylation [39], inhibits LC_{20} phosphatases [40], and has been implicated in the maintenance of contraction.

Mitogen-activated protein kinase (MAPK), also known as extracellular regulated kinase (ERK), is best characterised as the central signalling enzyme for the proliferative response of cultured ASM, but has recently been shown to phosphorylate caldesmon and increase the calcium sensitivity of the contractile apparatus in native ASM [41]. MAPK is activated by a wide range of bronchoconstrictor mediators.

Potassium channels

Potassium channels, of which there are many subtypes showing distinct activation and functional characteristics, play a key role in determining the membrane potential [42]. The two most important channel types in ASM appear to be the ATP-sensitive potassium channel (K^{+}_{ATP}) and the large conductance, calcium-activated potassium channel (BK^{+}_{Ca}) [43], although the delayed rectifier channel may also be expressed and be functionally important [44].

Potassium channel opening drugs (KCO), which activate K^{+}_{ATP} channels, suppress the spontaneous and agonist-induced tone of human isolated bronchial smooth muscle and counteract bronchoconstriction in anaesthetised guinea-pigs [45]. The KCO, SDZ PCO 400 has been shown to inhibit hyperreactivity induced by a variety of stimuli in guinea-pigs *in vivo* [46], but the importance of smooth muscle as a target for this effect is not clear.

Activation of BK^{+}_{Ca} has been implicated in β_2-adrenoceptor agonist-induced relaxation through both cAMP-dependent and independent mechanisms [47]. However, the involvement of K^+ efflux in the relaxant actions depends on the efficacy of the β-agonists and does not appear to be of any importance for low efficacy agonists such as salmeterol [48]. Moreover, KCO have shown only modest bronchodilator activity in asthmatics, suggesting that hyperpolarisation is not an efficacious relaxant mechanism.

Neural regulation

Parasympathetic innervation

Airways smooth muscle has a basal level of tone supplied by parasympathetic nerve activity [49], which releases acetylcholine to evoke contraction of airways smooth muscle by activating muscarinic cholinoceptors of the M_3-subtype (Fig. 4). Acetylcholine release from parasympathetic nerves is under autoinhibitory feedback control by prejunctional muscarinic cholinoceptors of the M_2-subtype [50].

In virus-infected humans, the increased responsiveness to histamine or cold air challenge, can be inhibited by muscarinic cholinoceptor antagonists such as atropine. This vagally-mediated, reflex bronchoconstriction results from dysfunction of autoinhibitory M_2-cholinoceptors [51]. Neuraminidase from parainfluenza virus inactivates M_2-cholinoceptors by cleaving sialic residues from glycoproteins and glycolipids, whereas inflammation following either antigen-challenge or ozone exposure results in eosinophil recruitment and release of cationic proteins, such as major basic protein, that allosterically antagonise the M_2-cholinoceptor [51]. Viral infection may also act indirectly by inducing epithelial damage, since epithelium exerts an inhibitory influence on the release of acetylcholine from parasympathetic nerves of guinea-pig trachea, possibly through the liberation of an epithelium-derived inhibitory substance [52].

Neuropeptides act as co-transmitters of classical autonomic nerves in the airways, limiting or prolonging the effect of the primary neurotransmitter [53]. However, in human airways *in vitro*, the neuropeptide tachykinins, VIP and neuropeptide Y (NPY) have no effect on cholinergic transmission. Nitric oxide (NO), released by electrical field stimulation inhibits cholinergic neurotransmission and functionally antagonises the contractile response to acetylcholine [54].

Pro-inflammatory cytokines, which play an important role in perpetuating the airway inflammatory response in asthma, including interleukin-1β (IL-1β) and tumour necrosis factor-α (TNFα) have been detected in bronchoalveolar lavage fluid from asthmatic patients [55]. Inhaled TNFα induces hyperresponsiveness and

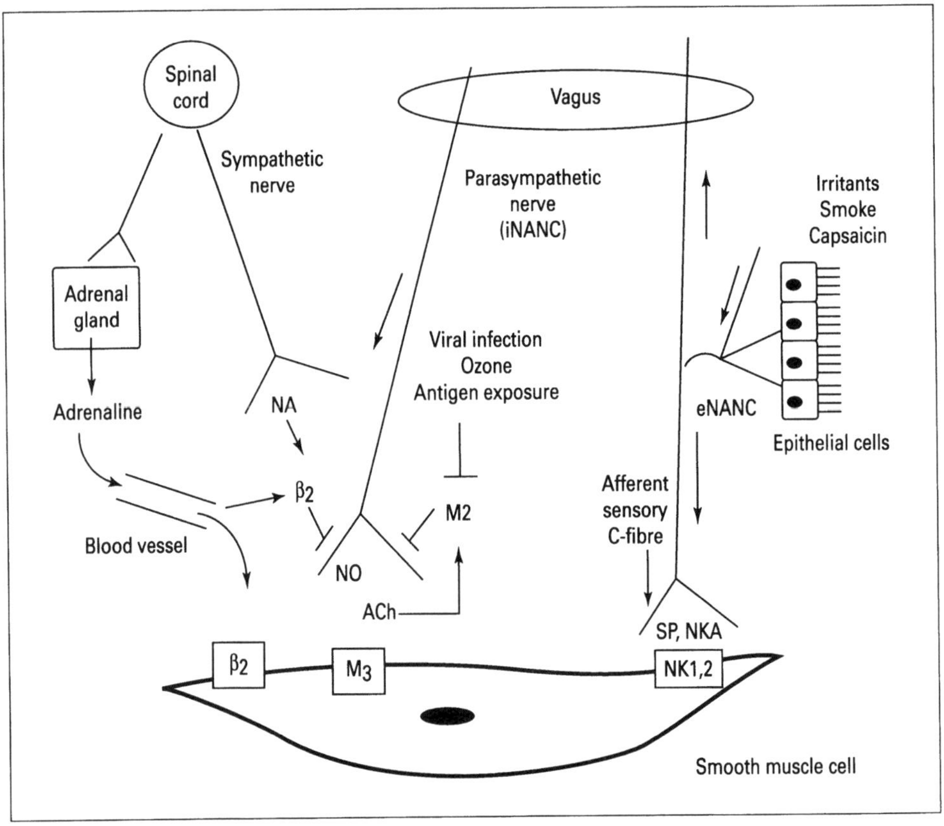

Figure 4
Neural influences on airway smooth muscle. β_2-Adrenoceptors mediate relaxation in response to circulating adrenaline. Sympathetic nerves may influence cholinergic function rather than directly relax airway smooth muscle and are sparse in human airways. M_3-cholinoceptors mediate contraction in response to acetylcholine (ACh) released from parasympathetic nerves which also release an inhibitory non-adrenergic, non-cholinergic (iNANC), neurotransmitter, most likely to be nitric oxide (NO). Autoinhibitory feedback of ACh release through activation of prejunctional M_2-cholinoceptors may be disrupted by viral infection, ozone exposure or antigen inhalation, resulting in excessive reflex cholinergic bronchomotor responses. The excitatory NANC (eNANC) pathway involves anti-dromic activation of afferent sensory C fibres which release neurokinin to elicit contractile responses following exposure to irritant stimuli.

acts prejunctionally to enhance cholinergic transmission in electrically field-stimulated human isolated bronchus [56]. Many other agents enhance cholinergic transmission in human airways including products of activated eosinophils [57] and endothelin-1 (ET-1) [58].

Sympathetic innervation

The extent and importance of sympathetic innervation of airways smooth muscle is species-dependent and appears to be sparse and inconsequential in humans [59]. β-Adrenoceptors are widely distributed throughout the airways, whereas α-adrenoceptors are not considered to play an important role in ASM [60]. β-Blocking drugs increase airways resistance in healthy subjects suggesting that circulating levels of adrenaline activate β_2-adrenoceptors to produce a dilator influence. Noradrenergic and cholinergic nerves have been found in close association in airways of guinea-pigs, canines and humans. Thus, noradrenaline may exert an indirect influence on ASM tone by modulating cholinergic neurotransmission [61].

Non-adrenergic, non-cholinergic innervation

Electrical field stimulation of isolated airway smooth muscle preparations elicits complex responses. The components of these responses which are not blocked by antagonists of classical autonomic neurotransmitters, designated non-adrenergic non-cholinergic (NANC), were originally ascribed to separate neural pathways coursing in the vagal nerve bundle. However, it is now established that the inhibitory NANC (iNANC) dilator tone is due to the release of co-transmitters from parasympathetic nerves, and the excitatory NANC (eNANC) system is associated with anti-dromic excitation in vagal afferent c-fibres [62].

iNANC mechanisms

Because of the sparsity of the sympathetic innervation of ASM, the iNANC system in humans is the primary neural bronchodilator pathway. There remains some uncertainty as to the identity of the neurotransmitter(s) subserving iNANC neurotransmission. The candidates include VIP and NO, although recent evidence argues against an important role for VIP. In human tracheal and bronchial smooth muscle, relaxations evoked by VIP are abolished by α-chymotrypsin, but iNANC responses are unaffected [63]. *In vivo*, inhaled VIP is a bronchodilator and attenuates histamine-induced bronchoconstriction in animals. However, in humans inhaled VIP has no detectable bronchodilator effect and provides little protection against histamine-induced bronchoconstriction [64]. These observations suggest that VIP is not the iNANC transmitter in human airways, but do not exclude the possibility that VIP has an important regulatory influence on other airway wall cell types or on other smooth muscle responses, such as proliferation [65].

Emerging evidence implicating NO as the neurotransmitter of iNANC nerves is best developed in guinea-pig airways. In human tracheal smooth muscle, the NOS inhibitor L-NAME produces a concentration-dependent inhibition of the iNANC response. Thus, NO may act as a brake on cholinergic bronchoconstriction [54,66], but the failure of NOS inhibitors to affect airways resistance in humans suggests that the iNANC system may be of limited importance [67], perhaps because it is less evident in intraparenchymal airways.

eNANC mechanisms

Lundberg and colleagues identified an ASM contractile response, particularly evident at high frequencies of excitation, which was mediated by activation of sensory nerves releasing tachykinins (substance P and neurokinin A) to act on neurokinin (NK) NK1 and NK2 receptors on ASM [68]. These sensory fibres may be activated anti-dromically by irritant stimuli such as cigarette smoke [69], leukotrienes and histamine [70,71]. The sensory C-fibres also contain calcitonin gene-related peptide (CGRP) which acts primarily to increase bronchial blood flow (69). Barnes and colleagues suggested that these sensory C-fibres function similarly to those in the skin which mediate the triple response *via* activation of mast cells by tachykinins. The term "neurogenic inflammation" was coined to describe the constellation of effects upon activation of this neuronal pathway, which include ASM constriction, increased bronchial blood flow and plasma exudation [72]. The importance of these neurogenic inflammatory responses is likely to be elucidated within the next few years as antagonists of neurokinin receptors are being evaluated for efficacy in asthma and other airway diseases.

Mediators

Phospholipid-derived mediators

Mediators derived from the hydrolysis of cell membrane phospholipid-esterified arachidonic acid, such as the prostaglandins (PGs) and the leukotrienes (LTs), have important pro-inflammatory actions in a variety of respiratory diseases including asthma, but have no clearly identified physiological functions in normal ASM. There are numerous cellular sources of eicosanoids in the airways. In asthmatics, release of eicosanoids from activated mast cells predominates in the early response to allergen-challenge [73]. The late phase response, which is associated with airways hyperresponsiveness that can last several days, is also accompanied by production of eicosanoids from cells infiltrating the airways [74].

Cyclo-oxygenase products

The levels of several cyclo-oxygenase products, including PGD_2, PGE_2, $PGF_{2\alpha}$, PGI_2, and thromboxane A_2 (TxA_2) are increased in broncho-alveolar lavage (BAL) fluid after antigen-challenge of asthmatics [75]. TxA_2, $PGF_{2\alpha}$, and PGD_2 are the predominant mast-cell derived bronchoconstrictors in asthma, activating smooth muscle constriction *via* the TP receptor [76, 77]. Subthreshold concentrations of a TxA_2-mimetic cause airway hyperresponsiveness to inhaled methacholine in asthmatics [78]. Prostacyclin and PGE_2 relax ASM by activating distinct receptors to elevate cAMP concentrations, but vasodilator and neural activities may limit the bronchoprotective actions of these eicosanoids.

Lipoxygenase products

The LTs are derived from arachidonic acid by the sequential actions of 5-lipoxygenase and glutathione transferase in eosinophils, mast cells and macrophages. Elevated levels of LTs are detected in BAL cells and fluids from asthmatic patients compared with normal subjects [79]. LTC_4 and LTD_4 are potent bronchoconstrictors (1000-fold greater than histamine) in both normal and asthmatic subjects activating $CysLT_1$ receptors to cause ASM contraction [80]. The persistence of the bronchomotor actions of LTs has been ascribed to the long-lived signalling mechanisms that these mediators activate and also to the presence of significant bronchoconstrictor activity of metabolites including LTE_4.

Platelet-activating factor

Platelet-activating factor (PAF) is synthesised by the action of phospholipase A_2 on alkyl-ether phosphatidylcholine followed by acetylation of the 2-position and is produced by inflammatory cells infiltrating the asthmatic airway including eosinophils [81]. Bronchoconstriction induced by PAF is likely to be largely indirectly mediated, although PAF produces a modest contractile response on human ASM [82]. The role of PAF as a mediator of airway hyperresponsiveness is well established in guinea-pigs, but remains controversial in human asthma [83].

Low molecular weight mediators

Nitric oxide

Increased NO concentrations have been detected in allergic airways disease due to induction of nitric oxide synthase (iNOS) in airway epithelial cells [84]. The large amounts of NO produced by epithelial cell iNOS as compared with endothelial NO production may result in a net pro-inflammatory action of NO in allergic airways disease, despite its relaxant actions on ASM [85]. In high concentrations, NO reacts with superoxide anions to generate toxic peroxynitrite and hydroxyl radicals, stimulates mucous secretion, amplifies T lymphocyte-driven inflammatory effects and stimulates plasma exudation by increasing pulmonary blood flow [86]. The potential anti-inflammatory actions of NO synthase inhibitors in asthma have not been been fully explored. Aminoguanidine, a selective inhibitor of iNOS, decreased NO production in asthmatics more effectively than the non-selective NOS inhibitor, L-NAME [67]. Importantly, however, no change in airway resistance was observed following a single bolus dose of these NOS inhibitors. Since L-NAME should block NO generation in response to iNANC activity, it appears that neither the latter system nor iNOS-derived NO exerts a dominant influence on bronchomotor tone.

Histamine

Histamine is released from degranulating mast cells during immediate hypersensitivity reactions. Histamine H_1-receptors, which mediate bronchoconstriction, predominate in the airway [87]. Activation of histamine H_2-receptors mediates bronchodilatation *via* an epithelial cell-derived relaxing factor, but this mechanism is relatively weak in humans [88]. Histamine receptor populations do not appear to be altered in asthmatic patients [89].

Adenosine

Adenosine, which is found in elevated concentrations in BAL fluid of asthmatics, causes airways obstruction in asthmatics and smokers, but not in healthy individuals [90]. A combination of histamine and leukotriene receptor antagonism completely inhibits the constrictor effects of adenosine in isolated human airways, suggesting that adenosine acts indirectly, possibly *via* stimulating mast cell degranulation [91]. However, recent studies suggest that activation of the A_1-receptor elicits bronchoconstriction in the absence of mast cells, possibly *via* an effect on NANC nerves or a direct constrictor action on smooth muscle [92].

Peptides

Endothelin

ET-1 levels are increased in inflamed airways in many respiratory diseases [93, 94]. ET-1 is a potent bronchoconstrictor in humans [95], and may elicit increased chronic ASM responsiveness by actions on smooth muscle ET_A- and ET_B-receptors [96], although the ET_B-receptor is desensitised by increased levels of airway ET-1 [97]. ET-1 does not appear to be involved in the early phase response to allergen exposure in asthmatics [94], and therefore might only be important for late-phase bronchoconstriction or the development of chronic hyperresponsiveness.

Tachykinins

The tachykinins are released from sub-epithelial sensory nerves in close proximity to the subjacent ASM indicating a potential role as constrictor mediators. Immunoreactive substance P levels are increased in BAL fluid obtained from asthmatic patients [98, 99]. Substance P and neurokinin A activate specific tachykinin receptors, NK1 and NK2, respectively, on ASM to cause contraction of human isolated airways [100], but the NK2 receptor is more important for constriction, while the NK1 receptor mediates neurogenic inflammation *via* actions on the microcirculation and the mucosa. NK2 receptor levels are increased four-fold in asthmatics relative to non-smoking controls, whereas there are no detectable changes to NK1 receptor levels [101]. In experimental animals, depletion of neuropeptides with the neurotoxin capsaicin protects against airways hyperresponsiveness which accompanies repeated antigen-challenge [102], virus infection [103], or delayed-type hypersensitivity reactions [104], consistent with a contribution of tachykinins to the development of airways hyperresponsiveness.

Cytokines and airway smooth muscle function

Pro-inflammatory cytokines act directly on ASM to modulate both contractile and relaxant responses. Incubation of guinea-pig [105] or rabbit [106] airways with IL-1β and TNFα reduces isoprenaline-induced relaxation of cholinoceptor-mediated contractile responses [105, 106]. IL-1β and TNFα, synergistically attenuate β-adrenoceptor-mediated airway relaxation, possibly as a result of enhanced muscarinic M_2-receptor/G_i protein coupling [106]. Intra-tracheal instillation of IL-1β in rats impaired relaxation of tracheal smooth muscle to isoprenaline *in vitro* associated with uncoupling of β-adrenoceptors from adenylate cyclase, a reduction in the number of β-adrenoceptors and a reduction in adenylate cyclase activity. IL-1β and TNFα significantly attenuated the decrease in cell stiffness induced by isoprenaline measured using magnetic twisting cytometry [7]. These observations suggest that the defect in β-adrenoceptor function established in asthma [107] may result from the release of proinflammatory cytokines. The glucocorticoid-sensitivity of these cytokine actions has not been established, nor has the possible relationship to PGE_2, a known regulator of β_2-adrenoceptors, been explored.

Epithelium

There appears to be a correlation between the degree of epithelial damage and airway hyperresponsiveness in asthmatics [108]. Removal of the epithelium in a variety of animal and human isolated airway preparations increases the responsiveness of the underlying ASM to histamine, serotonin and acetylcholine, and reduces the responsiveness to relaxant agonists such as isoprenaline [109]. Thus, the epithelium is thought to release a relaxant factor(s) which normally modulates the reactivity of the smooth muscle to both contractile and relaxant agents. The coaxial bioassay technique, in which open rings of precontracted, rat anococcygeus muscle or endothelial-denuded rabbit or rat aorta are inserted into the lumen of epithelium-intact guinea-pig trachea, has provided direct evidence for the release of an epithelium-derived relaxant factor(s) induced by muscarinic cholinoceptor agonists [110]. In addition, the superfusate from cylindrical preparations of acetylcholine-stimulated dog bronchus with intact epithelium relaxes both airway and vascular smooth muscle [111]. In tubular perfused bronchial segments, contractile agonist-sensitivity was the same after epithelium removal as that obtained when agonists were added to the serosal side of epithelium intact preparations [112]. Thus, the effect of epithelium removal on contractile agonists may also be a consequence of the loss of the physical barrier to diffusion thereby enhancing agonist access to the underlying smooth muscle.

Clinical pharmacology

Receptor antagonists/enzyme inhibitors

The bronchodilator PGE_2 is produced mainly by epithelial cells and may contribute to the general anti-inflammatory actions of the epithelium in asthma [112]. The lack of therapeutic benefit of cyclo-oxygenase inhibitors in asthma has been partly attributed to a reduction in bronchodilator prostanoids such as PGE_2 and PGI_2. Furthermore, the loss of bronchoprotective PGE_2 may contribute to the phenomenon of aspirin-sensitive asthma [113]. Although little success has been achieved using inhibitors of thromboxane synthesis such as OKY-046, and thromboxane receptor antagonists such as GR 32191B or BAY u3405 in the treatment of asthma [114], the advent of selective cyclo-oxygenase-2 inhibitors may shed new light on the contribution of prostanoids to the pathophysiology of airways disease.

LTC_4, LTD_4 and LTE_4 enhance bronchomotor responses to unrelated inhaled bronchactive agents and may therefore contribute to airway hyperresponsiveness [115, 116]. The development of antagonists to CysLT receptors has led to the emergence of a novel anti-asthma drug class [117]. In clinical studies of asthma, the CysLT receptor antagonists pranlukast, zafirlukast, and MK-679, reduce symptom scores, β_2-agonist usage, and improve spirometry measures associated with a reduced eosinophilia, mucous secretion, vascular permeability, and decreased release of tachykinins from sensory nerves [117]. In addition, long-term (12–24 weeks) treatment with LT receptor antagonists increases forced expired volume in 1 s (FEV_1) and decreases airway hyperresponsiveness to histamine [118].

H_1-Histamine receptor antagonists decrease the magnitude of the early phase of bronchoconstriction following allergen inhalation in asthmatic patients [119], but those antagonists without effects on mediator release are of no benefit clinically in asthma [120]. Despite initial enthusiasm based on extensive studies of allergic bronchoconstriction in experimental animals, results of trials of antagonists of PAF receptors have shown disappointing results in clinical asthma [121, 122].

The dual NK1 and NK2 tachykinin receptor antagonist, FK-224, provides protection against bradykinin-induced bronchoconstriction in asthmatic patients [123]. The advent of subtype-selective tachykinin receptor antagonists will provide a more definitive approach to understanding the role of tachykinins in asthma [124]. A NK1 selective antagonist inhibits exercise-induced airway narrowing in asthma [125]. However, NK1 and NK2 receptor antagonist studies do not support an important role for tachykinins in airways hyperresponsiveness in humans [126, 127].

β_2-Adrenoceptor agonists and phosphodiesterase inhibitors

There is an enormous amount of literature on the pharmacology of β_2-agonists in asthma which remain the drug of choice for the relief of acute bronchospasm (see [107] for a review). Although concerns have been raised about the safety of these agents, especially with regular usage, it appears that long-acting β_2-agonists do not exhibit any deleterious effects on the underlying asthmatic condition [128]. The original association between adverse outcome and short-acting β_2-agonists may have been the result of excessive usage and, in any case, remains controversial [129]. Tachyphylaxis to the bronchodilator effects of β_2-agonists develops with chronic use but the clinical impact may not be significant.

Theophylline is commonly used in the treatment of asthma at concentrations below those considered to have marked effects on PDE, as higher doses have limiting side-effects such as nausea. It remains to be established whether the advent of isoform-selective PDE inhibitors will circumvent these problems.

Glucocorticoids

The inhibitory effects of glucocorticoids on cytokine and inflammatory mediator release and the infiltration of inflammatory cells within the airway are well documented [130]. Glucocorticoids have largely indirect effects on ASM tone and hyperresponsiveness, reducing the levels of bronchoconstrictors and pro-inflammatory mediators available to the smooth muscle cells. However, glucocorticoids influence many contractile agonist receptor populations and signal transduction pathways in ASM, inhibit signal tranduction of smooth muscle cell proliferation [131], and regulate production of ASM-derived inflammatory mediators [132].

Glucocorticoids increase β_2-adrenoceptor gene transcription in the human lung *in vitro* [133], but the clinical relevance of this observation remains to be elucidated. Preincubation of ASM preparations with glucocorticoids reduces the contractile responses to acetylcholine and morphine, as well as reducing expression of muscarinic receptors [134, 135]. Glucocorticoids also negatively regulate histamine H_1-receptor coupling in human cultured ASM cells [136].

Non-contractile functions

Mediator production

Smooth muscle cells themselves produce mediators which contribute to the inflammatory response [132]. ASM generates increased levels of secretory phospholipase A_2 after cytokine challenge [137]. In addition, cytokines such as IL-1β, TNFα, and IFNγ increase the expression of inducible cyclo-oxygenase (COX-2) in human ASM *in vitro*, and elevate the cellular release of PGE_2 and $PGF_{2\alpha}$ [137–140]. Since bronchodilator PGE_2 is the main prostanoid produced by ASM, it could be argued that glucocorticoids are inhibiting bronchoprotective processes [138], such as ASM relaxation and inhibition of proliferation [141]. Nevertheless, immunohistochemical studies in bronchial mucosa of asthmatics demonstrate relatively small amounts of COX-2 or COX-1 in ASM compared with epithelial cells, suggesting that the influence of prostanoids generated by smooth muscle *in vivo* may be minor [142]. ASM not only responds to, but also produces a number of cytokines, including transforming growth factor β (TGFβ) [143], RANTES [144] and GM-CSF [145]. Glucocorticoids inhibit the production of GM-CSF [145] and the chemokine RANTES [144], but not TGFβ [143] from human ASM cells in culture.

Extracellular matrix

Cultured synthetic state smooth muscle cells produce and are able to modify their ECM. Release of proteases, including matrix metalloproteinase (MMP) may alter the collagen network in the cell microenvironment and be permissive for ASM proliferation [146]. TGFβ, which elicits complex growth patterns in many cell types including ASM [143, 147], also stimulates ASM production of hyaluronan which may lead to fibrosis and airway wall thickening due to water retention [143]. Growth factors such as thrombin, bFGF and TGFβ are sequestered in the ECM and may be mobilised upon its degradation by inflammatory cell-derived enzymes, resulting in ASM proliferation. Studies in vascular smooth muscle indicate that the synthetic state of ASM may be promoted by fibronectin, thrombospondin and type

I collagen and reinforced by smooth muscle production of these ECM components. Conversely, basement membrane collagen type IV and heparin promote the contractile phenotype and inhibit proliferation [22].

Airways hyperresponsiveness

Asthmatics have a characteristic increased sensitivity and reactivity to a wide range of of bronchoconstrictor stimuli, known as airway hyperresponsiveness (AHR). However, AHR has also been identified in other conditions, including chronic obstructive pulmonary disease (COPD), cystic fibrosis, heart failure, bronchopulmonary dysplasia, respiratory infections following exposure to environmental pollutants and even in some healthy individuals [148]. The contribution of ASM to airway hyperresponsiveness is still the subject of intense interest and diverse opinion [9]. In particular, the notion that there is no fundamental abnormality in asthmatic ASM, based on force measurements of isolated ASM preparations, is now being challenged by data suggesting that the velocity of asthmatic ASM contraction may be increased in association with larger amounts and activity of MLCK [9].

Measurements of airways hyperresponsiveness

Methacholine and histamine, which directly activate smooth muscle, are commonly used in assessment of airway responsiveness. Directly acting challenges elicit responses in healthy subjects, while challenges that act indirectly *via* neurones (bradykinin) or inflammatory cells (adenosine) only elicit bronchomotor responses in subjects with inflamed airways. Quantitative assessments of AHR have proved useful in investigations of the clinical status and pathophysiology of asthma. Many factors other than the underlying levels of AHR may influence the results of airway challenge including acute respiratory infections, recent allergen exposure, exposure to certain pollutants, current use of bronchodilators or anti-inflammatory medications [149]. Bradykinin, adenosine, LTs, ultrasonic nebulized distilled water (UNDW), exercise and cold-air hyperventilation may also be used to assess AHR [149]. Most of these challenges act indirectly on smooth muscle, and in some instances may better mimic naturally occurring asthma [150].

In healthy subjects, large airways make the major contribution to airways resistance, whereas in asthmatics, both large and small airway contributions are evident [151]. The sites of bronchomotor responses in humans can be determined by helium-oxygen flow-volume curves or by use of an anterograde catheter tip micromanometer [151]. High-resolution computed tomography (HRCT) is an emerging approach to the study of airway narrowing.

Airway wall remodelling in airways disease

The airways of asthmatic subjects are two to three times thicker than those of subjects with chronic obstructive pulmonary disease (COPD) and age and weight-matched controls with normal airway function [152]. Importantly, these studies also established that thickening of the airway wall is not merely the result of pre-terminal disease, since airways from mild to moderate asthmatics dying from unrelated causes also showed significant remodelling. Although these initial observations have been confirmed using sophisticated stereological techniques which identified both hyperplasia and hypertrophy of smooth muscle [153] transverse sectioning failed to identify a difference in ASM quantity between asthmatics and control subjects [154]. Nevertheless, the controls in the latter study had a history of tobacco smoking and several had COPD, which itself is associated with airway wall remodelling [155, 156].

Impact of remodelling on airways resistance increases induced by smooth muscle shortening

Normal smooth muscle shortening in an airway wall thickened by tissue remodelling may account for the reversible airway obstruction that characterises asthma [157]. The increase in smooth muscle mass contributes to the airway hyperresponsiveness by increasing the effect of minimal muscle shortening on the total increase in airway resistance [158]. Morphological and physiological studies have been designed to determine how increases in smooth muscle volume and changes in the contractile components of smooth muscle impact on smooth muscle shortening and total airway resistance (Fig. 5). Models of circumferential ASM contraction predict significantly greater narrowing of the airway lumen for a given percentage of ASM shortening in asthmatic compared with healthy airways [2, 159]. The relatively small changes in airway wall thickness have little effect on baseline resistance in airflow, but were predicted to decrease the diameter of airways sufficiently to occlude the airway lumen upon normal amounts of ASM shortening [157].

Airway narrowing responses are limited in non-asthmatic subjects which show a plateau in the dose-response curve for inhaled bronchoconstrictors, whereas asthmatic subjects inhaling safe concentrations of provocative stimuli do not reach a plateau response [160]. *In vivo* smooth muscle shortening is normally limited by the preload associated with attachment *via* connective tissue to parenchyma, whereas there is no preload on the smooth muscle *in vitro* allowing it to shorten by up to 80% of its resting length. Excessive shortening has been suggested to occur *in vivo* in asthmatics as a result of airway wall remodelling-induced unloading of smooth muscle. Intra-parenchymal airways are tethered to alveolar structures *via* the adventitial connnective tissue. Increases in the surface area of adventitia will decrease the strain against which smooth muscle shortens. This unloading may be significant

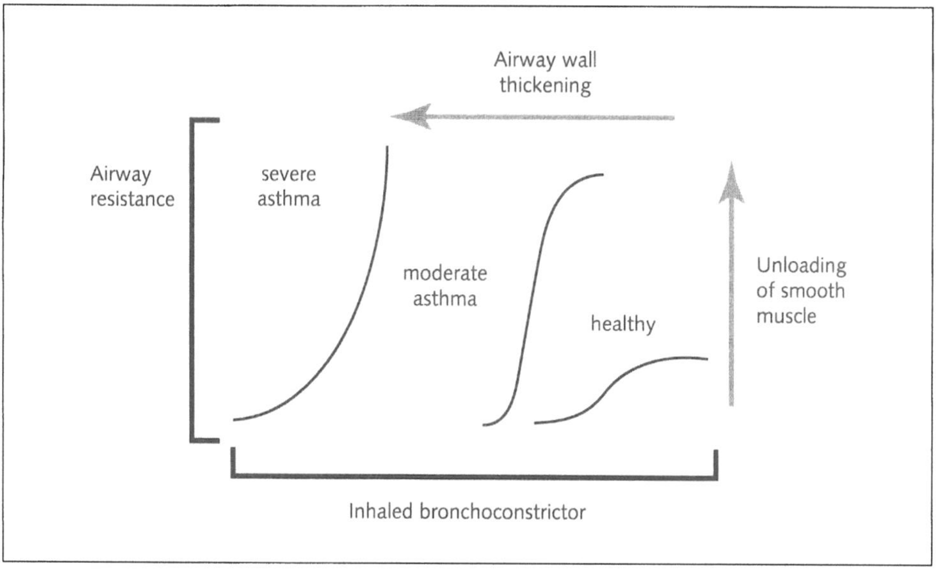

Figure 5
The relationship between airway wall remodelling and hyperresponsiveness may involve a combination of unloading of airway smooth muscle enhancing the capacity of muscle to shorten to lengths at which airway closure occurs, and airway wall thickening which increases airways resistance for a given amount of airway smooth muscle shortening.

enough to allow airway closure at physiological levels of smooth muscle shortening and could explain the absence of a plateau in the increase in airway resistance in response to inhalational challenge in asthmatic individuals [161]. Recent inhalational challenge studies performed at low lung volumes, at which the loading of smooth muscle is minimised have mimicked the hyperresponsive state in healthy subjects inhaling methacholine [162].

Animal models of airway wall remodelling

In vivo models of ASM growth have been developed in antigen-sensitised and chronically-challenged rats [163] and cats [164]. Reversible ASM volume increases have also been reported in hyperoxia-induced airway hyperresponsiveness [165]. In antigen-challenged Brown Norway rats, the area of smooth muscle in intraparenchymal airways was increased by 50–100% [166]. Leukotriene receptor antagonists protect against antigen-challenge induced airway wall remodelling and increases in airway responsiveness in these models [167]. In addition, strain differences between Fisher and Lewis rats in airway responsiveness have been linked to the volume of airway smooth muscle [168]. *In vitro* studies on proliferation of cultured ASM indicated that the Fisher strain, which is more responsive to bronchoconstrictors and has more ASM, is more sensitive to the mitogenic actions of $PDGF_{AB}$ than the Lewis strain [169]. This observation raises the possibility of a genetically determined link between airway hyperresponsiveness and ASM growth [169].

Growth responses of cultured airways smooth muscle

Over the last 8 years an increasing amount of attention has been directed towards identification of potential growth factors for ASM, the signal transduction mechanisms and the modulation of these growth responses by anti-asthma drugs [170].

Mediators regulating growth responses

Several bronchoconstrictors have been shown to elicit growth responses of cultured ASM. ET-1 alone weakly stimulates ASM DNA synthesis [171–173] and acts in synergy with other mitogens [174]. In a rat model of airway wall thickening, ET-1 had no effect on ASM proliferation *in vivo* [169]. However, the ET_A-receptor antagonist, BQ-610, inhibited rat airway wall mitogenesis stimulated by cigarette smoke [175]. Histamine stimulates proliferation of canine [176] and human cultured ASM cells [65], but its effects on chronic airway wall remodelling *in vivo* have yet to be investigated. Substance P and neurokinin A elicit growth of rabbit tracheal muscle *via* an NK1 receptor [177], but appear to be inactive on human airway muscle (Stewart, unpublished observations). LTs are relatively weak direct stimulants of human ASM proliferation, but act in synergy with powerful peptide growth factors [178]. In rabbit ASM, LT-induced proliferation is dependent on increases in insulin-like growth factor (IGF) availability [179]. TxA_2 mimetics have also been shown to stimulate DNA synthesis [141, 180] possibly through the secondary production of LTs [180]. Simulation of cyclical strain in cultured ASM stimulates both DNA synthesis and hypertrophy [181], the latter responses ocurring only when cells reach confluence [25]. Thus, the propensity of bronchoconstrictors to induce cell proliferation may be underestimated in cell culture studies, in which substrate attachment prevents the development of increased strain and there is no cyclical variation due to tidal breathing.

Established growth factors such as platelet-derived growth factor (PDGF) [176, 182], epidermal growth factor and basic fibroblast growth factor [141] are considerably more active and more potent than bronchoconstrictors in eliciting growth responses. The actions of serine proteases such as thrombin [141, 183] and mast cell-derived tryptase [184] are of increasing interest as knowledge of the protease-activated receptors (PARS) expands. The newly identified cleavage-dependent generation of a nascent amino terminus that acts as a tethered ligand for the PARS receptor, raises the possibility that transient exposure to these activated proteases could lead to sustained growth responses. The insulin-like growth factor (IGF) axis has been implicated in ASM mitogenesis: IGFs are secreted by ASM and stimulate proliferation when the concentration exceeds the binding capacity of IGF binding protein (IGF-BP) [185]. Matrix metalloproteinases (MMPs) metabolism of IGF-BP is stimulated by LTD_4 which is mitogenic in rabbit ASM [146, 179]. Interestingly, thrombin is known to stimulate the release of MMP2 from endothelial cells, raising the possibility of IGF involvement in thrombin-induced proliferative responses. Lysosomal hydrolases derived from inflammatory cells such as β-hexosaminidase have also been identified as ASM mitogens [186] acting *via* stimulation of a mannose receptor [187].

The growth-promoting actions of several cytokines have been evaluated. IL-1β elicits both proliferation and hypertrophy secondary to the release of PDGF [188, 189]. TNFα both stimulates [190, 191] and inhibits growth responses depending on the concentration and duration of incubation – short incubation periods at high concentrations result in inhibition of DNA synthesis [190]. In addition, our recent studies have shown that combinations of IL-1β and TNFα in human cultured ASM increase PGE_2 production to levels which have profound inhibitory effects on bFGF-stimulated DNA synthesis (Vlahos and Stewart, unpublished observations). T lymphocyte binding *via* integrins to cytokine-activated ASM induces proliferation by mechanisms which remain to be elucidated [192], but may involve signal through the MAPK pathway [193].

Mitogen signalling pathways

Signal transduction of proliferation is complex and incompletely understood (Fig. 6). The proximal signals activated by growth factors include phospholipase C [183, 194], elevation of $Ca^{2+}{}_i$, phosphoinositol-3-kinase, protein kinase C and tyrosine kinases [171, 195]. The elevation of $Ca^{2+}{}_i$ has been dissociated from the proliferative response by the use of G protein inhibitors [183] and separation of the concentration-response curves for growth responses and increases in $Ca^{2+}{}_i$ [171]. However, none of the growth factors yet investigated fails to activate MAPK (ERK), which is believed to play an obligatory role in the signalling cascade that leads to passage of cells through the restriction point of the cell cycle. In bovine tracheal muscle, persistent MAPK activation appears to be required for DNA synthesis [196] and similar observations have been made for human ASM. Specifically, inhibition of MAPK by PD98059, which prevents activation of the upstream kinase MEK1 and proliferation induced by thrombin, PDGF [197] and ET-1 [198], decreases levels of cyclin D1 (Ravenhall, Harris and Stewart, unpublished observations) which is required for passage through the restriction point of the cell cycle [199]. Cyclin D1 partners cyclin-dependent kinase 4 (cdk4) which phosphorylates the restriction protein, retinoblastoma (pRb) [200]. Upon phosphorylation pRb dissociates from and

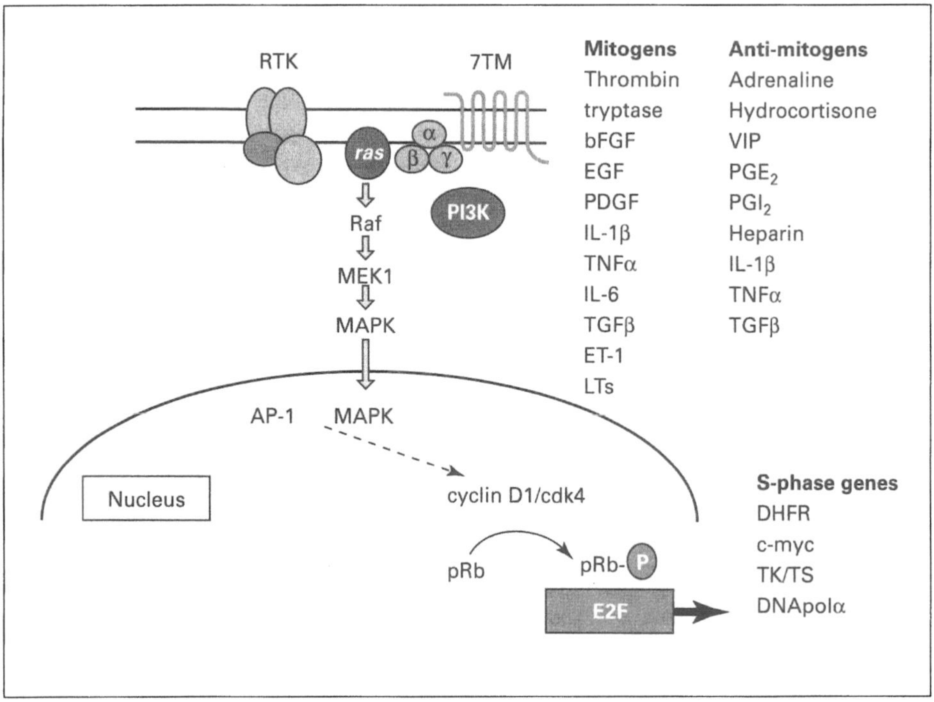

Figure 6
Identified elements of the signal transduction pathway for airway smooth muscle proliferation. Both G protein-coupled, seven transmembrane spanning region receptors (7TM) and growth factor receptor tyrosine kinases are linked through multiple pathways to the activation of the Ras/Raf pathway, upstream of mitogen-activated protein kinase (MAPK). The precise mechanisms regulating the expression of cyclin D1 in airway smooth muscle have not been established, but both MAPK subtrates and the AP-1 complex comprising Jun and Fos are candidate trancription factors. Cyclin D1 partners the cyclin-dependent kinase 4 (cdk4) which phosphorylates a number of essential S-phase genes including dihydrofolate reductase (DHFR), thymidine kinase (TK), thymidine synthetase (TS), the transcription factor c-myc and DNA polymerase α (DNApolα).

disinhibits the transcription factor complex E2F allowing the synthesis of genes essential for DNA synthesis and further cell cycle progression. Other obligatory signals for cell cycle progression are likely to be identified.

Influence of anti-asthma drugs on smooth muscle mitogenesis

Glucocorticoids inhibit proliferation of ASM *in vitro* in a mitogen-independent manner in human [131], rabbit [201], and bovine [202] species. The mechanism appears to involve suppression of cyclin D1 mRNA levels. There are no studies of the effects of glucocorticoids on ASM volumetric increases in animal models of chronic allergic responses.

Agents that elevated cAMP including β-adrenoceptor agonists [141, 201, 202], PGE_2 [141, 203, 204] and VIP [65] also inhibit ASM proliferation. The mechanism has yet to be fully elucidated, but does not appear to be related to regulation of $Ca^{2+}{}_i$ [205] or K^+ channels [206] and can occur late in G1 phase of the cell cycle indicating that regulation of passage through the restriction point may be the target [207]. Thus, salbutamol reduces the levels of cyclin D1 [208] and the phosphorylation of pRb without affecting cyclin D1 mRNA levels. Combinations of β-agonists and glucocorticoids have synergistic actions [201] as could be expected by their actions on distinct components of the mitogen signalling pathways. *In vivo* data is restricted to a study in guinea-pigs which suggested that the volume of ASM was increased by repeated exposure to fenoterol, but this was not associated with detectable increases in DNA synthesis and may therefore have resulted from hypertrophy [209].

Other endogenous anti-mitogens include TGFβ, which alone has small stimulatory effects on DNA synthesis, but with prolonged incubation (48 h) is mitogenic [143, 147]. Heparin inhibits DNA synthesis induced by FCS, but not by PDGF [204, 210] indicating that it acts on a proximal and mitogen-specific signalling mechanism, probably upstream of the common MAPK pathway.

Acknowledgements
The authors' work cited in this study was supported by grants from the NHMRC (Australia) and GlaxoWellcome UK. We thank John Bartolo and Drs John Wilson and Xun Li and the staff of the heart/lung transplant unit at the Alfred Hospital for assistance in the provision of human airway specimens.

References

1 Panettieri RA, Murray RK, DePalo LR, Yadvish PA, Kotlikoff MI (1989) A human airway smooth muscle cell line that retains physiological responsiveness. *Am J Physiol* 256: C329–335

2 Moreno RH, Hogg JC, Pare PD (1986) Mechanics of airway narrowing. *Am Rev Respir Dis* 133: 1171–1180

3 MA X, Li W, Stephens NL (1996) Detection of two clusters of mechanical properties of smooth muscle along the airway tree. *J Appl Physiol* 80: 857–861

4 Gabella G (1994) Anatomy of airways smooth muscle. In: D Raeburn D, MA Giembycz (eds): *Airways smooth muscle: structure, innervation and neurotransmission*. Birkhäuser Verlag, Basel, 1–29

5 Sparrow MP, McFawn PK, Omari TI, Mitchell HW (1992) Activation of smooth mus-

cle in the airway wall, force production, and airway narrowing. *Can J Physiol Pharmacol* 70: 607–614
6 Stephens NL, Jiang H, Halayko A (1993) Role of airway smooth muscle in asthma: possible relation to the neuroendocrine system. *Anatomical Record* 236: 152–163; discussion 163–167
7 Shore SA, Laporte J, Hall IP, Hardy E, Panettieri RA, Jr (1997) Effect of IL-1 beta on responses of cultured human airway smooth muscle cells to bronchodilator agonists. *Am J Respir Cell Mol Biol* 16: 702–712
8 Stephens NL, Seow CY, Halayko AJ, Jiang H (1992) The biophysics and biochemistry of smooth muscle contraction. *Can J Physiol Pharmacol* 70: 515–531
9 Solway J, Fredberg JJ (1997) Perhaps airway smooth muscle dysfunction contributes to asthmatic bronchial hyperresponsiveness after all. *Am J Respir Cell Mol Biol* 17: 144–146
10 Johnson JD, Snyder CH (1995) Calcium regulation of smooth muscle contractile proteins. In: AR Means (ed): *Advances in second messenger and phosphoprotein research.* Raven Press, New York, 153–174
11 Knighton DR, Pearson RB, Sowadski JM, Means AR, Ten Eyck LF, Taylor SS, Kemp BE (1992) Structural basis of the intrasteric regulation of myosin light chain kinases. *Science* 258: 130–135
12 Jiang H, Rao K, Liu X, Stephens NL (1992) Ragweed sensitization-induced increases of myosin light chain kinase content in canine airway smooth muscle. *Am J Respir Cell Mol Biol* 7: 567–573
13 Rembold CM, Murphy RA (1993) Models of the mechanism for cross-bridge attachment in smooth muscle. *J Muscle Res Cell Motil* 14: 325–333
14 Ikebe M, Reardon S (1988) Binding of caldesmon to smooth muscle myosin. *J Biol Chem* 263: 3055–3058
15 Walsh MP, Sutherland C (1989) A model for caldesmon in latch-bridge formation in smooth muscle. *Adv Exp Med Biol* 255: 337–346
16 Smith CWJ, Pritchard K, Marston SB (1987) The mechanism of calcium regulation of vascular smooth muscle thin filaments by caldesmon and calmodulin. *J Biol Chem* 262: 116–122
17 Gerthoffer WT (1994) Current concepts on mechanisms of force maintenance in airways smooth musle. In: D Raeburn, MA Giembycz (eds): *Airways smooth muscle: biochemical control of contraction and relaxation.* Birkhäuser Verlag, Basel, 117–136
18 Chamley-Campbell J, Campbell G, Ross R (1979) The smooth muscle cell in culture. *Physiol Rev* 85: 501–513
19 Halayko AJ, Stephens NL (1994) Potential role for phenotypic modulation of bronchial smooth muscle cells in chronic asthma. *Can J Physiol Pharmacol* 72: 1448–1457
20 Halayko AJ, Salari H, MA X, Stephens NL (1996) Markers of airway smooth muscle cell phenotype. *Am J Physiol* 270: L1040–51
21 Halayko AJ, Rector E, MA X, Stephens DL, Stephens NL (1997) Characterisation of airway smooth muscle cell phenotypes. *Am J Respir Crit Care Med* 155: A369

22 Hirst SJ (1996) Airway smooth muscle cell culture: application to studies of airway wall remodelling and phenotype plasticity in asthma. *Eur Respir J* 9: 808–820
23 Hirst SJ, Twort CH (1997) Effects of extracellular matrix on human airway smooth muscle cell proliferation and phenotype. *Am J Respir Crit Care Med* 155: A371
24 Smith PG, Tokui T, Ikebe M (1995) Mechanical strain increases contractile enzyme activity in cultured airway smooth muscle cells. *Am J Physiol* 268: L999–L1005
25 Smith PG, Moreno R, Ikebe M (1997) Strain increases airway smooth muscle contractile and cytoskeletal proteins *in vitro*. *Am J Physiol* 272: L20–L27
26 Schramm CM, Grunstein MM (1992) Assessment of signal transduction mechanisms regulating airway smooth muscle contractility. *Am J Physiol* 262: L119–39
27 Knox AJ, Tattersfield AE (1995) Airway smooth muscle relaxation. *Thorax* 50: 894–901
28 Marmy N, Mottas J, Durand J (1993) Signal transduction in smooth muscle cells from human airways. *Respir Physiol* 91: 295–306
29 Takahashi T, Belvisi MG, Patel H, Ward JK, Tadjkarimi S, Yacoub MH, Barnes PJ (1994) Effect of Ba 679 BR, a novel long-acting anticholinergic agent, on cholinergic neurotransmission in guinea pig and human airways. *Am J Respir Crit Care Med* 150: 1640–1645
30 Coburn RF, Baron CB (1990) Coupling mechanisms in airway smooth muscle. *Am J Physiol* 258: L119–L133
31 Advenier C, Cerrina J, Duroux P, Floch A, Rennier A (1984) Effects of five different calcium antagonists on guinea-pig isolated trachea. *Br J Pharmacol* 82: 727–733
32 Murray RK, Fleischmann BK, Kotlikoff MI (1993) Receptor-activated Ca influx in human airway smooth muscle: use of Ca imaging and perforated patch-clamp techniques. *Am J Physiol* 264: C485–90
33 Knox AJ, Baldwin DR, Cragoe EJ Jr, Ajao P (1993) The effect of sodium transport and calcium channel inhibitors on phorbol ester-induced contraction of bovine airway smooth muscle. *Pulmon Pharmacol* 6: 241–246
34 Hall IP, Donaldson J, Hill SJ (1989) Inhibition of histamine-stimulated inositol phospholipid hydrolysis by agents which increase cyclic AMP levels in bovine tracheal smooth muscle. *Br J Pharmacol* 97: 603–613
35 Jones KA, Lorenz RR, Warner DO, Katusic ZS, Sieck GC (1994) Changes in cytosolic cGMP and calcium in airway smooth muscle relaxed by 3-morpholinosydnonimine. *Am J Physiol* 266: L9–L16
36 Beavo JA, Conti M, Heaslip RJ (1994) Multiple cyclic nucleotide phosphodiesterases. *Mol Pharmacol* 46: 399–405
37 Webb BL, Lindsay MA, Barnes PJ, Giembycz MA (1997) Protein kinase C isoenzymes in airway smooth muscle. *Biochem J* 324: 167–175
38 Yang KX, Black JL (1996) Protein kinase C induced changes in human airway smooth muscle tone: the effects of Ca^{2+} and Na^{+} transport. *Eur J Pharmacol* 315: 65–71
39 Tajimi M, Hori M, Mitsui M, Ozaki H, Karaki H (1995) Inhibitory effect of forskolin

on myosin phosphorylation-dependent and independent contractions in bovine tracheal smooth muscle. *J Smooth Muscle Res* 31: 129–142
40 Peiper U, Knipp SC, Thies B, Henke R (1996) Activation of protein kinase C accelerates contraction kinetics of airway smooth muscle. *Eur J Physiol* 432: R47–R52
41 Gerthoffer WT, Yamboliev IAA, Pohl J, Haynes R, Dang S, McHugh J (1997) Activation of MAP kinases in airway smooth muscle. *Am J Physiol* 272: L244–L252
42 Edwards G, Weston AH (1995) The role of potassium channels in excitable cells. *Diabetes Res Clin Pract* 28 (Suppl): S57–S66
43 Snetkov VA, Hirst SJ, Twort CH, Ward JP (1995) Potassium currents in human freshly isolated bronchial smooth muscle cells. *Br J Pharmacol* 115: 1117–1125
44 Adda S, Fleischmann BK, Freedman BD, Yu M, Hay DW, Kotlikoff MI (1996) Expression and function of voltage-dependent potassium channel genes in human airway smooth muscle. *J Biol Chem* 271: 13239–13243
45 Buckle DR (1993) Prospects for potassium channel activators in the treatment of airways obstruction. *Pulmon Pharmacol* 6: 161–169
46 Chapman ID, Kristersson A, Mathelin G, Schaeublin E, Mazzoni L, Boubekeur K, Murphy N, Morley J (1992) Effects of a potassium channel opener (SDZ PCO 400) on guinea-pig and human pulmonary airways. *Br J Pharmacol* 106: 423–429
47 Kume H, Hall IP, Washabau RJ, Takagi K, Kotlikoff MI (1994) Beta-adrenergic agonists regulate KCa channels in airway smooth muscle by cAMP-dependent and -independent mechanisms. *J Clin Invest* 93: 371–379
48 Chiu P, Cook SJ, Small RC, Berry JL, Carpenter JR, Downing SJ, Foster RW, Miller AJ, Small AM (1993) β-Adrenoceptor subtypes and the opening of plasmalemmal K^+ channels in bovine trachealis muscle: studies of mechanical activity and ion fluxes. *Br J Pharmacol* 109: 1149–1156
49 Vincent NJ, Knudson R, Leith DF, Macklem PT, Mead J (1970) Factors influencing pulmonary resistance. *J Appl Physiol* 29: 236–243
50 Barnes PJ (1993) Muscarinic receptor subtypes in airways. *Life Sci* 52: 521–528
51 Fryer AD, Jacoby DB (1993) Effect of inflammatory cell mediators on M_2 muscarinic receptors in the lung. Life Sci 52: 529–536
52 Wessler, I, Helliwig D, Racke K (1990) Epithelium-derived inhibition of [^{3}H]-acetylcholine release from the isolated guinea-pig trachea. *Naunyn-Schmiedeberg's Arch Pharmacol* 342: 387–393
53 Barnes PJ, Baraniuk L, Belvisi MG (1991) Neuropeptides in the respiratory tract. *Am Rev Respir Dis* 144: 1187–1198
54 Ward JK, Belvisi MG, Fox AJ, Miura M, Tadjkarimi S, Yacoub MH, Barnes PJ (1993) Modulation of cholinergic neural bronchoconstriction by endogenous nitric oxide and vasoactive intestinal peptide in human airways *in vitro*. *J Clin Invest* 92: 736–742
55 Brodie DH, Lotz M, Cuomo AJ, Coburn DA, Federman EC, Wasserman SI (1992) Cytokines in symptomatic asthmatic airways. *J Allergy Clin Immunol* 89: 958–967
56 Anticevich SZ, Hughes JM, Black JL, Armour CL (1995) Induction of human airway hyperresponsiveness by tumour necrosis factor-alpha. *Eur J Pharmacol* 284: 221–225

57 Hallahan AR, Armour CL, Black JL (1990) Products of neutrophils and eosinophils increase the responsiveness of human isolated bronchial tissue. *Eur Respir J* 3: 554–558

58 Fernandes LB, Henry PJ, Rigby PJ, Goldie RG (1996) Endothelin B (ETB) receptor-activated potentiation of cholinergic nerve-mediated contraction in human bronchus. *Br J Pharmacol* 118: 1873–1874

59 Ind PW (1994) Role of the sympathetic nervous system and endogenous catecholamines in the regulation of airway smooth muscle tone. In: D Raeburn, MA Giembycz (eds): *Airways smooth muscle: structure, innervation and neurotransmission*. Birkhäuser Verlag, Basel, 29–41

60 Goldie RG (1990) Receptors in asthmatic airways. *Am Rev Respir Dis* 141: S151–S156

61 Bai TR, Lam R, Prasad FYF (1989) Effects of adrenergic agonists and adenosine on cholinergic neurotransmission in lung tracheal smooth muscle. *Pulmon Pharmacol* 1: 193–199

62 Barnes PJ (1994) Modulation of neurotransmitter release from airways nerves. In: D Raeburn, MA Giembycz (eds): *Airways smooth muscle: structure, innervation and neurotransmission*. Birkhäuser Verlag, Basel, 209–259

63 Belvisi MG, Stretton CD, Miura M, Verleden GM, Tadjarimi S, Yacoub MH, Barnes PJ (1992) Inhibitory NANC nerves in human tracheal smooth muscle: a quest for the neurotransmitter. *J Appl Physiol* 73: 2505–2510

64 Barnes PJ, Dixon CMS (1984) The effect of inhaled vasoactive intestinal peptide on bronchial hyperreactivity in man. *Am Rev Respir Dis* 130: 162–166

65 Maruno K, Absood A, Said SI (1995) VIP inhibits basal and histamine-stimulated proliferation of human airway smooth muscle cells. *Am J Physiol* 268: L1047–L1051

66 Belvisi MG, Stretton CD, Yacoub M, Barnes PJ (1992) Nitric oxide is the endogenous neurotransmitter of bronchodilator nerves in humans. *Eur J Pharmacol* 210: 221–222

67 Yates DH, Kharitonov SA, Thomas PS, Barnes PJ (1996) Endogenous nitric oxide is decreased in asthmatic patients by an inhibitor of inducible nitric oxide synthase. *Am J Respir Crit Care Med* 154: 247–250

68 Lundberg JM (1995) Tachykinins, sensory nerves, and asthma – an overview. *Can J Physiol Pharmacol* 73: 908–914

69 Lundberg JM, Martling CR, Lundblad L (1988) Cigarette smoke-induced irritation in the airways in relation to peptide-containing, capsaicin-sensitive sensory neurons. *Klinische Wochenschrift* 66 (Suppl 11): 151–160

70 Stewart AG, Thompson DC, Fennessy MR (1984) Involvement of capsaicin-sensitive afferent neurones in a vagal-dependent interaction between leukotriene D4 and histamine on bronchomotor tone. *Agents Actions* 15: 500–508

71 Ellis JL, Undem BJ (1991) Role of peptidoleukotrienes in capsaicin-sensitive sensory fibre-mediated responses in guinea-pig airways. *J Physiol* 436: 469–484

72 Barnes PJ (1986) Neural control of human airways in health and disease. *Am Rev Respir Dis* 134: 1289–1314

73 Henderson WR Jr (1994) Role of leukotrienes in asthma. *Ann Allergy* 72: 272–278

74 O'Byrne PM (1996) Airway inflammation and asthma. *Aliment Pharmacol Ther* 10 (Suppl 2): 18–24
75 Liu MC, Bleecker ER, Lichtenstein LM, Kagey-Sobotka A, Niv Y, McLemore, TL, Permutt S, Proud D, Hubbard WC (1990) Evidence for elevated levels of histamine, prostaglandin D2, and other bronchoconstricting prostaglandins in the airways of subjects with mild asthma. *Am Rev Respir Dis* 142: 126–132
76 Johnston SL, Bardin PG, Harrison J, Ritter W, Joubert JR, Holgate ST (1992) The effects of an oral thromboxane TP receptor antagonist BAY u 3405, on prostaglandin D2- and histamine-induced bronchoconstriction in asthma, and relationship to plasma drug concentrations. *Br J Clin Pharmacol* 34: 402–408
77 Aizawa H, Inoue H, Matsumoto K, Koto H, Nakano H, Hara N (1996) Thromboxane A2 antagonist inhibits leukotriene D4-induced smooth muscle contraction in guinea-pig lung parenchyma, but not in trachea. *Prostaglandins Leukot Essent Fatty Acids* 55: 437–440
78 Jones GL, Saroea HG, Watson RM, O'Byrne PM (1992) Effect of an inhaled thromboxane mimetic (U46619) on airway function in human subjects. *Am Rev Respir Dis* 145: 1270–1274
79 Sampson AP, Thomas RU, Costello JF, Piper PJ (1992) Enhanced leukotriene synthesis in leukocytes of atopic and asthmatic subjects. *Br J Clin Pharmacol* 33: 423–430
80 Chung KF (1995) Leukotriene receptor antagonists and biosynthesis inhibitors: potential breakthrough in asthma therapy. *Eur Respir J* 8:1203–1213
81 Stewart AG (1994) Biological properties of platelet-activating factor. In: FM Cunningham (ed): *Lipid mediators*. Academic Press, London, 223–296
82 Johnson PR, Black JL, Armour CL (1992) Platelet-activating factor-induced contraction of human isolated bronchus. *Eur Respir J* 5: 970–974
83 Spencer DA, Green SE, Evans JM, Piper PJ, Costello JF (1990) Platelet activating factor does not cause a reproducible increase in bronchial responsiveness in normal man. *Clin Exp Allergy* 20: 525–532
84 Kharitonov SA, Yates D, Barnes PJ (1995) Increased nitric oxide in exhaled air of normal human subjects with upper respiratory tract infections. *Eur Respir J* 8: 295–297
85 Barnes PJ, Liew FY (1995) Nitric oxide and asthmatic inflammation. *Immunol Today* 16: 128–130
86 Barnes PJ (1996) NO or no NO in asthma? *Thorax* 51: 218–220
87 Joad J, Casale TB (1988) Histamine and airway caliber. *Ann Allergy* 61: 1–7
88 Knight DA, Stewart GA, Thompson PJ (1992) Histamine tachyphylaxis in human airway smooth muscle. The role of H2-receptors and the bronchial epithelium. *Am Rev Respir Dis* 146: 137–140
89 White JP, Mills J, Eiser NM (1987) Comparison of the effects of histamine H1- and H2-receptor agonists on large and small airways in normal and asthmatic subjects. *Br J Dis Chest* 81: 155–169
90 Driver AG, Kukoly CA, Ali S, Mustafa SJ (1993) Adenosine in bronchoalveolar lavage fluid in asthma. *Am Rev Respir Dis* 148: 91–97

91 Bjorck T, Gustafsson LE, Dahlen SE (1992) Isolated bronchi from asthmatics are hyperresponsive to adenosine, which apparently acts indirectly by liberation of leukotrienes and histamine. *Am Rev Resp Dis* 145: 1087–1091

92 Meade CJ, Mierau J, Leon I, Ensinger HA (1996) *In vivo* role of the adenosine A_3 receptor: N6-2-(4-aminophenyl)ethyladenosine induces bronchospasm in BDE rats by a neurally mediated mechanism involving cells resembling mast cells. *J Pharmacol Exp Ther* 279: 1148–1156

93 Goldie RG, Knott PG, Carr MJ, Hay DW, Henry PJ (1996) The endothelins in the pulmonary system. *Pulmon Pharmacol* 9: 69–93

94 Barnes PJ (1994) Endothelins and pulmonary diseases. *J Appl Physiol* 77: 1051–1059

95 Takahashi T, Barnes PJ, Kawikova I, Yacoub MH, Warner TD, Belvisi MG (1997) Contraction of human airway smooth muscle by endothelin-1 and IRL 1620: effect of bosentan. *Eur J Pharmacol* 324: 219–222

96 Noguchi K, Ishikawa K, Yano M, Ahmed A, Cortes A, Abraham WM (1995) Endothelin-1 contributes to antigen-induced airway hyperresponsiveness. *J Appl Physiol* 79: 700–705

97 Goldie RG, Henry PJ, Knott PG, Self GJ, Luttmann MA, Hay DW (1995) Endothelin-1 receptor density, distribution, and function in human isolated asthmatic airways. *Am J Respir Crit Care Med* 152: 1653–1658

98 Tomaki M, Ichinose M, Miura M, Hirayama Y, Yamauchi H, Nakajima N, Shirato K (1995) Elevated substance P content in induced sputum from patients with asthma and patients with chronic bronchitis. *Am J Respir Crit Care Med* 151: 613–617

99 Nieber K, Baumgarten CR, Rathsack R, Furkert J, Oehme P, Kunkel G (1992) Substance P and beta-endorphin-like immunoreactivity in lavage fluids of subjects with and without allergic asthma. *J Allergy Clin Immunol* 90: 646–652

100 Advenier C, Naline E, Toty L, Bakdach H, Emonds-Alt X, Vilain P, Breliere JC, Le Fur G (1992) Effects on the isolated human bronchus of SR 48968, a potent and selective nonpeptide antagonist of the neurokinin A (NK2) receptors. *Am Rev Respir Dis* 146: 1177–1181

101 Bai TR, Zhou D, Weir T, Walker B, Hegele R, Hayashi S, McKay K, Bondy GP, Fong T (1995) Substance P (NK1)- and neurokinin A (NK2)-receptor gene expression in inflammatory airway diseases. *Am J Physiol* 269: L309–17

102 Matsuse T, Thomson RJ, Chen XR, Salari H, Schellenberg, RR (1991) Capsaicin inhibits airway hyperresponsiveness but not lipoxygenase activity or eosinophilia after repeated aerosolized antigen in guinea pigs. *Am Rev Respir Dis* 144: 368–372

103 Ladenius AR, Folkerts G, van der Linde HJ, Nijkamp FP (1995) Potentiation by viral respiratory infection of ovalbumin-induced guinea-pig tracheal hyperresponsiveness: role for tachykinins. *Br J Pharmacol* 115: 1048–1052

104 Buckley TL, Nijkamp FP (1994) Mucosal exudation associated with a pulmonary delayed-type hypersensitivity reaction in the mouse. Role for the tachykinins. *J Immunol* 153: 4169–4178

105 Wills-Karp M, Uchida Y, Lee JY, Jinot J, Hirata A, Hirata F (1993) Organ culture with

pro-inflammatory cytokines reproduces impairment of the β-adrenoceptor-mediated relaxation in traches of a guinea-pig antigen model. *Am J Respir Cell Mol Biol* 8: 153–159
106 Hakonarson H, Herrick DJ, Serrano PG, Grunstein MM (1996) Mechanism of cytokine-induced modulation of beta-adrenoceptor responsiveness in airway smooth muscle. *J Clin Invest* 97: 2593–2600
107 Barnes PJ (1995) Beta-adrenergic receptors and their regulation. *Am J Respir Crit Care Med* 152: 838–860
108 Laitinen LA, Laitinen A, Heino M, Kava T, Haahtela T (1985) Damage of the airway epithelium and bronchial reactivity in patients with asthma. *Am Rev Respir Dis* 131: 599–606
109 Goldie RG, Preuss JMH (1997) Epithelial function and airway responsiveness. In: AG Stewart (ed): *Airway wall remodelling in asthma*. CRC Press Inc, Boca Raton, 139–178
110 Fernandes LB, Goldie RG (1989) Co-axial bioassay of an epithelial relaxant factor from the guinea-pig trachea. *Br J Pharmacol* 97: 117–124
111 Vanhoutte PM (1988) Epithelium-derived relaxing factor(s) and bronchial reactivity. *Am Rev Respir Dis* 138: S24–S30
112 Sparrow MP, Omari TI, Mitchell HW (1995) The epithelial barrier and airway responsiveness. *Can J Physiol Pharmacol* 73: 180–190
113 Szczeklik A, Sladek K, Dworski R, Nizankowska E, Soja J, Sheller J, Oates J (1996) Bronchial aspirin challenge causes specific eicosanoid response in aspirin-sensitive asthmatics. *Am J Respir Crit Care Med* 154: 1608–1614
114 Finnerty JP, Twentyman OP, Harris A, Palmer JB, Holgate ST (1991) Effect of GR32191, a potent thromboxane receptor antagonist, on exercise induced bronchoconstriction in asthma. *Thorax* 46: 190–192
115 Fennessy MR, Stewart AG, Thompson DC (1986) Aerosolised and intravenously administered leukotrienes: effects on the bronchoconstrictor potency of histamine in the guinea-pig. *Br J Pharmacol* 87: 741–749
116 O'Hickey SP, Hawksworth RJ, Fong CY, Arm JP, Spur BW, Lee TH (1991) Leukotrienes C4, D4, and E4 enhance histamine responsiveness in asthmatic airways. *Am Rev Respir Dis* 144: 1053–1057
117 Ind PW (1996) Anti-leukotriene intervention: is there adequate information for clinical use in asthma? *Respir Med* 90: 575–586
118 Taki F, Suzuki R, Torii K, Matsumoto S, Taniguchi H, Takagi K (1994) Reduction of the severity of bronchial hyperresponsiveness by the novel leukotriene antagonist 4-oxo-8-[4-(4-phenyl-butoxy)benzoylamino]-2-(tetrazol-5-yl)-4H-1-benzopyran hemihydrate. *Arzneimittel-Forschung* 44: 330–333
119 Rafferty P (1990) Antihistamines in the treatment of clinical asthma. *J Allergy Clin Immunol* 86: 647–650
120 Malick A, Grant JA (1997) Antihistamines in the treatment of asthma. *Allergy* 52: 55–66
121 Evans DJ, Barnes PJ, Cluzel M, O'Connor BJ (1997) Effects of a potent platelet-acti-

vating factor antagonist, SR27417A, on allergen-induced asthmatic responses. *Am J Respir Crit Care Med* 156: 11–16

122 Kuitert LM, Angus RM, Barnes NC, Barnes, PJ, Bone MF, Chung KF, Fairfax AJ, Higenbotham TW, O'Connor BJ et al (1995) Effect of a novel potent platelet-activating factor antagonist, modipafant, in clinical asthma. *Am J Respir Crit Care Med* 151: 1331–1335

123 Ichinose M, Nakajima N, Takahashi T, Yamauchi H, Inoue H, Takishima, T (1992) Protection against bradykinin-induced bronchoconstriction in asthmatic patients by neurokinin receptor antagonist. *Lancet* 340: 1248–1251

124 Bertrand C, Geppetti P (1996) Tachykinin and kinin receptor antagonists: therapeutic perspectives in allergic airway disease. *Trends Pharmacol Sci* 17: 255–259

125 Ichinose M, Miura M, Yamauchi H, Kageyama N, Tomaki M, Oyake T, Ohuchi Y, Hida W, Miki H, Tamura G et al (1996) A neurokinin 1-receptor antagonist improves exercise-induced airway narrowing in asthmatic patients. *Am J Respir Crit Care Med* 153: 936–941

126 Joos GF, Van Schoor J, Kips JC, Pauwels RA (1996) The effect of inhaled FK224, a tachykinin NK-1 and NK-2 receptor antagonist, on neurokinin A-induced bronchoconstriction in asthmatics. *Am J Respir Crit Care Med* 153: 1781–1784

127 Fahy JV, Wong HH, Geppetti P, Reis JM, Harris SC, Maclean DB, Nadel, JA, Boushey HA (1995) Effect of an NK1 receptor antagonist (CP-99,994) on hypertonic saline-induced bronchoconstriction and cough in male asthmatic subjects. *Am J Respir Crit Care Med* 152: 879–884

128 Devoy MAB, Fuller RW, Palmer JBD (1995) Are there any detrimental effects of the use of long-acting β-agonists in the treatment of asthma? *Chest* 107: 1116–1124

129 Barrett TE, Strom BL (1995) Inhaled beta-adrenoceptor agonists in asthma: more harm than good? *Am J Respir Crit Care Med* 151: 574–577

130 Barnes PJ. (1995) Anti-inflammatory mechanisms of glucocorticoids. *Biochemical Society Transactions* 23: 940–945

131 Stewart AG, Fernandes D, Tomlinson PR (1995) The effect of glucocorticoids on proliferation of human cultured airway smooth muscle. *Br J Pharmacol* 116: 3219–3226

132 Johnson SR, Knox AJ (1997) Synthetic functions of airway smooth muscle in asthma. *Trends Pharmacol Sci* 18: 289–292

133 Mak JC, Nishikawa M, Barnes PJ (1995) Glucocorticosteroids increase beta 2-adrenergic receptor transcription in human lung. *Am J Physiol* 268: L41–L46

134 Nabishah BM, Morat PB, Kadir BA, Khalid BA (1991) Effect of steroid hormones on muscarinic receptors of bronchial smooth muscle. *Gen Pharmacol* 22: 389–392

135 Emala CW, Clancy J, Hirshman CA (1997) Glucocorticoid treatment decreases muscarinic receptor expression in canine airway smooth muscle. *Am J Physiol* 272: L745–L751

136 Hardy E, Farahani M, Hall IP (1996) Regulation of histamine H1 receptor coupling by dexamethasone in human cultured airway smooth muscle. *Br J Pharmacol* 118: 1079–1084

137 Vadas P, Stefanski E, Wloch M, Grouix B, Van Den Bosch H, Kennedy B (1996) Secretory non-pancreatic phospholipase A2 and cyclooxygenase-2 expression by tracheobronchial smooth muscle cells. *Eur J Biochem* 235: 557–563
138 Vigano T, Habib A, Hernandez A, Bonazzi A, Boraschi D, Lebret M, Cassina E, Maclouf J, Sala A, Folco G (1997) Cyclooxygenase-2 and synthesis of PGE2 in human bronchial smooth-muscle cells. *Am J Respir Crit Care Med* 155: 864–868
139 Belvisi MG, Saunders MA, Haddad el-B, Hirst SJ, Yacoub MH, Barnes PJ, Mitchell JA (1997) Induction of cyclo-oxygenase-2 by cytokines in human cultured airway smooth muscle cells: novel inflammatory role of this cell type. *Br J Pharmacol* 120: 910–916
140 Pang L, Knox AJ (1997) Effect of interleukin-1 beta, tumour necrosis factor-alpha and interferon-gamma on the induction of cyclo-oxygenase-2 in cultured human airway smooth muscle cells. *Br J Pharmacol* 121: 579–587
141 Tomlinson PR, Wilson JW, Stewart AG (1994) Inhibition by salbutamol of the proliferation of human airway smooth muscle cells grown in culture. *Br J Pharmacol* 111: 641–647
142 Demoly P, Jaffuel D, Lequeux N, Weksler B, Creminon C, Michel FB, Godard P, Bousquet J (1997) Prostaglandin H synthase 1 and 2 immunoreactivities in the bronchial mucosa of asthmatics. *Am J Respir Crit Care Med* 155: 670–675
143 Black PN, Young PG, Skinner SJ (1996) Response of airway smooth muscle cells to TGF-beta 1: effects on growth and synthesis of glycosaminoglycans. *Am J Physiol* 271: L910–L917
144 John M, Hirst SJ, Jose PJ, Robichaud A, Berkman N, Witt, C, Twort CH, Barnes PJ, Chung KF (1997) Human airway smooth muscle cells express and release RANTES in response to T helper 1 cytokines: regulation by T helper 2 cytokines and corticosteroids. *J Immunol* 158: 1841–1847
145 Saunders MA, Mitchell JA, Seldon PM, Yacoub MH, Barnes PJ, Giembycz MA, Belvisi MG (1997) Release of granulocyte-macrophage colony stimulating factor by human cultured airway smooth muscle cells: suppression by dexamethasone. *Br J Pharmacol* 120: 545–546
146 Rajah R, Nunn SE, Herrick DJ, Grunstein MM, Cohen P (1996) Leukotriene D4 induces MMP-1, which functions as an IGFBP protease in human airway smooth muscle cells. *Am J Physiol* 271: L1014–L1022
147 Cohen MD, Ciocca V, Panettieri RA Jr (1997) TGF-beta 1 modulates human airway smooth-muscle cell proliferation induced by mitogens. *Am J Respir Crit Care Med* 16: 85–90
148 Fish JE, Shaver JR, Peters SP (1995) Airway hyperresponsiveness in asthma. Is it unique? *Chest* 107: 154S–156S
149 Hopp RJ, Bewtra AK, Townley RG (1990) Clinical methods to evaluate airway reactivity. In: DK Agrawal, RG Townley (eds): *Airway smooth muscle modulation of receptors and response*. CRC Press Inc, Boca Raton, 167–179
150 Joos GF, Kips JC, Pauwels RA (1993) Direct and indirect bronchial responsiveness. *Respir Med* 87 (Suppl B): 31–36

151 Takashimi T, Yanai M, Sasaki H (1991) Site of airway hyperreactivity. *Am Rev Respir Dis* 143: S49–S51

152 Kuwano K, Bosken CH, Pare PD, Bai TR, Wiggs BR, Hogg, JC (1993) Small airways dimensions in asthma and in chronic obstructive pulmonary disease. *Am Rev Respir Dis* 148: 1220–1225

153 Ebina M, Takahashi T, Chiba T, Motomiya M (1993) Cellular hypertrophy and hyperplasia of airway smooth muscles underlying bronchial asthma: a 3-D morphometric study. *Am Rev Respir Dis* 148: 720–726

154 Thomson RJ, Bramley AM, Schellenberg RR (1996) Airway muscle stereology: implications for increased shortening in asthma. *Am J Respir Crit Care Med* 154: 749–757

155 Lambert RK, Wiggs BR, Kuwano K, Hogg JC, Pare PD (1993) Functional significance of increased airway smooth muscle in asthma and COPD. *J Appl Physiol* 74: 2771–2781

156 Bosken CH, Hards J, Gatter K, Hogg JC (1992) Characterization of the inflammatory reaction in the peripheral airways of cigarette smokers using immunocytochemistry. *Am Rev Respir Dis* 145: 911–917

157 James AL, Pare PD, Hogg JC (1989) The mechanics of airway narrowing in asthma. *Am Rev Respir Dis* 139: 242–246

158 Pare PD, Bai TR (1995) The consequences of chronic allergic inflammation. *Thorax* 50: 328–332

159 Wiggs BR, Bosken C, Pare PD, James A, Hogg JC (1992) A model of airway narrowing in asthma and in chronic obstructive pulmonary disease. *Am Rev Respir Dis* 145: 1251–1258

160 Woolcock AJ, Salome CM, Yan K (1984) The shape of the dose-reponse curve to histamine in asthmatic and normal subjects. *Am Rev Respir Dis* 130: 71–75

161 Macklem PT (1996) A theoretical analysis of the effect of airway smooth muscle load on airway narrowing. *Am J Respir Crit Care Med* 153: 83–89

162 Skloot G, Permutt S, Togias A (1995) Airway hyperresponsiveness in asthma: a problem of limited smooth muscle relaxation with inspiration. *J Clin Invest* 96: 2393–2403

163 Du T, Sapienza S, Wang CG, Renzi PM, Pantano R, Rossi P, Martin JG (1996) Effect of nedocromil sodium on allergen-induced airway responses and changes in the quantity of airway smooth muscle in rats. *J Allergy Clin Immunol* 98: 400–407

164 Padrid P, Snook S, Finucane T, Shiue P, Cozzi P, Solway J, Leff AR (1995) Persistent airway hyperresponsiveness and histologic alterations after chronic antigen challenge in cats. *Am J Respir Crit Care Med* 151: 184–193

165 Hershenson MB, Abe MK, Kelleher MD, Naureckas ET, Garland A, Zimmermann A, Rubinstein VJ, Solway J (1994) Recovery of airway structure and function after hyperoxic exposure in immature rats. *Am J Respir Crit Care Med* 149: 1663–1669

166 Sapienza S, Du T, Eidelman DH, Wang NS, Martin JG (1991) Structural changes in the airways of sensitized brown Norway rats after antigen challenge. *Am Rev Respir Dis* 144: 423–427

167 Wang CG, Du T, Xu LJ, Martin JG (1993) Role of leukotriene D4 in allergen-induced increases in airway smooth muscle in the rat. *Am Rev Respir Dis* 148: 413–417

168 Dandurand RJ, Xu LJ, Martin JG, Eidelman DH (1993) Airway-parenchymal interdependence and bronchial responsiveness in two highly inbred rat strains. *J Appl Physiol* 74: 538–544

169 Zacour ME, Martin JG (1996) Enhanced growth response of airway smooth muscle in inbred rats with airway hyperresponsiveness. *Am J Respir Cell Mol Biol* 15: 590–599

170 Stewart AG, Tomlinson PR, Wilson JW. (1995) Regulation of airway wall remodelling: prospects for the development of novel antiasthma drugs. In: JT August, MW Anders, F Murad, JT Coyle (eds): *Advances in pharmacology.* Academic Press, San Diego, 209–254

171 Stewart AG, Grigoriadis G, Harris T (1994) Mitogenic actions of endothelin-1 and epidermal growth factor in cultured airway smooth muscle. *Clin Exp Pharmacol Physiol* 21: 277–285

172 Glassberg MK, Ergul A, Wanner A, Puett D (1994) Endothelin-1 promotes mitogenesis in airway smooth muscle cells. *Am J Respir Cell Mol Biol* 10: 316–321

173 Noveral JP, Rosenberg SM, Anbar RA, Pawlowski NA, Grunstein MM (1992) Role of endothelin-1 in regulating proliferation of cultured rabbit airway smooth muscle cells. *Am J Physiol* 263: L317–L324

174 Panettieri RA, Jr., Goldie RG, Rigby PJ, Eszterhas AJ, Hay DW (1996) Endothelin-1-induced potentiation of human airway smooth muscle proliferation: an ETA receptor-mediated phenomenon. *Br J Pharmacol* 118: 191–197

175 Dadmanesh F, Wright JL (1997) Endothelin-A receptor antagonist BQ-610 blocks cigarette smoke-induced mitogenesis in rat airways and vessels. *Am J Physiol* 272: L614–L618

176 Panettieri RA, Yadvish PA, Kelly AM, Rubinstein NA, Kotlikoff MI (1990) Histamine stimulates proliferation of airway smooth muscle and induces c-fos expression. *Am J Physiol* 259: L365–L371

177 Noveral JP, Grunstein MM (1995) Tachykinin regulation of airway smooth muscle cell proliferation. *Am J Physiol* 269: L339–L343

178 Panettieri RA, Jr., Leonard T, Luttmann MA, Hay DWP (1997) Pranlukast, but not zafirlukast, inhibits LTD_4-induced potentation of human airway smooth muscle proliferation. *Am J Respir Crit Care Med* 155: A904

179 Cohen P, Noveral JP, Bhala A, Nunn SE, Herrick DJ, Grunstein MM (1995) Leukotriene D4 facilitates airway smooth muscle cell proliferation *via* modulation of the IGF axis. *Am J Physiol* 269: L151–L157

180 Noveral JP, Grunstein MM (1992) Role and mechanism of thromboxane-induced proliferation of cultured airway smooth muscle cells. *Am J Physiol* 263: L555–L561

181 Smith PG, Janiga KE, Bruce MC (1994) Strain increases airway smooth muscle cell proliferation. *Am J Respir Cell Mol Biol* 10: 85–90

182 Hirst SJ, Barnes PJ, Twort CH (1996) PDGF isoform-induced proliferation and receptor expression in human cultured airway smooth muscle cells. *Am J Physiol* 270: L415–L428

183 Panettieri RA, Jr., Hall IP, Maki CS, Murray RK (1995) alpha-Thrombin increases

cytosolic calcium and induces human airway smooth muscle cell proliferation. *Am J Respir Cell Mol Biol* 13: 205–216
184 Brown JK, Tyler CL, Jones CA, Ruoss SJ, Hartmann T, Caughey GH (1995) Tryptase, the dominant secretory granular protein in human mast cells, is a potent mitogen for cultured dog tracheal smooth muscle cells. *Am J Respir Cell Mol Biol* 13: 227–236
185 Noveral JP, Bhala A, Hintz RL, Grunstein MM, Cohen P (1994) Insulin-like growth factor axis in airway smooth muscle cells. *Am J Physiol* 267: L761–L765
186 Lew DB, Rattazzi MC (1991) Mitogenic effect of lysosomal hydrolases on bovine tracheal myocytes in culture. *J Clin Invest* 88: 1969–1975
187 Lew DB, Songu-Mize E, Pontow SE, Stahl PD, Rattazzi MC (1994) A mannose receptor mediates mannosyl-rich glycoprotein-induced mitogenesis in bovine airway smooth muscle cells. *J Clin Invest* 94: 1855–1863
188 De S, Zelazny ET, Souhrada JF, Souhrada M (1993) Interleukin-1 beta stimulates the proliferation of cultured airway smooth muscle cells *via* platelet-derived growth factor. *Am J Respir Cell Mol Biol* 9: 645–651
189 De S, Zelazny ET, Souhrada JF, Souhrada M (1995) IL-1 beta and IL-6 induce hyperplasia and hypertrophy of cultured guinea pig airway smooth muscle cells. *J Appl Physiol* 78: 1555–1563
190 Stewart AG, Tomlinson PR, Fernandes DJ, Wilson JW, Harris T (1995) Tumor necrosis factor alpha modulates mitogenic responses of human cultured airway smooth muscle. *Am J Respir Cell Mol Biol* 12: 110–119
191 Amrani Y, Panettieri RA, Frossard N, Bronner C (1996) Activation of the TNFa-p55 receptor induces myocyte proliferation and modulates agonist-evoked calcium transients in cultured human tracheal mast cells. *Am J Respir Cell Mol Biol* 15: 55–63
192 Lazaar AL, Albelda SM, Pilewski JM, Brennan B, Pure E, Panettieri RA, Jr (1994) T lymphocytes adhere to airway smooth muscle cells *via* integrins and CD44 and induce smooth muscle cell DNA synthesis. *J Exp Med* 180: 807–816
193 Heuertz RM, Hamann KJ, Hershenson MB, Leff AR (1997) Adhesion of bovine airway smooth muscle cells activates extracellular signal-regulated kinases. *Am J Respir Cell Mol Biol* 17: 456–461
194 De S, Zelazny ET, Souhrada JF, Souhrada M (1996) Role of phospholipase C and tyrosine kinase systems in growth response of human airway smooth muscle cells. *Am J Physiol* 270: L795–L802
195 Hirst SJ, Webb BL, Giembycz MA, Barnes PJ, Twort CH (1995) Inhibition of fetal calf serum-stimulated proliferation of rabbit cultured tracheal smooth muscle cells by selective inhibitors of protein kinase C and protein tyrosine kinase. *Am J Respir Cell Mol Biol* 12: 149–161
196 Kelleher MD, Abe MK, Chao TO, Jain M, Green JM, Solway J, Rosner MR, Hershenson MB (1995) Role of MAP kinase activation in bovine tracheal smooth muscle mitogenesis. *Am J Physiol* 268: L894–L901
197 Karpova AY, Abe MK, Li J, Liu PT, Rhee JM, Kuo WL, Hershenson MB (1997) MEK1

is required for PDGF-induced ERK activation and DNA synthesis in tracheal myocytes. *Am J Physiol* 272: L558–L565

198 Shapiro PS, Evans JN, Davis RJ, Posada JA (1996) The seven-transmembrane-spanning receptors for endothelin and thrombin cause proliferation of airway smooth muscle cells and activation of the extracellular regulated kinase and c-Jun NH2-terminal kinase groups of mitogen-activated protein kinases. *J Biol Chem* 271: 5750–5754

199 Xiong W, Pestell RG, Watanabe G, Li J, Rosner MR, Hershenson MB (1997) Cyclin D1 is required for S phase traversal in bovine tracheal myocytes. *Am J Physiol* 272: L1205–L1210

200 Sherr CJ (1996) Cancer cell cycles. *Science* 274: 1672–1677

201 Schramm CM, Omlor GJ, Quinn LM, Noveral JP (1996) Methylprednisolone and isoproterenol inhibit airway smooth muscle proliferation by separate and additive mechanisms. *Life Sci* 59: PL9–14

202 Young PG, Skinner SJ, Black PN (1995) Effects of glucocorticoids and beta-adrenoceptor agonists on the proliferation of airway smooth muscle. *Eur J Pharmacol* 273: 137–143

203 Florio C, Martin JG, Styhler A, Heisler S (1994) Antiproliferative effect of prostaglandin E2 in cultured guinea pig tracheal smooth muscle cells. *Am J Physiol* 266: L131–L137

204 Johnson PR, Armour CL, Carey D, Black JL (1995) Heparin and PGE2 inhibit DNA synthesis in human airway smooth muscle cells in culture. *Am J Physiol* 269: L514–L519

205 Tomlinson PR, Wilson JW, Stewart AG (1995) Salbutamol inhibits the proliferation of human airway smooth muscle cells grown in culture: relationship to elevated cAMP levels. *Biochem Pharmacol* 49: 1809–1819

206 Stewart AG, Gillzan KM The role of potassium channels in the inhibitory effects of β_2-adrenoceptor agonists on DNA synthesis in human cultured airway smooth muscle. *Pulmon Pharmacol; in press*

207 Stewart AG, Tomlinson PR, Wilson JW (1997) β_2-Adrenoceptor agonist-mediated inhibition of human airway smooth muscle cell proliferation: importance of the duration of β_2-adrenoceptor stimulation. *Br J Pharmacol* 121: 361–368

208 Stewart AG, Schachte LC, Tomlinson PR, Wilson JW (1997) Inhibition by salbutamol of changes in the levels of cyclin D and $p27^{Kip1}$ in thrombin-stimulated human cultured airway smooth muscle. *Pharmacol Rev Comm* 9: 37–40

209 Wang ZL, Walker BA, Weir TD, Yarema MC, Roberts CR, Okazawa M, Pare PD, Bai TR (1995) Effect of chronic antigen and beta 2 agonist exposure on airway remodeling in guinea pigs. *Am J Respir Crit Care Med* 152: 2097–2104

210 Kilfeather SA, Tagoe S, Perez AC, Okona-Mensa K, Matin R, Page CP (1995) Inhibition of serum-induced proliferation of bovine tracheal smooth muscle cells in culture by heparin and related glycosaminoglycans. *Br J Pharmacol* 114: 1442–1446

Drugs that reduce airways inflammation

Katharine H. Banner[1], Domenico Spina and Clive P. Page

The Sackler Institute of Pulmonary Pharmacology, King's College London, Bessemer Rd, London SE5 9PJ, UK; [1]present address: Pfizer Central Research, Ramsgate Rd, Sandwich, CT13 9NJ, UK

Introduction

It is clear from the preceding chapters that a number of inflammatory cells have the potential to contribute towards the pathology associated with asthma. The recognition that asthma is a chronic inflammatory disease of the airways has prompted recent guidelines being issued on the treatment of asthma, all of which have highlighted the need for earlier intervention with anti-inflammatory drugs. This chapter reviews the evidence that glucocorticosteroids, disodium cromoglycate (DSCG), nedocromil sodium and theophylline have anti-inflammatory activity in asthmatics and also considers new drugs which are under development as potential anti-inflammatory agents for the treatment of bronchial asthma.

Established anti-inflammatory drugs

Glucocorticosteroids

Adrenal extracts were first used to treat asthmatics in 1900 [1] with the active ingredient later identified as cortisone [2]. In an attempt to potentiate the anti-inflammatory effects and reduce the unwanted mineralocorticosteroid effects, orally active glucocorticosteroids were developed and proven to have therapeutic efficacy in asthma [3]. It soon became apparent that orally active glucocorticosteroids had a number of serious side-effects and thus attempts were made to develop drugs which could be delivered locally to the airways to achieve a higher local concentration with a lower dosage than would be required for systemic administration. The first inhaled glucocorticosteroids to be developed were beclomethasone diproprionate [4] and betamethasone valerate [5]. Inhaled glucocorticosteroid therapy for asthma has enabled the well known toxicity of sys-

Cellular Mechanisms in Airways Inflammation, edited by Clive P. Page, Katharine H. Banner and Domenico Spina

temic side-effects to be reduced. Oral and inhaled glucocorticosteroids taken acutely, have no effect on the early asthmatic response [6, 7], although when taken prophylactically over longer periods, it is possible to demonstrate an inhibitory effect of glucocorticosteroids on the early asthmatic response [8, 9]. Acute treatment with glucocorticosteroids can inhibit the development of the late asthmatic response following inhalation of antigen [6, 7, 10] and have variable effects on the increase in airways responsiveness to spasmogens [10, 11]. However, prolonged treatment with glucocorticosteroids has been shown to reduce increased airways responsiveness to carbachol during the pollen season in allergic asthmatics [12] and following 12-week treatment in stable asthmatics [13]. Furthermore, glucocorticosteroids also reduce the level of the maximal response to carbachol following 4 weeks treatment with budesonide in mild asthmatics [14] and following 12 weeks treatment with budesonide in asthmatics who did not achieve a maximum response to carbachol prior to treatment [13]. The beneficial effect of glucocorticosteroids upon the slope and maximum response to inhaled spasmogen is thought to reflect suppression of the inflammatory response.

Glucocorticosteroids suppress almost every step of the inflammatory process in asthma. They are thought to achieve this by a variety of mechanisms including inhibiting the transcription of genes for a wide range of cytokines [15]; inhibiting enzymes involved in the formation of lipid mediators (e.g. PLA2 and COX) [16, 17]; inhibiting the expression of adhesion molecules (e.g. ICAM-1 and E selectin) [18]; inhibiting inducible nitric oxide synthetase [19], increasing the transcription of β_2 receptors [20], lipocortin [21] and neutral endopeptidases [22]; suppressing eosinophil colony formation and chemotaxis [23], macrophage activation and mediator release [24] and inhibiting lymphocyte proliferation and lymphokine release [25]. The precise molecular mechanism(s) to which glucocorticosteroids owe their therapeutic efficacy in asthma remains unclear, but recent studies have shown that the glucocorticosteroid/glucocorticosteroid receptor complex may bind to AP-1 transcription factor, thereby inhibiting the expression of pro-inflammatory genes [26] and/or reduce the expression of transcription factors AP-1 and NFκB [27] which would lead to a reduction in the transcription of pro-inflammatory genes and synthesis of pro-inflammatory enzymes and mediators.

Inhaled glucocorticosteroids are currently the most effective anti-inflammatory agents available to alleviate the symptoms of chronic asthma. However, despite the efficacy and improved safety of inhaled compared to oral glucocorticosteroids, there is still concern about safety of inhaled glucocorticosteroids in paediatric asthmatics. Furthermore, compliance with inhaled drugs is less than for oral drugs [28] and a number of patients still have poorly controlled asthma and a poor quality of life despite regular treatment with glucocorticosteroids. These limitations have prompted the search for more orally effective anti-inflammatory agents for the treatment of asthma.

Disodium cromoglycate and nedocromil sodium

Disodium cromoglycate (DSCG) was developed as a result of investigations into the properties of khellin, an isolate from the seeds of a Mediterranean herb which possesses prophylactic properties [29]. Nedocromil sodium is chemically unrelated to DSCG and exhibits similar properties, and is at least two orders of magnitude more potent than DSCG [30].

DSCG attenuates the early and late asthmatic response following inhalation of antigen [6, 10, 31]. Prophylactic 28-day treatment of allergic asthmatics with DSCG reduced eosinophil numbers in bronchoalveolar lavage (BAL) fluid [32] consistent with the effect of this drug on the late asthmatic response. Exacerbations of bronchial hyperresponsiveness following antigen challenge are also abrogated by DSCG [10, 31] and DSCG suppressed bronchial hyperresponsiveness to histamine during [33], but not outside [34], of the pollen season in atopic asthmatics, suggesting that DSCG is beneficial against acute exacerbations of bronchial hyperresponsiveness. This is consistent with clinical studies demonstrating the ability of DSCG to suppress bronchoconstriction induced by non-allergic stimuli including exercise, sulphur dioxide, distilled water, cold air and adenosine (reviewed in [35]).

Nedocromil sodium inhibits the early and late asthmatic response [36] and the subsequent increase in airway responsiveness to inhaled spasmogens [36, 37] when administered prior to antigen challenge. Similarly, prophylactic treatment with nedocromil sodium reduced exacerbation of airways responsiveness to histamine during the pollen season in atopic asthmatics [38]. Nedocromil sodium also afforded protection against bronchoconstriction induced by cold air, exercise, sulphur dioxide, distilled water, adenosine and neurokinin A, and in many cases nedocromil sodium was more potent than DSCG (reviewed in [35]).

The mechanism of action of DSCG and nedocromil sodium has long been thought of as a consequence of mast cell stabilisation. However DSCG is a relatively weak inhibitor of histamine release from human lung mast cells following immunological challenge [39] and it is clear that DSCG inhibits the activation of a number of other inflammatory cells related to the pathogenesis of asthma including macrophages, eosinophils, platelets and neutrophils [40]. In addition, inhalation of DSCG in asthmatics inhibited neutrophil and monocyte activation [41] and reduced the number of eosinophils and epithelial ICAM-1 expression in bronchial biopsies [42]. Nedocromil sodium has also been shown to have other effects unrelated to mast cell stabilization including inhibiting the release of 15-hydroxyeicosatetraenoic acid [43], IL-8 [44, 45] and chemotactic factors [46] from human bronchial epithelial cells. Nedocromil sodium has also been reported to inhibit eosinophil activity *in vitro* [47], although conflicting results have been observed concerning reduction in eosinophil number in bronchial biopsies following 12–16 week treatment of asthmatics with nedocromil sodium [48, 49].

The precise molecular mechanisms responsible for the action of DSCG and nedocromil sodium remain to be established but may be due to inhibition of calcium influx into cells [50]. Alternatively there is evidence to suggest that these drugs can reduce the sensitivity of nerve endings in the airways thus abolishing local reflexes which can stimulate inflammation [51], an effect which may be attributable to their ability to block the activity of a chloride channel on the mucosal surface of airway epithelial cells as well as intermediate conductance chloride channels in cultured mucosal mast cells [52].

Theophylline

In 1886, Henry Hyde Salter described the efficacious use of strong coffee taken on an empty stomach as a treatment for asthma [53] and the principle agent in coffee which produced bronchodilation is known to be caffeine. Theophylline has a similar chemical structure to caffeine and was first used in the treatment of asthma as early as 1922, when theophylline was found to be effective in the treatment of three asthmatics and has been used since the turn of the century for the treatment of diseases of the airways [54]. Theophylline is well known for its bronchodilator activity, although, it is becoming increasingly apparent that this drug also possesses anti-inflammatory and immunomodulatory activity.

The intravenous administration of theophylline and enprophylline prior to allergen challenge inhibited the development of the late asthmatic response [55, 56] without any effect on the acute bronchoconstrictor response and associated bronchial hyperresponsiveness to methacholine [57]. Thus, neither functional antagonism of airway smooth muscle shortening nor mast cell degranulation accounted for the attenuated late asthmatic response by theophylline and enprofylline, although, in allergic rhinitis, 1-week treatment with theophylline reduced histamine release during pollen exposure [58] which indicated that theophylline inhibited mast cell and basophil degranulation in this disorder.

Individuals exposed for long periods of time to certain industrial chemicals develop asthma-like symptoms that can be duplicated in the clinical laboratory following aerosol challenge with the inciting agent. Thus, susceptible individuals demonstrate acute bronchospasm, late asthmatic responses and bronchial hyperresponsiveness following inhalation of toluene di-isocyanate (TDI) [59]. The inflammatory nature of this response has been confirmed by its sensitivity to inhibition by the glucocorticosteroid, beclomethasone. Theophylline partially modified the acute response and attenuated the late asthmatic response induced by TDI but was ineffective against bronchial hyperresponsiveness [59, 60]. This latter finding is consistent with the inability of theophylline to modulate allergen-induced bronchial hyperresponsiveness in asthmatics [57, 61]. The inhibitory effect of theophylline against the late asthmatic response in asthma may be a consequence of a restoration of T-suppressor cell function since it has long been recognised that theophylline can increase T-suppressor cell function [62-65] and impair graft rejection *in vitro* [65] and *in vivo* [66]. Individuals who do not develop a late asthmatic response have been shown to recruit a greater proportion of $CD8^+$ (suppressor) than $CD4^+$ (helper) T lymphocytes in BAL fluid [67].

Recent clinical studies have confirmed the anti-inflammatory properties of theophylline. In two randomised, placebo controlled studies [61, 68], the effect of theophylline or placebo was investigated on various inflammatory indices following once and twice daily treatment for 1 and 5 weeks, respectively. The late asthmatic response was reduced in those subjects treated with theophylline after 5 weeks [61] despite a mean plasma concentration of only 7.8 µg/ml. The lack of effect of theophylline on the acute response is presumably due to the low plasma levels in these subjects. Inhibition of the late asthmatic response therefore, was unlikely to be due to functional antagonism of airway smooth muscle shortening or inhibition of mast cell degranulation [61]. Analysis of bronchial biopsies taken from mild asthmatics treated with low dose theophylline over 6 weeks revealed a significant reduction in $EG2^+$ staining cells (activated eosinophils) and total number of eosinophils [69], which may be a consequence of the ability of theophylline to induce apoptosis of human eosinophils [70]. Similarly, a reduction in $CD3^+$ T lymphocytes and expression of various activation markers on $CD4^+$ T lymphocytes including HLA-DR and VLA-1 was observed in BAL fluid [71]. Furthermore, a reduction in $CD4^+$, $CD8^+$ T lymphocytes and IL-4 and IL-5 containing cells was observed in bronchial biopsies from asthmatics who were taking theophylline over a 6-week period [72]. In other studies, withdrawing theophylline from asthmatics who were taking glucocorticosteroids resulted in a significant deterioration of their disease [73, 74], together with a concomitant rise in the number of $CD4^+$, and $CD8^+$ T lymphocytes in bronchial biopsies [74].

Together, these studies document the ability of theophylline to impair lymphocyte trafficking in the airways at sub-bronchodilator doses. Furthermore, 10-day treatment with theophylline also reduced neutrophil and monocyte chemotaxis *ex vivo* [75]. In another study alveolar macrophages were shown to generate less superoxide *ex vivo* after *in vivo* oral theophylline treatment [76]. In this study a reduction in alveolar macrophage intracellular, bactericidal killing and H_2O_2 release was also found which correlated well with BAL theophylline concentrations.

Recently, two studies have demonstrated that in asthmatics who were poorly controlled on existing glucocorticosteroid therapy, a significant improvement in a number of clinical outcomes including, peak expiratory flow, FEV_1, symptom scores and reduced rescue medication was observed when patients were taking theophylline together with low dose glucocorticosteroid compared with high glucocorticosteroid treatment [77, 78]. In both studies, the plasma levels of theophylline measured were unlikely to be sufficient to induce bronchodilation (median 7.8 µg/ml [77] and mean 10.1 µg/ml [78]).

The mechanism by which theophylline suppresses inflammation is the subject of much controversy and detailed hypotheses are beyond the scope of this article. Suffice to say that a number of mechanisms have been proposed which include adenosine A_{2b} receptor antagonism [79], alteration of intracellular calcium mobilisation [80], stimulation of endogenous catecholamine release [81], prostaglandin antagonism [82] and phosphodiesterase inhibition (PDE) [83]. However, inhibition of PDE remains a popular theory to explain much of the clinical effects of theophylline, although, a recent study has shown that the ability of theophylline to promote apoptosis of human eosinophils may be unrelated to PDE inhibition [70]. The possibility that the anti-inflammatory activity of theophylline may be attributable to inhibition of PDE has led to many pharmaceutical companies pursuing selective PDE inhibitors for the treatment of asthma.

Novel anti-inflammatory drugs

Selective phosphodiesterase inhibitors

A variety of pharmacological, biochemical and molecular biological studies have revealed the existence of eleven diverse PDE families which are comprised of at least 15 gene products with further diversity occurring as a consequence of differential splicing and post-translational processing [84, 85]. Of particular interest is the role of PDE4 in regulating the function of a variety of cells thought to participate in the inflammatory process and there is considerable interest in the development of PDE4 inhibitors for the treatment of inflammatory diseases such as asthma.

The PDE4 inhibitors rolipram [86–88], Ro201724 [86], RP73401 [87, 88] and CDP840 [88] were all effective at inhibiting pulmonary eosinophilia induced by allergen challenge in the guinea-pig. This effect is not a feature peculiar to the guinea-pig since rolipram and CDP840 can also attenuate the allergen-induced eosinophilia in allergic rabbits [89, 90], whilst rolipram [91–93] and RP73401 [87] can inhibit allergen-induced pulmonary eosinophilia in allergic rats and primates. In allergic mice, the mixed PDE3/PDE4 inhibitor, benzafentrine and the PDE4 inhibitor, rolipram attenuated macrophage and eosinophil accumulation in BAL fluid [94]. Moreover, in addition to the ability of rolipram, Ro201724 and CDP840 [86, 88, 95] to inhibit pulmonary recruitment of eosinophils following allergen challenge, there is some evidence to suggest that these inhibitors as well as the PDE4 selective inhibitor, CP80633 [96] can attenuate the activation of eosinophils recruited to the lung, as assessed by measurements of eosinophil peroxidase (EPO) contained in and/or secreted by the eosinophil.

The PDE3 inhibitor, siguazodan has been shown to attenuate ovalbumin-induced pulmonary eosinophilia in guinea-pigs [97], although in other studies, the PDE3 inhibitors, siguazodan [86, 95] and milrinone [95, 98] were ineffective. These discrepancies could be attributed to differences in the degree of sensitisation and/or dose of allergen employed to challenge the animals. Interestingly, the PDE3 inhibitor milrinone also inhibited pulmonary eosinophilia in allergic rats [93]. The PDE5 inhibitor zaprinast appeared to have no effect on allergen-induced eosinophilia in the rat [93] or the guinea-pig [86, 98]. The mixed PDE3/4 inhibitors zardaverine [95, 97, 99] and ORG20421 [92] inhibited pulmonary eosinophilia in the guinea-pig and neutrophilia in the rat, respectively. Furthermore, pulmonary neutrophilia and the attendant increase in elastase and TNFα in BAL fluid following exposure to LPS in the rat was significantly reduced by zardaverine [100].

The ability of PDE inhibitors to impair the development of bronchial hyperresponsiveness following allergen exposure in sensitised animals has also been investigated. For example, the mixed PDE3/4 inhibitor, ORG20241 [101] and the PDE4 inhibitor, rolipram [98, 101] attenuated bronchial hyperresponsiveness to spasmogens following allergen challenge in guinea-pigs. Similarly, inhalation of pollutants such as ozone caused an 8–10-fold increase in airway sensitivity to histamine that was significantly attenuated by CDP840 [102]. Similarly, rolipram [90] and CDP840 [89] significantly inhibited bronchial hyperresponsiveness induced by *Alternaria tenuis* in the rabbit. The mixed PDE3/4 inhibitor zardaverine attenuated the LPS-induced bronchial hyperresponsiveness to serotonin in the rat [100]. Similarly, rolipram inhibited bronchial hyperresponsiveness following repeated antigen challenge of atopic cynomolgus monkeys [91].

PDE inhibitors are currently being developed for the treatment of asthma although side-effects including nausea and vomiting have halted the development of some examples of this class of drug into the clinic. To date, there are a limited number of clinical studies investigating the efficacy of PDE inhibitors in the treatment of asthma.

Inhalation of zardaverine was shown to produce a modest bronchodilator effect in patients with asthma, although unacceptable side-effects of nausea and emesis were reported in a significant number of patients [103], while oral administration of cilostazol (PDE3 inhibitor) caused bronchodilation and bronchoprotection against methacholine challenge in healthy subjects at the expense of mild to severe headache [104]. AH-2132 (benzafentrine) has also been reported to have significant bronchodilator activity in normal volunteers [105]; ibudilast significantly improved baseline airways responsiveness to spasmogen by two-fold after 6 months treatment [106] and MKS492 (PDE3 inhibitor) attenuated the early and late asthmatic response in atopic asthmatics [107].

Recently, the PDE4 selective inhibitor, CDP840 has been demonstrated to modestly attenuate the development of the late asthmatic response in mild asthmatics whilst having no effect on the acute response and no side-effects were reported [108]. The ability of CDP840 to inhibit the late asthmatic response was not associated with bronchodilation, suggesting other actions than smooth muscle relaxation. In contrast, another PDE4 inhibitor RP73401, had no significant effect on allergen-induced bronchoconstriction in allergic asthmatics [109].

Drugs affecting leukotriene synthesis and action

Cysteinyl leukotrienes (LT) including LTC_4, D_4 and E_4 are endogenous bioactive lipid mediators which are known to posses potent pro-inflammatory actions including vascular permeability, mucus secretion, bronchial hyperresponsiveness as well as activation and recruitment of inflammatory cells, in addition to being very potent spasmogens of human airway smooth muscle. Leukotrienes are derived from the 5-lipoxygenase (5-LO) pathway of arachidonic acid metabolism and two approaches have been explored to inhibit the pharmacological activity of leukotrienes; inhibition of the 5-LO enzyme and leukotriene receptor antagonism.

The 5-lipoxygenase inhibitor zileuton was effective against bronchoconstriction induced by exercise [110], cold air [111] and reduced airways responsiveness to distilled water and histamine [112], but was ineffective against bronchoconstriction following antigen challenge [113] in asthmatics. Furthermore, in a small study, zileuton attenuated both airways and blood eosinophilia in nocturnal asthmatics [114]. Similarly, the FLAP inhibitors, MK-0591 [115] and MK-886 [116] attenuated the early and late asthmatic response following antigen challenge but not the attendant increase in airway responsiveness to spasmogen.

The leukotriene antagonists zafirlukast (ICI 204,219), montelukast (MK-0476) and pranlukast (SB 205312, ONO 1078) have also been assessed clinically. Zafirlukast potently inhibited bronchoconstriction to inhaled LTD_4 challenge, attenuated early and late phase bronchoconstriction to inhaled allergen [117, 118] and following exercise [119] and attenuated bronchoconstriction to inhaled sulphurdioxide [120]. Similarly, pranlukast a potent antagonist of LTD_4 induced bronchoconstriction [121], attenuated aspirin induced asthma [122], antigen-induced acute bronchoconstriction [123] and had a modest effect against airways responsiveness to methacholine following 1 week of treatment [124]. Montelukast [125, 126] and pranlukast [127, 128] improve pulmonary function and clinical symptoms are well tolerated and appear to be safe.

Thromboxane A_2 receptor antagonists and synthetase inhibitors

Thromboxane $(TX)A_2$ is a potent bronchoconstrictor agent which is released in asthma [129] and has been implicated as a potential mediator in this disease [130].

The TXA_2 antagonist BAY u3405 produced a modest decrease in airways responsiveness to methacholine following 2-week treatment in asthmatics [131] but was ineffective against bradykinin induced bronchoprovocation following a single oral administration [132]. Similarly, the TXA_2 antagonist, GR32191 was ineffective against methacholine responsiveness in adult asthmatics following 3-week treatment [133]. These studies suggest that TXA_2 antagonists are unlikely to suppress baseline airways hyperresponsiveness in asthmatics.

The TXA_2 synthetase inhibitor ozagrel (OKY-046) reduced cough sensitivity to capsaicin [104], and bronchoconstriction to acetaldehyde [134] in asthmatics, indicating a possible role for TXA_2 in sensitisation of afferent nerves. In contrast, airways responsiveness to methacholine was not significantly altered following 1-week treatment with UK-38,485 [135]. Similarly, whilst acute treatment with CGS 13080 attenuated the acute bronchoconstrictor response to antigen, the late asthmatic response and attendant bronchial hyperresponsiveness was not inhibited [136]. In a phase III study, ozagrel was reported to have a significantly greater effect in ameliorating asthma symptoms than azelastine hydrochloride and reduced the dose of concomitant steroid therapy [137]. It is clear that TXA_2 antagonists and TXA_2 synthetase inhibitors may have a greater beneficial effect against acute exacerbations of asthma induced by stimulants of afferent nerves.

Monoclonal antibodies

One of the hallmark features of atopic disease is the presence of IgE which has been suggested to play a pivotal role in the pathogenesis of the atopic state [138]. Crosslinking of antigen to high affinity IgE receptors (FcεRI) on various inflammatory cells including mast cells and basophils is a critical step in mediating many of the acute symptoms of asthma. The development of novel peptides which can inhibit the binding of IgE to FcεRI may therefore have beneficial effects in the treatment of atopic diseases [139]. Recently, asthmatics were treated with the monoclonal antibody, rhuMAb-25, which binds to the FcεRI binding domain of IgE. A reduction in serum IgE levels, early and late asthmatic response to inhaled antigen, reduced sputum eosinophil numbers and reduced airways hyperresponsiveness to antigen and methacholine was observed following 9-week treatment with rhuMAb-25 [140, 141].

The low affinity IgE receptor FcεRII (CD23) is thought to mediate a number of effects including inhibition of IgE synthesis, antigen presentation; proliferation and differentiation of B cells; and activation of monocytes, effects which can be ascribed to the membrane and soluble conformers of CD23 [138]. A recent study has shown that antibodies directed against CD23 attenuated eosinophil recruitment to the airways following antigen challenge in a murine model of inflammation [142]. The development of peptides and other drugs which target this receptor may also provide a novel therapeutic approach to the treatment of asthma.

The cytokine interleukin (IL)-5 is important in the differentiation, migration and activation of eosinophils. Monoclonal antibodies directed against IL-5 including TRFK-5, attenuated eosinophil recruitment and bronchial hyperresponsiveness in allergic mice [143–146], guinea-pigs [147] and primates [148]. In the primate study, the ameliorating effect of TRFK-5 on antigen induced eosinophilia and hyperresponsiveness was evident 3 months after treatment [148]. Recently, inhalation of human recombinant IL-5 in asthmatics was associated with a three-fold increase in airways sensitivity to methacholine, a six-fold increase in sputum eosinophil number and a three-fold increase in sputum ECP levels, 24 h following antigen challenge [149]. The effect of antibodies to IL-5 in asthma are currently under investigation.

Eotaxin receptor blockers

Chemokines are a group of small molecular weight peptides (8–10 kDa) which have a number of biological effects including chemotaxis, immunoregulation, and cell growth and are classified into CXC, CC and C families [150]. Of particular interest is the role of the CC chemokine, eotaxin, a potent chemoattractant for eosinophils [151–153] and basophils [154] mediated *via* selective activation of the G protein coupled CC chemokine receptor (CCR) 3 [152, 155]. In a murine model of tissue eosinophilia, targeted disruption of the eotaxin gene resulted in an attenuation of the early (18 h) but not late (48 h) phase recruitment of eosinophils to the lung following antigen challenge [156], suggesting that substances additional to eotaxin are involved in the recruitment of eosinophils to the airways. Furthermore, antibodies directed against eotaxin suppressed constitutive and allergen-induced chemoattractant activity in BAL fluid [157]. Treatment of skin sites with antisera to eotaxin, or following desensitisation of CCR3 with eotaxin and blockade of the receptor with RANTES, inhibited the accumulation of radiolabelled eosinophils following antigen challenge [158]. More recently, a monoclonal antibody (7B11) directed against CCR3 inhibited binding, chemotaxis and calcium influx of eosinophils induced by eotaxin, RANTES, monocyte chemotactic protein (MCP)-2, MCP-3 and MCP-4 [159] and suggests the possibility of developing receptor antagonists for the CCR3 receptor.

Drugs affecting cell trafficking

Proteoglycans

There is now considerable evidence that proteoglycans such as heparin have a wide range of biological properties beyond their well known activities as anti-coagulants. Proteoglycans are a family of structurally distinct, polyanionic complex carbohydrates compose of repeating disaccharide units. Naturally occurring proteoglycans include heparin, heparan sulphate, chondroitin 6-sulphate and dermatan sulphate. Heparin is found exclusively in mast cell granules where it binds various mediators including histamine and can influence the activities of a number of mast cell derived enzymes such as tryptase [160]. Heparan sulphate has a much wider distribution in the body, being associated with stromal matrices, basement membrane and many cell surfaces, including endothelial cells.

There is now substantial evidence showing that heparin and related proteoglycans can inhibit the various phases of leukocyte adherence to the vascular endothelium and the subsequent trafficking of these cells into tissues, including the lung [160]. As such proteoglycans may serve as useful molecules to interfere with the inflammatory process, and indeed have recently been shown to be of benefit in a number of inflammatory conditions clinically, including rheumatoid arthritis [161], ulcerative colitis [162, 163] and interstitial cystitis [164]. Given the importance of inflammatory cells in the pathogenesis of asthma, and the important role played by adhesion molecules in the migration of inflammatory cells into the airways (see above), it is of considerable interest that heparin can bind to both L- and P-selectin [165] and that heparan sulphate derived from pulmonary artery endothelial cells will interact with a chimera of L-selectin [166]. A number of proteoglycans, including heparin and heparan, have been shown to inhibit the rolling and adhesion of neutrophils to vascular endothelial cells, and to inhibit the migration of neutrophils [167] and eosinophils into tissues, including the lung [168, 169]. An interesting recent development in this area is the identification of non-anticoagulant proteoglycans such as O-desulphated heparin that retain anti-inflammatory activities [170], including the ability to inhibit eosinophil infiltration into the airways [171]. This raises the real possibility of developing novel anti-inflammatory drugs based on proteoglycans that do not have unwanted side-effects related to other actions of proteoglycans.

Another interesting effect of heparin of relevance to the trafficking of inflammatory cells is the inhibition of the enzyme heparinase, an enzyme secret by a number of inflammatory cells that can degrade heparan sulphate on the endothelial cell surface [172]. Increased levels of heparinases have been reported in the sputum from subjects with asthma [173] and loss of GAGs on the surface of endothelium has been reported to be an important mechanism contributing to inflammatory changes in other clinical conditions [174]. Heparan and chronically modified heparin have been reported to inhibit the degradation of heparan sulphate by inflammatory cells [175] and to inhibit T cell trafficking by an action on heparinases [176]. The clinical potential of the actions of proteoglycans are not yet fully understood, but it has now been shown clinically that heparin can inhibit allergen [177] and exercise-induced asthma [178, 179], as well as allergen-induced eosinophil infiltration into the nose of allergic subjects [180], suggesting that indeed proteoglycans may well provide anti-inflammatory activities in the treatment of respiratory disease in man.

Anti-adhesion therapy

A number of studies have used antibodies directed against selected adhesion molecules including ICAM-1 [181], LFA-1 [182, 183], VLA-4 [182, 184] and shown that bronchial hyperresponsiveness and attendant pulmonary eosinophilia following antigen challenge is abrogated in a variety of species including, primates, guinea-pig and mice.

A number of studies have shown that treatment with antibodies directed against leukocyte integrin CD18 [185] or ICAM-1 [186] did not reduce the recruitment of eosinophils into the airways yet bronchial hyperresponsiveness was reduced. In contrast, inhibition of the late response, eosinophil recruitment to the lung and bronchial hyperresponsiveness was reduced in an allergic rabbit model [187]. Similarly, an antibody directed against VLA-4 reduced the number of eosinophils recovered in BAL and reduced eosinophil peroxidase levels, however, bronchial hyperresponsiveness following antigen challenge was not affected [188]. The discrepancies in the results might be a consequence of the selectivity of the antibodies since antibodies directed against the β_2 integrin CD18 abolished the accumulation of neutrophils in the skin but not the lung [189].

Tryptase inhibitors

Tryptase is a mast cell serine protease released following IgE stimulation of mast cells [190]. The physiological role for tryptase is unclear but it is known to affect fibroblast proliferation, degrade fibrinogen, generate C3a [191], stimulate mucus secretion [192] and degrade sensory neuropeptides [193, 194]. Thus, mast cell tryptase could play a role in regulation of haemostasis, mucus secretion and vascular permeability.

Elevated tryptase levels are evident in asthma, even in the absence of deliberate antigen challenge [195, 196], which may contribute toward bronchial hyperresponsiveness since incubation of tracheal smooth muscle with canine tryptase augments smooth muscle contractility *in vitro* [197] as well as airways responsiveness to carbachol in sheep following aerosolization of tryptase [198].

The mast cell tryptase inhibitor, APC-366 inhibited antigen induced late phase response and bronchial hyperresponsiveness to carbachol in sheep [199] and bronchial hyperresponsiveness to aerosolised tryptase [198]. Similarly, lactoferrin, which disrupts the quaternary structure of tryptase, also attenuated antigen-induced late response and bronchial hyperresponsiveness in allergic sheep [200].

H_1 receptor antagonists and anti-allergic drugs

H_1 receptor antagonists

Anti-histamines are widely used in the treatment of allergic diseases where the release of histamine is thought to play an important role in the symptoms associated with hayfever, urticaria, and mild asthma [201].

However, it is clear that a number of H_1 receptor antagonists including cetirizine, terfenadine, ebastine, oxatimide, loratidine and ketotifen demonstrate anti-inflammatory activity unrelated to H_1 receptor blockade. For example, cetirizine inhibits

FMLP- and PAF-induced chemotaxis of [202–204], and superoxide generation by eosinophils [204]; inhibits FMLP-, LTB_4-induced chemotaxis of lymphocytes and monocytes [205] and inhibited eosinophil survival *in vitro* [206]. Similarly, oxatimide inhibited antigen induced degranulation of human lung mast cells and basophils *in vitro* [207]. The mechanism by which these drugs inhibit inflammatory cell function is unclear but may relate to stabilisation of cell membranes and interference with intracellular calcium mobilisation.

A number of clinical studies have reported that cetirizine can attenuate the wheal and flare response following antigen, whilst having no effect on the late cutaneous response nor the attendant eosinophilia and deposition of ECP [208, 209]. Similarly, 3-week treatment with cetirizine failed to attenuate early and late phase response but caused conflicting effects on bronchial hyperresponsiveness following antigen challenge [210, 211]. Nonetheless, expression of ICAM-1 and eosinophil number in scrapings from nasal mucosa was significantly reduced following 15-day treatment of children sensitive to house dust mite with cetirizine [212]. Following 26 weeks treatment, cetirizine has also been shown to reduce a number of clinical symptoms in patients with perennial asthma [213]. Thus, while acute studies have reported a lack of beneficial effect of cetirizine on a number of inflammatory indices, it is clear that cetirizine may be useful when taken prophylactically in some asthmatics.

Ketotifen

Ketotifen is an orally active drug used mainly as a prophylactic against asthma attacks particularly in the treatment of paediatric asthmatics [214, 215]. Ketotifen is a potent H_1 receptor antagonist, but has a number of other pharmacological actions of relevance to its efficacy in asthma, including the ability to stabilise mast cells, upregulate β_2-adrenoceptors [216] and to inhibit eosinophil recruitment *in vivo* [217]. This latter action of ketotifen is unrelated to its action as a H_1-receptor antagonist, as its action against eosinophil recruitment is not shared by other H_1-receptor antagonists except cetirizine. The anti-eosinophilic action of ketotifen may be central to its ability to alter allergic asthma and contribute to its efficacy in other allergic diseases.

Suplatast

Suplatast tosilate (IPD-1151T) is a dimethylsulfonium substance which displays a number of anti-allergic properties. For example, suplatast inhibits IgE production from B-cell clones from a patient allergic to Japanese cedar pollen [218]; expression of IL-4 in mononuclear cells [218]; IL-4 and IL-5 production from murine T lymphocytes [219]; and differentiation of mast cells from murine splenocytes and proliferation of mast cell progenitor cells [220].

In animal studies, suplatast inhibited airway hyperresponsiveness and infiltration of eosinophils, macrophages and $CD4^+$ T lymphocytes following antigen challenge in sensitised guinea-pigs [221]. In one clinical study, a significant increase in peak expiratory flow and improvement in bronchial hyperresponsiveness was observed in mild asthmatics following 6 weeks of treatment with suplatast. Furthermore, a significant reduction in the number of eosinophils and $EG2^+$ staining cells was observed in bronchial biopsies from these patients [222].

Cell activation inhibitor (CI-949)

The benzothiophene compound, CI-959 inhibits the activation of a number of inflammatory cells including eosinophils, neutrophils and lung mast cells. For example, the respiratory burst from human eosinophils [223] and neutrophils [224]; enzyme release from human macrophages and neutrophils [223]; and release of leukotrienes, histamine and thromboxane from human lung [224, 225] are inhibited by CI-959. Similarly, CI-959 has been shown to inhibit IL-2 production from human lymphocytes as well as proliferation stimulated by conconavalin A but not phytohaemagluttinin. CI-959 had minimal effect on IL-1 and TNFα release from human monocytes [226], suggesting that this drug has little action on monocytes. Whilst the mechanism of action of CI-959 remains to be established, it appears to be more effective at inhibiting respiratory burst in neutrophils *via* receptor coupled mechanisms as opposed to mechanisms which involve calcium entry or activation of protein kinase C suggesting that CI-959 may inhibit calcium-regulated signalling mechanisms [227].

Conclusion

Asthma remains a major burden to healthcare systems world-wide. While significant improvements have been made in asthma therapy over the last decade, the prevalence and severity of asthma continues to rise in many Western countries, despite more prescriptions being written. Compliance remains a major problem with many existing anti-asthma drugs as they have to be administered by inhalation. There is a therefore a real need for the introduction of a novel orally acting anti-inflammatory drug for the treatment of asthma.

References

1 Solis-Cohen S (1900) The use of adrenal substance in the treatment of asthma. *J Am Med Assoc* 34: 1164–1166

2 Mason HL, Myers CS, Kendall EC (1936) The chemistry of crystalline substances isolated from the supradrenal gland. *J Biol Chem* 114: 613–631

3 Barach AL, Bickerman HA, Beck GJ (1955) Clinical and physiological studies on the use of metacortandracin in respiratory disease. I. Bronchial asthma. *Br J Dis Chest* 27: 515–527

4 Clark TJ (1972) Effect of beclomethasone dipropionate delivered by aerosol in patients with asthma. *Lancet* 1: 1361–1364

5 Brown HM, Storey G, George WHS (1971) Beclomethasone dipropionate: A new steroid aerosol for the treatment of allergic asthma. *Br Med J* 1: 585–590

6 Booij Noord H, Orie NG, De Vries K (1971) Immediate and late bronchial obstructive reactions to inhalation of house dust and protective effects of disodium cromoglycate and prednisolone. *J Allergy Clin Immunol* 48: 344–354

7 Pepys J, Davies RJ, Breslin AB, Hendrick DJ, Hutchcroft BJ (1974) The effects of inhaled beclomethasone dipropionate (Becotide) and sodium cromoglycate on asthmatic reactions to provocation tests. *Clin Allergy* 4: 13–24

8 Burge PS (1982) The effects of corticosteroids on the immediate asthmatic reaction. *Eur J Respir Dis* (Suppl) 122: 163–166

9 Dahl R, Johansson SA (1982) Importance of duration of treatment with inhaled budesonide on the immediate and late bronchial reaction. *Eur J Respir Dis* (Suppl) 122: 167–175

10 Cockcroft DW, Murdock KY (1987) Comparative effects of inhaled salbutamol, sodium cromoglycate, and beclomethasone dipropionate on allergen-induced early asthmatic responses, late asthmatic responses, and increased bronchial responsiveness to histamine. *J Allergy Clin Immunol* 79: 734–740

11 Kidney JC, Boulet LP, Hargreave FE, Deschesnes F, Swystun VA, O'Byrne PM, Choudry N, Morris MM, Jennings B, Andersson N, Andreasson A, Cockcroft DW (1997) Evaluation of single-dose inhaled corticosteroid activity with an allergen challenge model. *J Allergy Clin Immunol* 100: 65–70

12 Sotomayor H, Badier M, Vervloet D, Orehek J (1984) Seasonal increase of carbachol airway responsiveness in patients allergic to grass pollen. Reversal by corticosteroids. *Am Rev Respir Dis* 130: 56–58

13 Booms P, Cheung D, Timmers MC, Zwinderman AH, Sterk PJ (1997) Protective effect of inhaled budesonide against unlimited airway narrowing to methacholine in atopic patients with asthma. *J Allergy Clin Immunol* 99: 330–337

14 Bel EH, Timmers MC, Zwinderman AH, Dijkman JH, Sterk PJ (1991) The effect of inhaled corticosteroids on the maximal degree of airway narrowing to methacholine in asthmatic subjects. *Am Rev Respir Dis* 143: 109–113

15 Guyre PM, Girard MT, Morganelli PM, Manganiello PD (1988) Glucocorticoid effects on the production and actions of immune cytokines. *J Steroid Biochem* 30: 89–93

16 Schalkwijk C, Vervoordeldonk M, Pfeilschifter J, Marki F, van den Bosch H (1991) Cytokine- and forskolin-induced synthesis of group II phospholipase A2 and

prostaglandin E2 in rat mesangial cells is prevented by dexamethasone. *Biochem Biophys Res Commun* 180: 46–52

17 O'Banion MK, Winn VD, Young DA (1992) cDNA cloning and functional activity of a glucocorticoid- regulated inflammatory cyclooxygenase. *Proc Natl Acad Sci USA* 89: 4888–4892

18 Cronstein BN, Kimmel SC, Levin RI, Martiniuk F, Weissmann G (1992) A mechanism for the antiinflammatory effects of corticosteroids: the glucocorticoid receptor regulates leukocyte adhesion to endothelial cells and expression of endothelial-leukocyte adhesion molecule 1 and intercellular adhesion molecule 1. *Proc Natl Acad Sci USA* 89: 9991–9995

19 Radomski MW, Palmer RM, Moncada S (1990) Glucocorticoids inhibit the expression of an inducible, but not the constitutive, nitric oxide synthase in vascular endothelial cells. *Proc Natl Acad Sci USA* 87: 10043–10047

20 Collins S, Caron MG, Lefkowitz RJ (1988) Beta-adrenergic receptors in hamster smooth muscle cells are transcriptionally regulated by glucocorticoids. *J Biol Chem* 263: 9067–9070

21 Flower RJ (1988) Eleventh Gaddum memorial lecture. Lipocortin and the mechanism of action of the glucocorticoids. *Br J Pharmacol* 94: 987–1015

22 Sont JK, van Krieken JH, van Klink HC, Roldaan AC, Apap CR, Willems LN, Sterk PJ (1997) Enhanced expression of neutral endopeptidase (NEP) in airway epithelium in biopsies from steroid- versus nonsteroid-treated patients with atopic asthma. *Am J Respir Cell Mol Biol* 16: 549–556

23 Wallen N, Kita H, Weiler D, Gleich GJ (1991) Glucocorticoids inhibit cytokine-mediated eosinophil survival. *J Immunol* 147: 3490–3495

24 Joyce DA, Steer JH, Abraham LJ (1997) Glucocorticoid modulation of human monocyte/macrophage function: control of TNF-alpha secretion. *Inflamm Res* 46: 447–451

25 Wilckens T, De-Rijk R (1997) Glucocorticoids and immune function: unknown dimensions and new frontiers. *Immunol Today* 18: 418–424

26 Barnes PJ, Adcock I (1993) Anti-inflammatory actions of steroids: molecular mechanisms [see comments]. *Trends Pharmacol Sci* 14: 436–441

27 LeVan TD, Behr FD, Adkins KK, Miesfeld RL, Bloom JW (1997) Glucocorticoid receptor signaling in a bronchial epithelial cell line. *Am J Physiol* 272: L838–43

28 Kelloway JS, Wyatt RA, Adlis SA (1994) Comparison of patients' compliance with prescribed oral and inhaled asthma medications. *Arch Intern Med* 154: 1349–1352

29 Cox JS, Beach JE, Blair AM, Clarke AJ, King J, Lee TB, Loveday DE, Moss GF, Orr TS, Ritchie JT, Sheard P (1970) Disodium cromoglycate (Intal). *Adv Drug Res* 5: 115–196

30 Holgate ST (1986) Clinical evaluation of nedocromil sodium in asthma. *Eur J Respir Dis* (Suppl) 147: 149–159

31 Mattoli S, Foresi A, Corbo GM, Valente S, Ciappi G (1987) Effects of two doses of cromolyn on allergen-induced late asthmatic response and increased responsiveness. *J Allergy Clin Immunol* 79: 747–754

32 Diaz P, Galleguillos FR, Gonzalez MC, Pantin CF, Kay AB (1984) Bronchoalveolar

lavage in asthma: the effect of disodium cromoglycate (cromolyn) on leukocyte counts, immunoglobulins, and complement. *J Allergy Clin Immunol* 74: 41–48
33 Lowhagen O, Rak S (1985) Modification of bronchial hyperreactivity after treatment with sodium cromoglycate during pollen season. *J Allergy Clin Immunol* 75: 460–467
34 Lowhagen O, Rak S (1985) Bronchial hyperreactivity after treatment with sodium cromoglycate in atopic asthmatic patients not exposed to relevant allergens. *J Allergy Clin Immunol* 75: 343–347
35 Spina D, Page CP (1996) Airway sensory nerves in asthma – targets for therapy? *Pulm Pharmacol* 9: 1–18
36 Aalbers R, Kauffman HF, Groen H, Koeter GH, de Monchy JG (1991) The effect of nedocromil sodium on the early and late reaction and allergen-induced bronchial hyperresponsiveness. *J Allergy Clin Immunol* 87: 993–1001
37 Crimi E, Brusasco V, Crimi P (1989) Effect of nedocromil sodium on the late asthmatic reaction to bronchial antigen challenge. *J Allergy Clin Immunol* 83: 985–990
38 Dorward AJ, Roberts JA, Thomson NC (1986) Effect of nedocromil sodium on histamine airway responsiveness in grass-pollen sensitive asthmatics during the pollen season. *Clin Allergy* 16: 309–315
39 Butchers PR, Fullarton JR, Skidmore IF, Thompson LE, Vardey CJ, Wheeldon A (1979) A comparison of the anti-anaphylactic activities of salbutamol and disodium cromoglycate in the rat, the rat mast cell and in human lung tissue. *Br J Pharmacol* 67: 23–32
40 Kay AB, Walsh GM, Moqbel R, Macdonald AJ, Nagakura T, Carroll MP, Richerson HB (1987) Disodium cromoglycate inhibits activation of human inflammatory cells *in vitro*. *J Allergy Clin Immunol* 80: 1–8
41 Moqbel R, Walsh GM, Macdonald AJ, Kay B (1986) Effect of disodium cromoglycate on activation of human eosinophils and neutrophils following reversed (anti-IgE) anaphylaxis. *Clin Allergy* 16: 73–83
42 Hoshino M, Nakamura Y, Shin Z, Fukushima Y (1997) Effects of ketotifen on symptoms and on bronchial mucosa in patients with atopic asthma. *Allergy* 52: 814–820
43 Mattoli S, Mezzetti M, Fasoli A, Patalano F, Allegra L (1990) Nedocromil sodium prevents the release of 15- hydroxyeicosatetraenoic acid from human bronchial epithelial cells exposed to toluene diisocyanate *in vitro*. *Int Arch Allergy Appl Immunol* 92: 16–22
44 Vittori E, Sciacca F, Colotta F, Mantovani A, Mattoli S (1992) Protective effect of nedocromil sodium on the interleukin-1-induced production of interleukin-8 in human bronchial epithelial cells. *J Allergy Clin Immunol* 90: 76–84
45 Devalia JL, Rusznak C, Abdelaziz MM, Davies RJ (1996) Nedocromil sodium and airway inflammation *in vivo* and *in vitro*. *J Allergy Clin Immunol* 98: S51–7
46 Abdelaziz MM, Devalia JL, Khair OA, Rusznak C, Calderon M, Sapsford RJ, Bayram H, Davies RJ (1997) The effect of nedocromil sodium on human airway epithelial cell-induced eosinophil chemotaxis and adherence to human endothelial cell *in vitro*. Eur Respir J 10: 851–857
47 Sedgwick JB, Bjornsdottir U, Geiger KM, Busse WW (1992) Inhibition of eosinophil

density change and leukotriene C4 generation by nedocromil sodium. *J Allergy Clin Immunol* 90: 202–209

48 Manolitsas ND, Wang J, Devalia JL, Trigg CJ, McAulay AE, Davies RJ (1995) Regular albuterol, nedocromil sodium, and bronchial inflammation in asthma. Am J Respir Crit Care Med 151: 1925–1930

49 Altraja A, Laitinen A, Meriste S, Marran S, Martson T, Sillastu H, Laitinen LA (1996) Effect of regular nedocromil sodium or albuterol on bronchial inflammation in chronic asthma. *J Allergy Clin Immunol* 98: S58–64

50 Foreman JC, Garland LG (1976) Cromoglycate and other antiallergic drugs: a possible mechanism of action. Br Med J 1: 820–821

51 Dixon M, Jackson DM, Richards IM (1980) The action of sodium cromoglycate on 'C' fibre endings in the dog lung. *Br J Pharmacol* 70: 11–13

52 Romanin C, Reinsprecht M, Pecht I, Schindler H (1991) Immunologically activated chloride channels involved in degranulation of rat mucosal mast cells. *EMBO J* 10: 3603–3608

53 Persson CGA, Pauwels R (1991) Pharmacology of anti-asthma xanthines. In: CP Page, PJ Barnes (eds): *Pharmacology of asthma.* Springer-Verlag, Berlin, 207

54 Becker AB, Simons KJ, Gillespie CA, Simons FE (1984) The bronchodilator effects and pharmacokinetics of caffeine in asthma. *N Engl J Med* 310: 743–746

55 Pauwels R, van Renterghem D, van der Straeten M, Johannesson N, Persson CG (1985) The effect of theophylline and enprofylline on allergen-induced bronchoconstriction. *J Allergy Clin Immunol* 76: 583–590

56 Crescioli S, Spinazzi A, Plebani M, Pozzani M, Mapp CE, Boschetto P, Fabbri LM (1991) Theophylline inhibits early and late asthmatic reactions induced by allergens in asthmatic subjects. *Ann Allergy* 66: 245–251

57 Cockcroft DW, Murdock KY, Gore BP, O'Byrne PM, Manning P (1989) Theophylline does not inhibit allergen-induced increase in airway responsiveness to methacholine. *J Allergy Clin Immunol* 83: 913–920

58 Naclerio RM, Bartenfelder D, Proud D, Togias AG, Meyers DA, Kagey Sobotka A, Norman PS, Lichtenstein LM (1986) Theophylline reduces histamine release during pollen-induced rhinitis. *J Allergy Clin Immunol* 78: 874–876

59 Mapp C, Boschetto P, dal Vecchio L, Crescioli S, de Marzo N, Paleari D, Fabbri LM (1987) Protective effect of antiasthma drugs on late asthmatic reactions and increased airway responsiveness induced by toluene diisocyanate in sensitized subjects. *Am Rev Respir Dis* 136: 1403–1407

60 Crescioli S, de Marzo N, Boschetto P, Spinazzi A, Plebani M, Mapp CE, Fabbri LM, Ciaccia A (1992) Theophylline inhibits late asthmatic reactions induced by toluene diisocyanate in sensitised subjects. *Eur J Pharmacol* 228: 45–50

61 Ward AJ, McKenniff M, Evans JM, Page CP, Costello JF (1993) Theophylline – an immunomodulatory role in asthma? *Am Rev Respir Dis* 147: 518–523

62 Shohat B, Volovitz B, Varsano I (1983) Induction of suppressor T cells in asthmatic children by theophylline treatment. *Clin Allergy* 13: 487–493

63 Lahat N, Nir E, Horenstien L, Colin AA (1985) Effect of theophylline on the proportion and function of T- suppressor cells in asthmatic children. *Allergy* 40: 453–457
64 Zocchi MR, Pardi R, Gromo G, Ferrero E, Ferrero ME, Besana C, Rugarli C (1985) Theophylline induced non specific suppressor activity in human peripheral blood lymphocytes. *J Immunopharmacol* 7: 217–234
65 Fink G, Mittelman M, Shohat B, Spitzer SA (1987) Theophylline-induced alterations in cellular immunity in asthmatic patients. *Clin Allergy* 17: 313–316
66 Guillou PJ, Ramsden C, Kerr M, Davison AM, Giles GR (1984) A prospective controlled clinical trial of aminophylline as an adjunctive immunosuppressive agent. *Transplant Proc* 16: 1218–1220
67 Gonzalez MC, Diaz P, Galleguillos FR, Ancic P, Cromwell O, Kay AB (1987) Allergen-induced recruitment of bronchoalveolar helper (OKT4) and suppressor (OKT8) T-cells in asthma. Relative increases in OKT8 cells in single early responders compared with those in late-phase responders. *Am Rev Respir Dis* 136: 600–604
68 Hendeles L, Harman E, Huang D, O'Brien R, Blake K, Delafuente J (1995) Theophylline attenuation of airway responses to allergen: comparison with cromolyn metered-dose inhaler. *J Allergy Clin Immunol* 95: 505–514
69 Sullivan P, Bekir S, Jaffar Z, Page C, Jeffery P, Costello J (1994) Anti-inflammatory effects of low-dose oral theophylline in atopic asthma. *Lancet* 343: 1006–1008
70 Yasui K, Hu B, Nakazawa T, Agematsu K, Komiyama A (1997) Theophylline accelerates human granulocyte apoptosis not *via* phosphodiesterase inhibition. *J Clin Invest* 100: 1677–1684
71 Jaffar ZH, Sullivan P, Page CP, Costello J (1996) Low-dose theophylline modulates T-lymphocyte activation in allergen-challenged asthmatics. *Eur Respir J* 9: 456–462
72 Finnerty JP, Lee C, Wilson S, Madden J, Djukanovic R, Holgate ST (1996) Effects of theophylline on inflammatory cells and cytokines in asthmatic subjects: a placebo-controlled parallel group study. *Eur Respir J* 9: 1672–1677
73 Brenner M, Berkowitz R, Marshall N, Strunk RC (1988) Need for theophylline in severe steroid-requiring asthmatics. *Clin Allergy* 18: 143–150
74 Kidney J, Dominguez M, Taylor PM, Rose M, Chung KF, Barnes PJ (1995) Immunomodulation by theophylline in asthma. Demonstration by withdrawal of therapy. *Am J Respir Crit Care Med* 151: 1907–1914
75 Condino Neto A, Vilela MM, Cambiucci EC, Ribeiro JD, Guglielmi AA, Magna LA, De Nucci G (1991) Theophylline therapy inhibits neutrophil and mononuclear cell chemotaxis from chronic asthmatic children. *Br J Clin Pharmacol* 32: 557–561
76 O'Neill SJ, Sitar DS, Klass DJ, Taraska VA, Kepron W, Mitenko PA (1986) The pulmonary disposition of theophylline and its influence on human alveolar macrophage bactericidal function. *Am Rev Respir Dis* 134: 1225–1228
77 Evans DJ, Taylor DA, Zetterstrom O, Chung KF, O'Connor BJ, Barnes PJ (1997) A comparison of low-dose inhaled budesonide plus theophylline and high-dose inhaled budesonide for moderate asthma. *N Engl J Med* 337: 1412–1418
78 Ukena D, Harnest U, Sakalauskas R, Magyar P, Vetter N, Steffen H, Leichtl S, Rathgeb

F, Keller A, Steinijans VW (1997) Comparison of addition of theophylline to inhaled steroid with doubling of the dose of inhaled steroid in asthma. *Eur Respir J* 10: 2754–2760

79 Feoktistov I, Biaggioni I (1995) Adenosine A2b receptors evoke interleukin-8 secretion in human mast cells. An enprofylline-sensitive mechanism with implications for asthma. *J Clin Invest* 96: 1979–1986

80 Kolbeck RC, Speir WA Jr, Carrier GO, Bransome ED Jr (1979) Apparent irrelevance of cyclic nucleotides to the relaxation of tracheal smooth muscle induced by theophylline. *Lung* 156: 173–183

81 Higbee MD, Kumar M, Galant SP (1982) Stimulation of endogenous catecholamine release by theophylline: a proposed additional mechanism of action for theophylline effects. *J Allergy Clin Immunol* 70: 377–382

82 Horrobin DF, Manku MS, Franks DJ, Hamet P (1977) Methyl xanthine phosphodiesterase inhibitors behave as prostaglandin antagonists in a perfused rat mesenteric artery preparation. *Prostaglandins* 13: 33–40

83 Nicholson CD, Shahid M (1994) Inhibitors of cyclic nucleotide phosphodiesterase isoenzymes – their potential utility in the therapy of asthma. *Pulm Pharmacol* 7: 1–17

84 Beavo JA (1995) Cyclic nucleotide phosphodiesterases: functional implications of multiple isoforms. *Physiol Rev* 75: 725–748

85 Muller T, Engels P Fozard JR (1996) Subtypes of the type 4 cAMP phosphodiesterases: structure, regulation and selective inhibition. *Trends Pharmacol Sci* 17: 294–298

86 Lagente V, Moodley I, Perrin S, Mottin G Junien JL (1994) Effects of isozyme-selective phosphodiesterase inhibitors on eosinophil infiltration in the guinea-pig lung. *Eur J Pharmacol* 255: 253–256

87 Raeburn D, Underwood SL, Lewis SA, Woodman VR, Battram CH, Tomkinson A, Sharma S, Jordan R, Souness JE, Webber SE et al (1994) Anti-inflammatory and bronchodilator properties of RP 73401, a novel and selective phosphodiesterase type IV inhibitor. *Br J Pharmacol* 113: 1423–1431

88 Hughes B, Howat D, Lisle H, Holbrook M, Tames T, Gozzard N, Blease K, Hughes P, Kingaby R, Warrellow G et al (1996) The inhibition of antigen-induced eosinophilia and bronchoconstriction by CDP840, a novel stereo-selective inhibitor of phosphodiesterase type 4. *Br J Pharmacol* 118: 1183–1191

89 Gozzard N, El-Hashim A, Herd CM, Blake SM, Holbrook M, Hughes B, Higgs GA, Page CP (1996) Effect of the glucocorticosteroid budesonide and a novel phosphodiesterase type 4 inhibitor CDP840 on antigen-induced airway responses in neonatally immunised rabbits. *Br J Pharmacol* 118: 1201–1208

90 Gozzard N, Herd CM, Blake SM, Holbrook M, Hughes B, Higgs GA, Page CP (1996) Effects of theophylline and rolipram on antigen-induced airway responses in neonatally immunized rabbits. *Br J Pharmacol* 117: 1405–1412

91 Turner CR, Andresen CJ, Smith WB, Watson JW (1994) Effects of rolipram on responses to acute and chronic antigen exposure in monkeys. *Am J Respir Crit Care Med* 149: 1153–1159

92 Elwood W, Sun J, Barnes PJ, Giembycz MA, Chung KF (1995) Inhibition of allergen-induced lung eosinophilia by type-III and combined type III- and IV-selective phosphodiesterase inhibitors in brown-Norway rats. *Inflamm Res* 44: 83–86
93 Howell RE, Jenkins LP, Fielding LE, Grimes D (1995) Inhibition of antigen-induced pulmonary eosinophilia and neutrophilia by selective inhibitors of phosphodiesterase types 3 or 4 in Brown Norway rats. *Pulm Pharmacol* 8: 83–89
94 Nagai H, Takeda H, Iwama T, Yamaguchi S, Mori H (1995) Studies on anti-allergic action of AH 21-132, a novel isozyme- selective phosphodiesterase inhibitor in airways. *Jap J Pharmacol* 67: 149–156
95 Banner KH, Marchini F, Buschi A, Moriggi E, Semeraro C, Page CP (1995) The effect of selective phosphodiesterase inhibitors in comparison with other anti-asthma drugs on allergen-induced eosinophilia in guinea-pig airways. *Pulm Pharmacol* 8: 37–42
96 Turner CR, Cohan VL, Cheng JB, Showell HJ, Pazoles CJ, Watson JW (1996) The *in vivo* pharmacology of CP-80,633, a selective inhibitor of phosphodiesterase 4. *J Pharmacol Exp Ther* 278: 1349–1355
97 Underwood DC, Kotzer CJ, Bochnowicz S, Osborn RR, Luttmann MA, Hay DW, Torphy TJ (1994) Comparison of phosphodiesterase III, IV and dual III/IV inhibitors on bronchospasm and pulmonary eosinophil influx in guinea pigs. *J Pharmacol Exp Ther* 270: 250–259
98 Ortiz JL, Valles JM, MartiCabrera M, Cortijo J, Morcillo EJ (1996) Effects of selective phosphodiesterase inhibitors on platelet- activating factor- and antigen-induced airway hyperreactivity, eosinophil accumulation, and microvascular leakage in guinea pigs. *Naunyn-Schmiedeberg's Arch Pharmacol* 353: 200–206
99 Schudt C, Winder S, Eltze M, Kilian U, Beume R (1991) Zardaverine: a cyclic AMP specific PDE III/IV inhibitor. *Agents Actions* (Suppl) 34: 379–402
100 Kips JC, Joos GF, Peleman RA, Pauwels RA (1993) The effect of zardaverine, an inhibitor of phosphodiesterase isoenzymes III and IV, on endotoxin-induced airway changes in rats. *Clin Exp Allergy* 23: 518–523
101 Santing RE, Olymulder CG, van der Molen K, Meurs H, Zaagsma J (1995) Phosphodiesterase inhibitors reduce bronchial hyperreactivity and airway inflammation in unrestrained guinea pigs. *Eur J Pharmacol* 275: 75–82
102 Holbrook M, Gozzard N, James T, Higgs G, Hughes B (1996) Inhibition of bronchospasm and ozone-induced airway hyperresponsiveness in the guinea-pig by CDP840, a novel phosphodiesterase type 4 inhibitor. *Br J Pharmacol* 118: 1192–1200
103 Brunnee T, Engelstatter R, Steinijans VW, Kunkel G (1992) Bronchodilatory effect of inhaled zardaverine, a phosphodiesterase III and IV inhibitor, in patients with asthma. *Eur Respir J* 5: 982–985
104 Fujimura M, Kamio Y, Kasahara K, Bando T, Hashimoto T, Matsuda T (1995) Prostanoids and cough response to capsaicin in asthma and chronic bronchitis. *Eur Respir J* 8: 1499–1505
105 Foster RW, Rakshi K, Carpenter JR, Small RC (1992) Trials of the bronchodilator activ-

ity of the isoenzyme-selective phosphodiesterase inhibitor AH 21-132 in healthy volunteers during a methacholine challenge test. *Br J Clin Pharmacol* 34: 527–534

106 Kawasaki A, Hoshino K, Osaki R, Mizushima Y, Yano S (1992) Effect of ibudilast: a novel antiasthmatic agent, on airway hypersensitivity in bronchial asthma. *J Asthma* 29: 245–252

107 Bardin PG, Dorward MA, Lampe FC, Franke B, Holgate ST (1998) Effect of selective phosphodiesterase 3 inhibition on the early and late asthmatic responses to inhaled allergen. *Br J Clin Pharmacol* 45: 387–391

108 Harbinson PL, MacLeod D, Hawksworth R, O'Toole S, Sullivan PJ, Heath P, Kilfeather S, Page CP, Costello J, Holgate ST, Lee TH (1997) The effect of a novel orally active selective PDE4 isoenzyme inhibitor CDP840 on allergen-induced responses in asthmatic subjects. *Eur Respir J* 10: 1008–1014

109 Jonker GJ, Tijhuis GJ, de Menchey JGR (1996) RP 73401 (a phosphodiesterase IV inhibitor) single does not prevent allergen induced bronchoconstriction during the early phase reaction in asthmatics. *Eur Respir J* 9: 82s

110 Meltzer SS, Hasday JD, Cohn J, Bleecker ER (1996) Inhibition of exercise-induced bronchospasm by zileuton: a 5-lipoxygenase inhibitor. *Am J Respir Crit Care Med* 153: 931–935

111 Israel E, Dermarkarian R, Rosenberg M, Sperling R, Taylor G, Rubin P, Drazen JM (1990) The effects of a 5-lipoxygenase inhibitor on asthma induced by cold, dry air [see comments]. *N Engl J Med* 323: 1740–1744

112 Dekhuijzen PNR, Bootsma GP, Wielders PLML, Van den Berg LRM, Festen J, van Herwaarden CLA (1997) Effects of single-dose zileuton on bronchial hyperresponsiveness in asthmatic patients with inhaled corticosteroids. *Eur Respir J* 10: 2749–2753

113 Hui KP, Taylor IK, Taylor GW, Rubin P, Kesterson J, Barnes NC, Barnes PJ (1991) Effect of a 5-lipoxygenase inhibitor on leukotriene generation and airway responses after allergen challenge in asthmatic patients. *Thorax* 46: 184–189

114 Wenzel SE, Trudeau JB, Kaminsky DA, Cohn J, Martin RJ, Westcott JY (1995) Effect of 5-lipoxygenase inhibition on bronchoconstriction and airway inflammation in nocturnal asthma. *Am J Respir Crit Care Med* 152: 897–905

115 Diamant Z, Timmers MC, van der Veen H, Friedman BS, De Smet M, Depre M, Hilliard D, Bel EH, Sterk PJ (1995) The effect of MK-0591, a novel 5-lipoxygenase activating protein inhibitor, on leukotriene biosynthesis and allergen-induced airway responses in asthmatic subjects *in vivo*. *J Allergy Clin Immunol* 95: 42–51

116 Friedman BS, Bel EH, Buntinx A, Tanaka W, Han YH, Shingo S, Spector R, Sterk P (1993) Oral leukotriene inhibitor (MK-886) blocks allergen-induced airway responses. *Am Rev Respir Dis* 147: 839–844

117 Taylor IK, O'Shaughnessy KM, Fuller RW, Dollery CT (1991) Effect of cysteinyl-leukotriene receptor antagonist ICI 204.219 on allergen-induced bronchoconstriction and airway hyperreactivity in atopic subjects [see comments]. *Lancet* 337: 690–694

118 Dahlen B, Zetterstrom O, Bjorck T, Dahlen SE (1994) The leukotriene-antagonist ICI-

204,219 inhibits the early airway reaction to cumulative bronchial challenge with allergen in atopic asthmatics. *Eur Respir J* 7: 324–331
119 Finnerty JP, Wood Baker R, Thomson H, Holgate ST (1992) Role of leukotrienes in exercise-induced asthma. Inhibitory effect of ICI 204219, a potent leukotriene D4 receptor antagonist. *Am Rev Respir Dis* 145: 746–749
120 Lazarus SC, Wong HH, Watts MJ, Boushey HA, Lavins BJ, Minkwitz MC (1997) The leukotriene receptor antagonist zafirlukast inhibits sulfur dioxide-induced bronchoconstriction in patients with asthma. *Am J Respir Crit Care Med* 156: 1725–1730
121 O'Shaughnessy TC, Georgiou P, Howland K, Dennis M, Compton CH, Barnes NC (1997) Effect of pranlukast, an oral leukotriene receptor antagonist, on leukotriene D4 (LTD4) challenge in normal volunteers. *Thorax* 52: 519–522
122 Yamamoto H, Nagata M, Kuramitsu K, Tabe K, Kiuchi H, Sakamoto Y, Yamamoto K, Dohi Y (1994) Inhibition of analgesic-induced asthma by leukotriene receptor antagonist ONO-1078. *Am J Respir Crit Care Med* 150: 254–257
123 Taniguchi Y, Tamura G, Honma M, Aizawa T, Maruyama N, Shirato K, Takishima T (1993) The effect of an oral leukotriene antagonist, ONO-1078, on allergen-induced immediate bronchoconstriction in asthmatic subjects. *J Allergy Clin Immunol* 92: 507–512
124 Fujimura M, Sakamoto S, Kamio Y, Matsuda T (1993) Effect of a leukotriene antagonist, ONO-1078, on bronchial hyperresponsiveness in patients with asthma. *Respir Med* 87: 133–138
125 Reiss TF, Altman LC, Chervinsky P, Bewtra A, Stricker WE, Noonan GP, Kundu S, Zhang J (1996) Effects of montelukast (MK-0476), a new potent cysteinyl leukotriene (LTD4) receptor antagonist, in patients with chronic asthma. *J Allergy Clin Immunol* 98: 528–534
126 De Lepeleire I, Reiss TF, Rochette F, Botto A, Zhang J, Kundu S, Decramer M (1997) Montelukast causes prolonged, potent leukotriene D4-receptor antagonism in the airways of patients with asthma. *Clin Pharmacol Ther* 61: 83–92
127 Oosaki R, Mizushima Y, Kashii T, Kawasaki A, Kobayashi M (1997) Therapeutic effect of pranlukast, a selective cysteinyl leukotriene receptor antagonist, on bronchial asthma. *Int Arch Allergy Immunol* 114: 97–100
128 Grossman J, Faiferman I, Dubb JW, Tompson DJ, Busse W, Bronsky E, Montanaro A, Southern L, Tinkelman D (1997) Results of the first U.S. double-blind, placebo-controlled, multicenter clinical study in asthma with pranlukast, a novel leukotriene receptor antagonist. *J Asthma* 34: 321–328
129 Shephard EG, Malan L, Macfarlane CM, Mouton W, Jourbert JR (1985) *Br J Clin Pharmacol* 19: 459–470
130 Devillier P, Bessard G (1997) Thromboxane A2 and related prostaglandins in airways. *Fundam Clin Pharmacol* 11: 2–18
131 Aizawa H, Shigyo M, Nogami H, Hirose T, Hara N (1996) BAY u3405, a thromboxane A2 antagonist, reduces bronchial hyperresponsiveness in asthmatics. *Chest* 109: 338–342

132 Rajakulasingam K, Johnston SL, Ducey J, Ritter W, Howarth PH, Holgate ST (1996) Effect of thromboxane A2-receptor antagonist on bradykinin-induced bronchoconstriction in asthma. *J Appl Physiol* 80: 1973–1977

133 Stenton SC, Young CA, Harris A, Palmer JB, Hendrick DJ, Walters EH (1992) The effect of GR32191 (a thromboxane receptor antagonist) on airway responsiveness in asthma. *Pulm Pharmacol* 5: 199–202

134 Myou S, Fujimura M, Nishi K, Ohka T, Masuda T (1994) Inhibitory effect of a selective thromboxane synthetase inhibitor, OKY-046, on acetaldehyde-induced bronchoconstriction in asthmatic patients. *Chest* 106: 1414–1418

135 Gardiner PV, Young CL, Holmes K, Hendrick DJ, Walters EH (1993) Lack of short-term effect of the thromboxane synthetase inhibitor UK-38,485 on airway reactivity to methacholine in asthmatic subjects. *Eur Respir J* 6: 1027–1030

136 Manning PJ, Stevens WH, Cockcroft DW, O'Byrne PM (1991) The role of thromboxane in allergen-induced asthmatic responses. *Eur Respir J* 4: 667–672

137 Kurosawa M (1995) Role of thromboxane A2 synthetase inhibitors in the treatment of patients with bronchial asthma. *Clin Ther* 17: 2–11

138 Sutton BJ, Gould HJ (1993) The human IgE network. *Nature* 366: 421–428

139 McDonnell JM, Beavil AJ, Mackay GA, Henry AJ, Cook JP, Gould HJ, Sutton BJ (1997) Structure-based design of peptides that inhibit IgE binding to its high-affinity receptor Fc epsilon RI. *Biochem Soc Trans* 25: 387–392

140 Boulet LP, Chapman KR, Cote J, Kalra S, Bhagat R, Swystun VA, Laviolette M, Cleland LD, Deschesnes F, Su JQ, DeVault A, Fick RB Jr, Cockcroft DW (1997) Inhibitory effects of an anti-IgE antibody E25 on allergen- induced early asthmatic response. *Am J Respir Crit Care Med* 155: 1835–1840

141 Fahy JV, Fleming HE, Wong HH, Liu JT, Su JQ, Reimann J, Fick RB Jr, Boushey HA (1997) The effect of an anti-IgE monoclonal antibody on the early- and late-phase responses to allergen inhalation in asthmatic subjects. *Am J Respir Crit Care Med* 155: 1828–1834

142 Coyle AJ, Wagner K, Bertrand C, Tsuyuki S, Bews J Heusser C (1996) Central role of immunoglobulin (Ig) E in the induction of lung eosinophil infiltration and T helper 2 cell cytokine production: inhibition by a non-anaphylactogenic anti-IgE antibody. *J Exp Med* 183: 1303–1310

143 Nakajima H, Iwamoto I, Tomoe S, Matsumura R, Tomioka H, Takatsu K, Yoshida S (1992) $CD4^+$ T-lymphocytes and interleukin-5 mediate antigen-induced eosinophil infiltration into the mouse trachea. *Am Rev Respir Dis* 146: 374–377

144 Eum SY, Haile S, Lefort J, Huerre M, Vargaftig BB (1995) Eosinophil recruitment into the respiratory epithelium following antigenic challenge in hyper-IgE mice is accompanied by interleukin 5-dependent bronchial hyperresponsiveness. *Proc Natl Acad Sci USA* 92: 12290–12294

145 Foster PS, Hogan SP, Ramsay AJ, Matthaei KI, Young IG (1996) Interleukin 5 deficiency abolishes eosinophilia, airways hyperreactivity, and lung damage in a mouse asthma model. *J Exp Med* 183: 195–201

146 Hamelmann E, Oshiba A, Loader J, Larsen GL, Gleich G, Lee J, Gelfand EW (1997) Antiinterleukin-5 antibody prevents airway hyperresponsiveness in a murine model of airway sensitization. *Am J Respir Crit Care Med* 155: 819–825
147 Underwood DC, Osborn RR, Newsholme SJ, Torphy TJ, Hay DW (1996) Persistent airway eosinophilia after leukotriene (LT) D4 administration in the guinea pig: modulation by the LTD4 receptor antagonist, pranlukast, or an interleukin-5 monoclonal antibody. *Am J Respir Crit Care Med* 154: 850–857
148 Mauser PJ, Pitman AM, Fernandez X, Foran SK, Adams GK, Kreutner W, Egan RW, Chapman RW (1995) Effects of an antibody to interleukin-5 in a monkey model of asthma. *Am J Respir Crit Care Med* 152: 467–472
149 Shi H-Z, Xiao C-Q, Zhong D, Qin S-M, Liu Y, Liang G-R, Xu H, Chen Y-Q, Long X-M, Xie Z-F (1998) Effect of inhaled interleukin-5 on airway hyperreactivity and eosinophilia in asthmatics. *Am J Respir Crit Care Med* 157: 204–209
150 Alam R (1997) Chemokines in allergic inflammation. *J Allergy Clin Immunol* 99: 273–277
151 Ponath PD, Qin S, Ringler DJ, Clark Lewis I, Wang J, Kassam N, Smith H, Shi X, Gonzalo JA, Newman W, Gutierrez Ramos JC, Mackay CR (1996) Cloning of the human eosinophil chemoattractant, eotaxin. Expression, receptor binding, and functional properties suggest a mechanism for the selective recruitment of eosinophils. *J Clin Invest* 97: 604–612
152 Kitaura M, Nakajima T, Imai T, Harada S, Combadiere C, Tiffany HL, Murphy PM, Yoshie O (1996) Molecular cloning of human eotaxin, an eosinophil-selective CC chemokine, and identification of a specific eosinophil eotaxin receptor, CC chemokine receptor 3. *J Biol Chem* 271: 7725–7730
153 Garcia Zepeda EA, Rothenberg ME, Ownbey RT, Celestin J, Leder P, Luster AD (1996) Human eotaxin is a specific chemoattractant for eosinophil cells and provides a new mechanism to explain tissue eosinophilia. *Nat Med* 2: 449–456
154 Yamada H, Hirai K, Miyamasu M, Iikura M, Misaki Y, Shoji S, Takaishi T, Kasahara T, Morita Y, Ito K (1997) Eotaxin is a potent chemotaxin for human basophils. *Biochem Biophys Res Commun* 231: 365–368
155 Daugherty BL, Siciliano SJ, DeMartino JA, Malkowitz L, Sirotina A, Springer MS (1996) Cloning, expression, and characterization of the human eosinophil eotaxin receptor. *J Exp Med* 183: 2349–2354
156 Rothenberg ME, MacLean JA, Pearlman E, Luster AD, Leder P (1997) Targeted disruption of the chemokine eotaxin partially reduces antigen-induced tissue eosinophilia. *J Exp Med* 185: 785–790
157 Humbles AA, Conroy DM, Marleau S, Rankin SM, Palframan RT, Proudfoot AE, Wells TN, Li D, Jeffery PK, Griffiths Johnson DA, Williams TJ, Jose PJ (1997) Kinetics of eotaxin generation and its relationship to eosinophil accumulation in allergic airways disease: analysis in a guinea pig model *in vivo*. *J Exp Med* 186: 601–612
158 Teixeira MM, Wells TN, Lukacs NW, Proudfoot AE, Kunkel SL, Williams TJ, Hellewell

PG (1997) Chemokine-induced eosinophil recruitment. Evidence of a role for endogenous eotaxin in an *in vivo* allergy model in mouse skin. *J Clin Invest* 100: 1657–1666
159 Heath H, Qin S, Rao P, Wu L, LaRosa G, Kassam N, Ponath PD, Mackay CR (1997) Chemokine receptor usage by human eosinophils. The importance of CCR3 demonstrated using an antagonistic monoclonal antibody. *J Clin Invest* 99: 178–184
160 Tyrell DJ, Kilfeather S, Page CP (1995) Therapeutic uses of heparin beyond its traditional role as anticoagulant. *Trends Pharmacol Sci* 16: 198–204
161 Gaffney A, Gaffney P (1996) Rheumatoid arthritis and heparin. *Brit J Rheumatol* 35: 808–809
162 Gaffney PR, Doyle CT, Gaffney A, Hogan J, Hayes DP, Annis P (1995) Paradoxical response to heparin in 10 patients with ulcerative colitis. *Am J Gastroenterol* 90: 220–223
163 Dwarakanath AD, Yu LG, Brookes C, Pryce D, Rhodes JM (1995) 'Sticky' neutrophils, pathergic arthritis, and response to heparin in pyodema gangrenosum complicating ulcerative colitis. *Gut* 37: 585–588
164 Parsons CL, Housley T, Schmidt JD, Lebow D (1994) Treatment of interstitial cycstitis with intravesical heparin. *Br J Urol* 73: 504–507
165 Asa D, Gant T, Oda Y, Brandley BK (1992) Evidence for two classes of carbohydrate binding sites on selectins. *Glycobiol* 2: 395–400
166 Norgard-Sumnicht KE, Varki NM, Varki A (1993) Calcium-dependent heparin-like ligands for L-selectin in nonlymphoid endothelial cells. *Science* 261: 480–483
167 Ley K, Cerrito M, Arfors KE (1991) Sulfated polysaccharides inhibit leukocyte rolling in rabbit mesentery venules. *Am J Physiol* 260: H1667–H1673
168 Seeds EA, Hanss J, Page CP (1993) The effect of heparin and related proteoglycans on allergen and PAF-induced eosinophil infiltration. *J Lipid Mediat* 7: 269–278
169 Seeds EA, Horne AP, Tyrrell DJ, Page CP (1995) The effect of inhaled heparin and related glycosaminoglycans on allergen-induced eosinophil infiltration in guinea-pigs. *Pulm Pharmacol* 8: 97–105
170 Fryer A, Huang YC, Rao G, Jacoby D, Mancilla E, Whorton R, Piantadosi CA, Kennedy T, Hoidal J (1997) Selective O-desulfation produces nonanticoagulant heparin that retains pharmacological activity in the lung. *J Pharmacol Exp Ther* 282: 208–219
171 Seeds EAM, Kennedy T, Hoidal J, Page CP (1998) The effect of O-desulphated heparin on allergen induced eosinophil infiltration in the guinea-pig. *Am J Respir Crit Care Med* 157: A825
172 Vlodavsky I, Eldor A, Haimovitz FA, Matzner Y, Ishai MR, Lider O, Naparstek Y, Cohen IR, Fuks Z (1992) Expression of heparanase by platelets and circulating cells of the immune system: possible involvement in diapedesis and extravasation. *Invasion Metastasis* 12: 112–127
173 Ramdin LSP, Shute JK (1997) The heparin/heparinase balance in the airways: A modulator of inflammation? *Eur Respir J* 10: 135s
174 Murch SH, MacDonald TT, Walker SJ, Levin M, Lionetti P, Klein NJ (1993) Disruption of sulphated glycosaminoglycans in intestinal inflammation. *Lancet* 341: 711–714

175 Willenborg DO, Parish CR (1988) Inhibition of allergic encephalomyelitis in rats by treatment with sulfated polysaccharides. *J Immunol* 140: 3401–3405

176 Lider O, Mekori YA, Miller T, Bar TR, Vlodavsky I, Baharav E, Cohen IR, Naparstek Y (1990) Inhibition of T lymphocyte heparanase by heparin prevents T cell migration and T cell-mediated immunity. *Eur J Immunol* 20: 493–499

177 Diamant Z, Timmers MC, van der Veen H, Page CP, van-der-Meer FJ, Sterk PJ (1996) Effect of inhaled heparin on allergen-induced early and late asthmatic responses in patients with atopic asthma. *Am J Respir Crit Care Med* 153: 1790–1795

178 Ahmed T, Garrigo J, Danta I (1993) Preventing bronchoconstriction in exercise-induced asthma with inhaled heparin. *N Engl J Med* 329: 90–95

179 Garrigo J, Danta I, Ahmed T (1996) Time course of the protective effect of inhaled heparin on exercise-induced asthma. *Am J Respir Crit Care Med* 153: 1702–1707

180 Crimi N, Armato F, Lamicela M, Magri S, Pisotorio MP, Mastruzzo C, Vancheri C (1995) Inhibitory effect of heparin on eosinophil recruitment after nasal allergen challenge. *Eur Respir J* 8: 10s

181 Wegner CD, Gundel RH, Reilly P, Haynes N, Letts LG, Rothlein R (1990) Intercellular adhesion molecule-1 (ICAM-1) in the pathogenesis of asthma. *Science* 247: 456–459

182 Laberge S, Rabb H, Issekutz TB, Martin JG (1995) Role of VLA-4 and LFA-1 in allergen-induced airway hyperresponsiveness and lung inflammation in the rat. *Am J Respir Crit Care Med* 151: 822–829

183 Bloemen PG, Buckley TL, van den Tweel MC, Henricks PA, Redegeld FA, Koster AS, Nijkamp FP (1996) LFA-1, and not Mac-1, is crucial for the development of hyperreactivity in a murine model of nonallergic asthma. *Am J Respir Crit Care Med* 153: 521–529

184 Pretolani M, Ruffie C, Lapa S-JR, Joseph D, Lobb RR, Vargaftig BB (1994) Antibody to very late activation antigen 4 prevents antigen-induced bronchial hyperreactivity and cellular infiltration in the guinea pig airways. *J Exp Med* 180: 795–805

185 Milne AA, Piper PJ (1994) The effects of two anti-CD18 antibodies on antigen-induced airway hyperresponsiveness and leukocyte accumulation in the guinea pig. *Am J Respir Cell Mol Biol* 11: 337–343

186 Sun J, Elwood W, Haczku A, Barnes PJ, Hellewell PG, Chung KF (1994) Contribution of intercellular-adhesion molecule-1 in allergen-induced airway hyperresponsiveness and inflammation in sensitised brown-Norway rats. *Int Arch Allergy Immunol* 104: 291–295

187 El-Hashim AZ, Jacques CA, Herd CM, Lee TH, Page CP (1997) The effect of R 15.7/HO, an anti-CD18 antibody, on the late airway response and airway hyperresponsiveness in an allergic rabbit model. *Br J Pharmacol* 121: 671–678

188 Milne AA, Piper PJ (1995) Role of the VLA-4 integrin in leucocyte recruitment and bronchial hyperresponsiveness in the guinea-pig. *Eur J Pharmacol* 282: 243–249

189 Hellewell PG, Young SK, Henson PM, Worthen GS (1994) Disparate role of the beta 2-integrin CD18 in the local accumulation of neutrophils in pulmonary and cutaneous inflammation in the rabbit. *Am J Respir Cell Mol Biol* 10: 391–398

190 Schwartz LB, Lewis RA, Seldin D, Austen KF (1981) Acid hydrolases and tryptase from secretory granules of dispersed human lung mast cells. *J Immunol* 126: 1290–1294
191 Harvima RJ, Schwartz LB (1993) Mast cell-derived mediators. In: JC Foreman (ed): *Immunopharmacology of mast cells and basophils*. Academic Press, London, 115
192 Sommerhoff CP, Caughey GH, Finkbeiner WE, Lazarus SC, Basbaum CB, Nadel JA (1989) Mast cell chymase. A potent secretagogue for airway gland serous cells. *J Immunol* 142: 2450–2456
193 Caughey GH, Leidig F, Viro NF, Nadel JA (1988) Substance P and vasoactive intestinal peptide degradation by mast cell tryptase and chymase. *J Pharmacol Exp Ther* 244: 133–137
194 Tam EK, Caughey GH (1990) Degradation of airway neuropeptides by human lung tryptase. *Am J Respir Cell Mol Biol* 3: 27–32
195 Wenzel SE, Fowler AA 3rd, Schwartz LB (1988) Activation of pulmonary mast cells by bronchoalveolar allergen challenge. *In vivo* release of histamine and tryptase in atopic subjects with and without asthma. *Am Rev Respir Dis* 137: 1002–1008
196 Bousquet J, Chanez P, Lacoste JY, Enander I, Venge P, Peterson C, Ahlstedt S, Michel FB, Godard P (1991) Indirect evidence of bronchial inflammation assessed by titration of inflammatory mediators in BAL fluid of patients with asthma. *J Allergy Clin Immunol* 88: 649–660
197 Sekizawa K, Caughey GH, Lazarus SC, Gold WM, Nadel JA (1989) Mast cell tryptase causes airway smooth muscle hyperresponsiveness in dogs. *J Clin Invest* 83: 175–179
198 Molinari JF, Scuri M, Moore WR, Clark J, Tanaka R, Abraham WM (1996) Inhaled tryptase causes bronchoconstriction in sheep *via* histamine release. *Am J Respir Crit Care Med* 154: 649–653
199 Clark JM, Abraham WM, Fishman CE, Forteza R, Ahmed A, Cortes A, Warne RL, Moore WR, Tanaka RD (1995) Tryptase inhibitors block allergen-induced airway and inflammatory responses in allergic sheep. *Am J Respir Crit Care Med* 152: 2076–2083
200 Elrod KC, Moore WR, Abraham WM, Tanaka RD (1997) Lactoferrin, a potent tryptase inhibitor, abolishes late-phase airway responses in allergic sheep. *Am J Respir Crit Care Med* 156: 375–381
201 Holgate ST, Finnerty JP (1989) Antihistamines in asthma. *J Allergy Clin Immunol* 83: 537–547
202 Michel L, De Vos C, Rihoux JP, Burtin C, Benveniste J, Dubertret L (1988) Inhibitory effect of oral cetirizine on *in vivo* antigen-induced histamine and PAF-acether release and eosinophil recruitment in human skin. *J Allergy Clin Immunol* 82: 101–109
203 Charlesworth EN, Kagey Sobotka A, Norman PS, Lichtenstein LM (1989) Effect of cetirizine on mast cell-mediator release and cellular traffic during the cutaneous late-phase reaction. *J Allergy Clin Immunol* 83: 905–912
204 Okada C, Eda R, Miyagawa H, Sugiyama H, Hopp RJ, Bewtra AK, Townley RG (1994) Effect of cetirizine on human eosinophil superoxide generation, eosinophil chemotaxis and eosinophil peroxidase *in vitro*. *Int Arch Allergy Immunol* 103: 384–390
205 Jinquan T, Reimert CM, Deleuran B, Zachariae C, Simonsen C, Thestrup Pedersen K

(1995) Cetirizine inhibits the *in vitro* and *ex vivo* chemotactic response of T lymphocytes and monocytes. *J Allergy Clin Immunol* 95: 979–986
206 Sedgwick JB, Busse WW (1997) Inhibitory effect of cetirizine on cytokine-enhanced *in vitro* eosinophil survival. *Ann Allergy Asthma Immunol* 78: 581–585
207 Patella V, de Crescenzo G, Marino O, Spadaro G, Genovese A, Marone G (1996) Oxatomide inhibits the release of proinflammatory mediators from human basophils and mast cells. *Int Arch Allergy Immunol* 111: 23–29
208 Atkins PC, Zweiman B, Moskovitz A, von Allmen C, Ciliberti M (1997) Cellular inflammatory responses and mediator release during early developing late-phase allergic cutaneous inflammatory responses: effects of cetirizine. *J Allergy Clin Immunol* 99: 806–811
209 Zweiman B, Atkins PC, Moskovitz A, von Allmen C, Ciliberti M, Grossman S (1997) Cellular inflammatory responses during immediate, developing, and established late-phase allergic cutaneous reactions: effects of cetirizine. *J Allergy Clin Immunol* 100: 341–347
210 de Bruin Weller MS, Rijssenbeek Nouwens LH, de Monchy JG (1994) Lack of effect of cetirizine on early and late asthmatic response after allergen challenge. *J Allergy Clin Immunol* 94: 231–239
211 Bentley AM, Walker S, Hanotte F, De Vos C, Durham SR (1996) A comparison of the effects of oral cetirizine and inhaled beclomethasone on early and late asthmatic responses to allergen and the associated increase in airways hyperresponsiveness. *Clin Exp Allergy* 26: 909–917
212 Fasce L, Ciprandi G, Pronzato C, Cozzani S, Tosca MA, Grimaldi I, Canonica GW (1996) Cetirizine reduces ICAM-I on epithelial cells during nasal minimal persistent inflammation in asymptomatic children with mite-allergic asthma. *Int Arch Allergy Immunol* 109: 272–276
213 Aaronson DW (1996) Evaluation of cetirizine in patients with allergic rhinitis and perennial asthma. *Ann Allergy Asthma Immunol* 76: 440–446
214 Bustos GJ, Bustos D, Romero O (1995) Prevention of asthma with ketotifen in preasthmatic children: a three-year follow-up study. *Clin Exp Allergy* 25: 568–573
215 Canny GJ, Reisman J, Levison H (1997) Does ketotifen have a steroid-sparing effect in childhood asthma? *Eur Respir J* 10: 65–70
216 Craps LP, Greenwood C, Ney UM (1985) Ketotifen and asthma. In:EB Weiss, MS Segal, M Stein (eds): *Bronchial asthma. Mechanisms and therapeutics*. Little, Brown and Company (Inc), Boston, 734
217 Arnoux B, Denjean A, Page CP, Nolibe D, Morley J, Benveniste J (1988) Accumulation of platelets and eosinophils in baboon lung after paf-acether challenge. Inhibition by ketotifen. *Am Rev Respir Dis* 137: 855–860
218 Yanagihara Y, Kiniwa M, Ikizawa K, Shida T, Matsuura N, Koda A (1993) Suppression of IgE production by IPD-1151T (suplatast tosilate), a new dimethylsulfonium agent: (2). Regulation of human IgE response. *Jpn J Pharmacol* 61: 31–39
219 Yamaya H, Basaki Y, Togawa M, Kojima M, Kiniwa M, Matsuura N (1995) Down-reg-

ulation of Th2 cell-mediated murine peritoneal eosinophilia by antiallergic agents. *Life Sci* 56: 1647–1654

220 Konno S, Adachi M, Asano K, Gonogami Y, Ikeda K, Okamoto K, Takahashi T (1994) Suppressive effects of IPD-1151T (suplatast-tosilate) on induction of mast cells from normal mouse splenocytes. *Eur J Pharmacol* 259: 15–20

221 Taniguchi H, Togawa M, Ohwada K, Kiniwa M, Matsuura N, Nagai H, Koda A (1996) Suplatast tosilate, a new type of antiallergic agent, prevents the expression of airway hyperresponsiveness in guinea pigs. *Eur J Pharmacol* 318: 447–454

222 Sano Y, Miyamoto T, Makino S (1997) Anti-inflammatory effect of suplatast tosilate on mild asthma [letter]. *Chest* 112: 862–863

223 Wright CD, Devall LJ, Aker DO, Thueson DO, Conroy MC (1990) Differential regulation of the activation of human eosinophils, macrophages, and neutrophils: effect of the allergic mediator release inhibitor CI-949. *Agents Actions* 31: 11–15

224 Connor DT, Cetenko WA, Mullican MD, Sorenson RJ, Unangst PC, Weikert RJ, Adolphson RL, Kennedy JA, Thueson DO, Wright CD et al (1992) Novel benzothiophene-, benzofuran-, and naphthalenecarboxamidotetrazoles as potential antiallergy agents. *J Med Chem* 35: 958–965

225 Adolphson RL, Schellenberg RR, Thueson DO, Conroy MC (1990) CI-959, a new, potential antiallergic drug, inhibits mediator release from lung and contractions of human airways *in vitro*. *Int Arch Allergy Appl Immunol* 93: 267–271

226 Dong MK, Wilburn DJ, Conroy MC, Gilbertsen RB (1991) Inhibition of interleukin-2 production and lymphocyte responsiveness by the cell activation inhibitor, CI-959. *Agents Actions* 34: 53–55

227 Wright CD, Stewart SF, Kuipers PJ, Hoffman MD, Devall LJ, Kennedy JA, Ferin MA, Thueson DO, Conroy MC (1994) Selective regulation of human neutrophil functions by the cell activation inhibitor CI-959. *J Leukoc Biol* 55: 443–451

T cells in the lung

David M. Kemeny[1] *and Brian J. O'Connor*[2]

Departments of [1]Immunology and [2]Respiratory Medicine, Guys, King's and St Thomas's School of Medicine and Dentistry, Rayne Institute, 123 Coldharbour Lane, London SE5 9NU, UK

Introduction

Because of the requirement for efficient gas exchange, the respiratory tract is particularly vulnerable to opportunistic infection. The immune system, therefore, plays a particularly vital role in protecting the respiratory mucosa from infection. The cells that orchestrate this response are immune T cells. The respiratory mucosa contains large numbers of T cells and a network of dendritic cells that present antigen to them. For many years it was thought that IgE-mediated inflammation was the only precipitating factor in asthma. Mast cells sensitised with IgE antibodies were triggered following contact with aeroallergens which caused immediate and subsequent late phase inflammatory events leading to airway narrowing and subsequently to asthma. However, studies by Kay and colleagues have shown that T cells are also directly important in asthma [1–4] as they are in the allergen-induced late phase response in the skin [5]. The airways of asthmatic patients are rich in T cells. In experimental animals, adoptive transfer of antigen-specific Th2 T cells and subsequent aerosol challenge are sufficient to induce inflammation and increase bronchial hyperresponsiveness [6, 7]. The cytokines produced by immune T cells and their contribution to allergic inflammation and asthma is the subject of this chapter.

CD4 and CD8 T cells

Immune T cells provide defence against intra and extracellular pathogens. CD8 T cells are MHC class-I restricted while CD4 T cells respond to antigenic peptides presented in the MHC class II cleft. The MHC I pathway collects antigen such as viral or self proteins present in the cytosol of the cell that have been broken down into small peptides by an organelle called the proteosome. It is now known that there are two types of proteosome. The first is termed the proteosome, and degrades a wide range of proteins. The second, called the immunoproteosome, is restricted to the breakdown of a narrower range of proteins [8]. The small peptides produced by the

Cellular Mechanisms in Airways Inflammation, edited by Clive P. Page, Katharine H. Banner and Domenico Spina

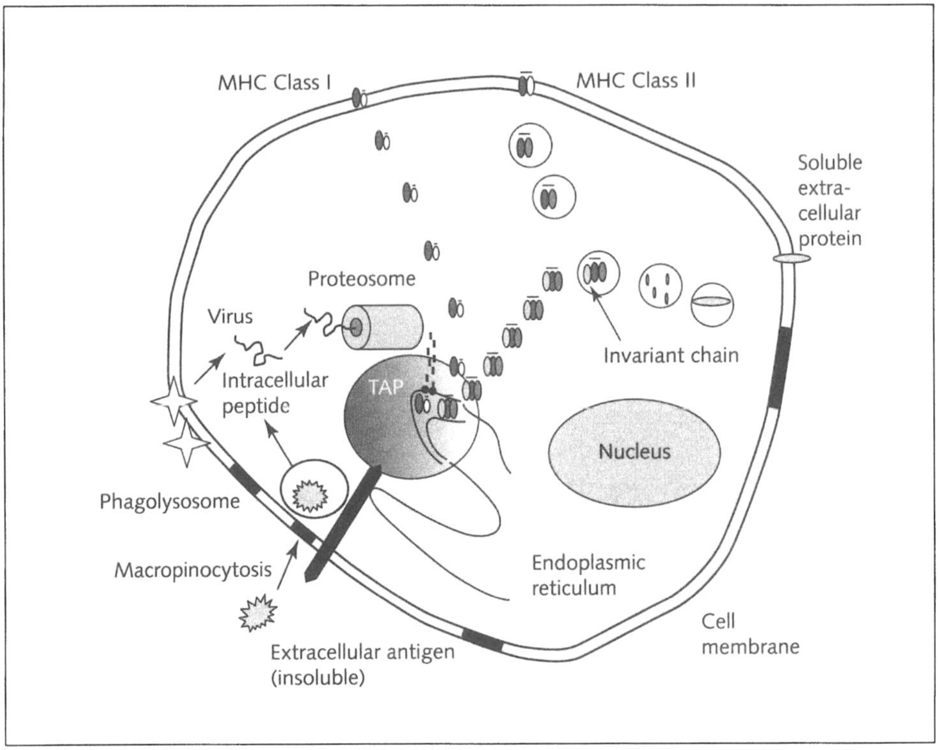

Figure 1

MHC class I and II antigen processing pathways. Most soluble antigen enters via the endosomal compartment. Some enters by phagocytosis or macropinocytosis. Viruses are able to infect antigen-presenting cells via coated pits. MHC molecules are synthesized in the endoplasmic reticulum (ER). Small (7–8 amino acid) peptides are derived from the proteosome and are assembled into the MHC I complex of a chain and β2 microglobulin. MHC II molecules are also synthesised in the ER. To prevent them from binding peptides destined for MHC I they have an extra chain (invariant chain) that binds to the α and β chains of the MHC II complex. Part of this molecule obscures the peptide-binding cleft (clip peptide). Once in the endosome the invariant chain is degraded by enzymes revealing the MHC II peptide binding groove which picks up 15–17 amino acid peptides and migrates to the cell surface where they are presented to T cells.

proteosome are inserted in the peptide-binding groove between the first and second domains of the MHC class I α chain. A specialized molecule called the transporter of peptide (TAP) [9–13] facilitates this. Soluble protein antigens normally enter the MHC class II pathway *via* endosomes that contain proteases that degrade the antigen into peptides (Fig. 1). MHC class II molecules are prevented from binding to peptides in the endoplasmic reticulum (ER) by a molecule called invariant chain which

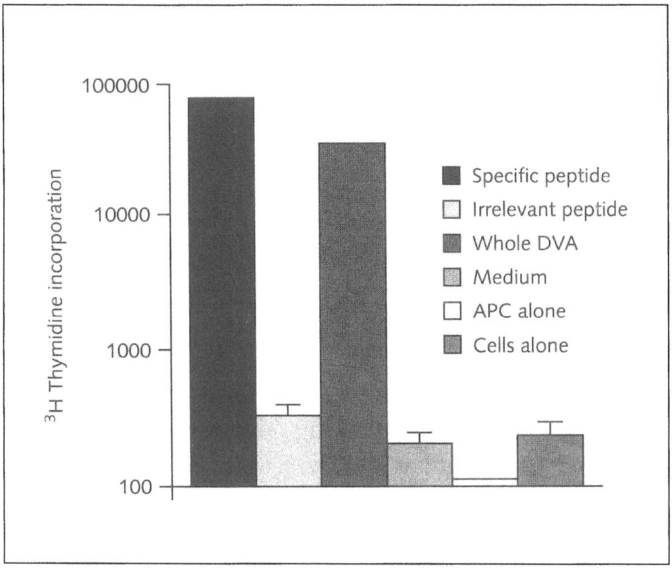

Figure 2
Proliferation of CD8 vβ5.2 TcR transgenic T cells following culture with adherent splenic antigen presenting cells pulsed with OVA peptide or whole ovalbumin.

blocks the peptide binding groove and is cleaved in the endosomes. However these two pathways are not completely exclusive and when antigen presenting cells, such as macrophages are activated, for example by binding to plastic, their ability to process soluble antigen *via* the MHC I pathway is greatly enhanced (Fig. 2).

In addition to CD4 T cells, CD8 T cells are also involved in lung immunity. CD8 T cells recognise antigen presented by MHC class 1 as stated above. As above, whole proteins can get into the MHC class I pathway once inside the cell. They are broken down by some but not all proteosomes. The immunoproteosome does not process soluble antigen that enters the cell as well as the proteosome and is present in a higher proportion in B cells. This may explain why these cells are poor targets for CD8 T cells [8]. The immunoproteosome is also present in DCs and this may explain why peptide is more readily processed into class I than whole protein [25, 26].

Th1 and Th2 CD4 T-cell subsets

Until 1986 it was unclear how the different effector functions of CD4 T cells were mediated [14]. In 1986 Mosmann and colleagues published a seminal study in

Table 1 - The cytokine profile of mouse CD4 and human CD8 T-cell subsets

Subset	IL-2	IFNγ	TNFβ	IL-4	IL-5	IL-6	IL-10	IL-13
Th1/Tc1	+++	+++	+++	–	–	–	–	–
Th0/Tc0	+++	+++	+++	+++	+++	+++	+++	+++
Th2/Tc2	–	–	–	+++	+++	+++	+++	+++

which well-established mouse CD4 T-cell clones were classified according to the cytokines they produced (Tab. 1). They observed that the clones were polarized into those that secreted IFNγ, IL-2 and TNFβ but not IL-4, IL-5, IL-6, IL-10 or p600 (IL-13), which they termed T-helper 1 (Th1), and those that made IL-4, IL-5, IL-6, IL-10 or p600 (IL-13), but not IFNγ, IL-2 or TNFβ, which they called T-helper 2 (Th2). Some cytokines, interleukin-3 (IL-3), tumour necrosis factor α (TNFα) and granulocyte-macrophage colony stimulating factor (GM-CSF) are secreted in similar amounts by both subsets. It soon became evident that Th1 cells were associated with immunity to bacterial and viral pathogens while Th2 responses were associated with nematode and other parasitic infections and with allergy as discussed below. A third category termed Th0, which made all cytokines, was later described [15].

Th1/Th2 T-cell surface markers

In addition to cytokines, cell surface ligands may distinguish different types of T cell. Putative Th1 cell markers include the signaling lymphocytic activation molecule (SLAM), a 70-kDa costimulatory molecule belonging to the immunoglobulin superfamily. SLAM mediates CD28-independent proliferation of human T cells and IFNγ production by human Th1 and Th2 clones. SLAM is expressed on primary mouse T and B cells. Following Th1 and Th2 differentiation, its expression is restricted to mouse Th1 but not Th2 CD4 T cells [16]. Another molecule termed LAG-3 is also reported to be associated with Th1 cells [17, 18].

There are also a number of potential Th2 cell makers. ST2L (also known as T1, DER4, or Fit) is expressed on Th2 but not Th1 cells [19]. CD30 is expressed at a higher level on Th2 cells, and reflects their ability to respond to IL-4 [20]. Indeed signaling *via* CD30 promotes Th2-cell formation [21]. For CD8 T-cell subsets, established Tc1 cells (6–8 weeks into culture) fail to induce CD30, CD40L following activation [22]. Tc1 cells constitutively express lower levels of CD28 than Tc2 cells. After activation, CD28 levels on Tc1 CD8 T cells fall while CD28 on Tc2 cells does not. Th1 cells do not express the β chain of the IFNγ receptor [23]. Mice in whom the IFNγR2 gene has been inactivated have defective Th1 differentiation, are defective in contact hypersensitivity and are highly susceptible to infection by *Listeria monocytogenes* [24].

Regulatory T-cell subsets

For many years *in vitro* and *in vivo* studies of T cells have shown that these cells can inhibit as well as enhance specific immune function. However attempts to define suppressor factors have been elusive. A number of processes have now been defined. As is shown below, the cytokines made by Th1 cells (specifically IFNγ) inhibit Th2 cells and cytokines made by Th2 cells (especially IL-4) inhibit Th1 cells. Thus the balance of the developing Th1/Th2 immune response can be directed down one or other of these pathways. This process has been termed immune deviation [27, 28]. At mucosal surfaces another immune regulatory process has been described as immunological tolerance in which immune T cells are inhibited rather than redirected. The cells that mediate these effects have been termed regulatory T cells. The first to be reported were Th3 cells. These cells predominantly secrete TGFβ [29–32] (Fig. 3b). A second regulatory subset termed Tr1 that mainly makes IL-10 has since been described [33]. Tr1 cells inhibit Th1 cells [34] and prevent Th1 inflammatory disorders such as colitis [33, 35, 36]. They have two possible phenotypes: CD45RB^{high} [35–38] and CD45RB^{low}/CD38^{+} [39]. Th3 cells are found following induction of oral tolerance [30–32, 40]. There may be further subsets [41] that have yet to be defined. IL-10 induces Tr1 cells [33]; it is not known what specific signals induce Th3 cells.

Available evidence indicates that the cytokine profile of human T-cell clones resembles that seen in the mouse although there are some notable exceptions. T-cell clones prepared from atopic donors are Th2 like [42–47] while the majority, derived from non-atopic individuals, were closer to Th1. Some human Th1 clones, however, make appreciable amounts of IL-6 [48] and both Th1 and Th2 human CD4 T-cell clones can make IL-10.

Th1 and Th2 differentiation and growth

A number of factors control the differentiation and subsequent growth of Th1 and Th2 cells including the cytokines present and the type of stimulus delivered. As so often in immunology, the effects of cytokines can be both autocrine and paracrine. IL-4, for example, promotes the generation of IL-4 producing Th2 cells. As these cells make IL-4 this, in turn, promotes differentiation into additional Th2 cells [49–51]. IL-4 also inhibits differentiation into Th1 cells and reduces Th1 cell growth [52]. Cytokines can also act synergistically – for example a combination of IL-4 and IL-10 inhibits cell-mediated immunity [53, 54].

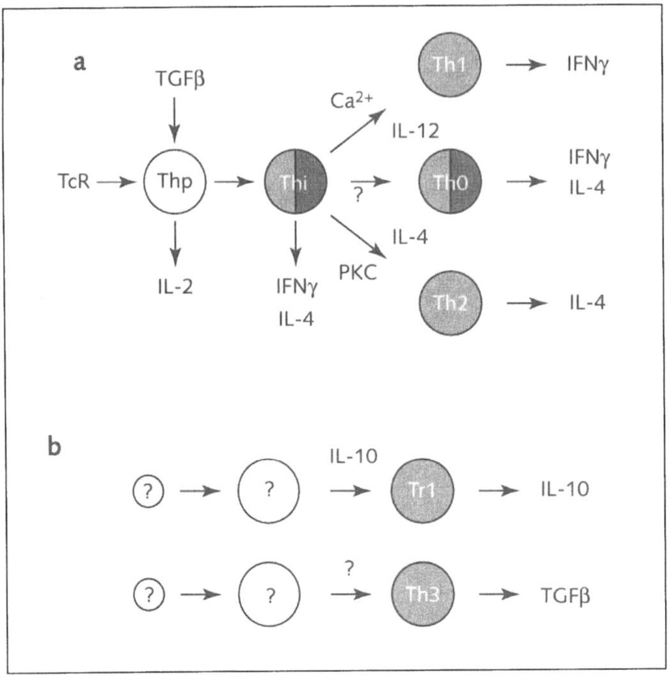

Figure 3
The contribution of cytokines and TcR delivered signals to CD4 T cell differentiation.
(a) Following T cell receptor (TcR) engagement naïve CD4 T cells (Thp) make IL-2. TGFβ maintains cells in this state. Subsequent engagement of co-stimulatory molecules, such as CD28, induces cytokine gene expression via an intermediate (Thi) that makes both IFNγ and IL-4 into Th1, Th2 or Th0 effector cells. The formation of these different cells is regulated by the presence of key cytokines. IL-12 promotes Th1 cells and IL-4 Th2 cells. It is unclear what causes Th0 cell formation. In addition to these cytokine delivered signals the balance of TcR delivered signals that activate the calcium (Ca^{2+}) and protein kinase c (PKC) pathways are capable of overriding the effects of cytokines.
(b) In addition to the above T cell subsets are regulatory T cells (Tr1) that are induced by IL-10 and make IL-10 and Th3 cells that mainly make TGFβ.

Following T-cell receptor (TcR) engagement, naïve CD4 T cells (Thp) make IL-2. TGFβ maintains cells in this state [53], which may be important for clonal expansion (Fig. 3a). Subsequent engagement of co-stimulatory molecules, such as CD28, induces cytokine gene expression, *via* an intermediate (Thi) that makes both IFNγ and IL-4 [55], into Th1, Th2 or Th0 effector cells. The formation of these different cells is regulated by the presence of key cytokines. IL-12 promotes formation of Th1 cells [56] and IL-4 is required for Th2 cells [49]. It is unclear what causes Th0 cell formation or what is their function (see below).

As well as cytokines, different stimuli delivered *via* the T-cell receptor influence Th1 and Th2 cell formation. O'Garra and colleagues have shown that both strong and weak stimuli favour mouse Th2 formation *in vitro* [57]. *In vivo* we have found that the optimum dose of antigen for IgE responses in the mouse today is 1 mg/ml. This contrasts with previous studies showing microgram [58–60] and even nanogram [61] quantities worked best. What appears to have happened is that as animal colonies have become free of certain pathogens, such as the pin worm syphacea, they have lost the ability to respond to low antigen dose but still respond to high doses.

By contrast, Bottomly has shown that increased interaction (valency) between T cell and antigen presenting cell favors Th1 over Th2. Transgenic CD4 T cells produced IFNγ when exposed to high antigen doses, while low doses of the same peptide induced Th2-like cells that produced IL-4 [62]. Priming by altered peptide ligands (APLs) for both IL-4 production and IFNγ production does not require two different types of APCs [63]. Indeed the nature of the signals sent by the T cell receptor (TcR) can influence the type of T cell with high affinity antigen peptides favoring Th1 and low affinity peptides favoring Th2 [64–66]. High affinity TcR delivered signals activate the calcium (Ca^{2+}) pathway [67] while low affinity TcR signals favor the protein kinase c (PKC) pathway [66]. Such TcR delivered signals are able to override the effects of cytokines such as IL-4 and IL-12.

Tc1 and Tc2 CD8 T cells

CD8 T cells are regulated by the same cytokines but it is generally more difficult to make Tc2 CD8 T cells as compared with Th2 CD4 T cells [50, 68–70]. In common with CD4 T cells, IL-4 enhances differentiation into Tc2 cells and inhibits Tc1 cell formation while IL-12 promotes differentiation into Tc1 cells [71] and inhibits Tc2 cell formation. As for CD4 T cells, growth of Tc1 but not Tc2 cells is inhibited by IL-4 while IL-12 enhances Tc1 but not Tc2 cell proliferation [22]. *In vivo*, polarized T cell subsets persist. Transgenic CD8 T cells, polarised into Th1 or Th2-like subsets *in vitro*, then adoptively transferred into wild type mice revert to a naïve (resting), $CD45RB^{high}$ phenotype. When re-challenged with antigen 13 weeks later the transgenic cells produced the same pattern of cytokines [72]. It is not known, but is expected, that similarly polarised CD4 T-cell subsets too retain the same pattern of cytokine secretion.

IgE regulation

Shortly after IgE was discovered it became clear that IgE production by B cells was regulated by T cells. Tada showed that rat IgE responses could be inhibited by Lyt2

(CD8α) bearing T cells [73–75]. Katz and others showed that CD4 T-cell help was also required [76, 77]. For many years different theories were advanced and specific immunoregulatory molecules proposed. In 1986 the speculation ended when Coffman and Carty [78] using BCSF-1 and in 1987 Snapper and Paul using its new name, IL-4 [79] showed that this molecule regulated B-cell IgE class switching. Subsequently p600 (IL-13) was shown to posses the same IgE promoting properties as IL-4 [80].

During antibody synthesis, the genes encoding the variable part of the IgE molecule (VDJ) are rearranged to yield different affinity antibodies. B cells making the highest affinity antibody are selected by rescue from apoptosis. The heavy chain of the immunoglobulin gene is spliced onto the VDJ complex that encodes the combining site. In the case of IgE, a sterile transcript that does not contain the full length sequences produced first. This regulates expression of the full-length sequence. The combining site is joined to the heavy chain by looping out intervening DNA. This produces a circle of DNA containing the intervening heavy chain genes analysis of these switch circles has shown that switching can occur in stages, in a single jump, up and down the gene. This process is regulated by an obligatory signal delivered by CD40L on the CD4 helper T cell and specific cytokines.

The process of class switching can be followed through a series of distinct steps shown in Figure 4. In step 1, IgM antibody bearing B cells take up antigen *via* their surface antibody. This antigen is then processed and presented *via* MHC class II molecules in step 2 to CD4 T helper T cells. Ligation of the T-cell receptor in this way upregulates expression of CD40L (CD154) (Step 3) which binds to CD40 on the surface of the B cell which is constitutively expressed. Ligation of CD40 stimulates the B cell which the expresses CD80 (B7.1) in step 4. CD80 binds to CD28, which is constitutively expressed on some CD4 T cells, and in step 5 together with the T-cell receptor-MHC interaction stimulates IL-4/IL-13 synthesis and secretion. These cytokines bind in turn to receptors on B cells (Step 6) and initiate class switching to IgE, which is secreted in step 7.

Th1 vs Th2 pathology

Following exposure to antigen CD4 Th2 cells infiltrate the lung of asthmatic patients. These cells can readily be found in the late phase response both in the lung [81, 82] and following intradermal injection of antigen into the skin [5] of allergic patients. The cytokines secreted by these cells have direct pro inflammatory effects. IL-4 and IL-5, for example, promote the recruitment and survival of eosinophils [83] and mast cells. Eosinophilia, airway hyperreactivity, and lung damage failed to occur in ovalbumin aerosol sensitised, IL-5 knockout mice [84]. Human IL-6, when over-expressed in mouse lung epithelial cells causes a T-cell infiltrate but reduces lung hyperresponsiveness [85]. IL-11 similarly over expressed can cause airway remodeling with subepithelial airway fibrosis [86]. IL-13, when targeted to the lung,

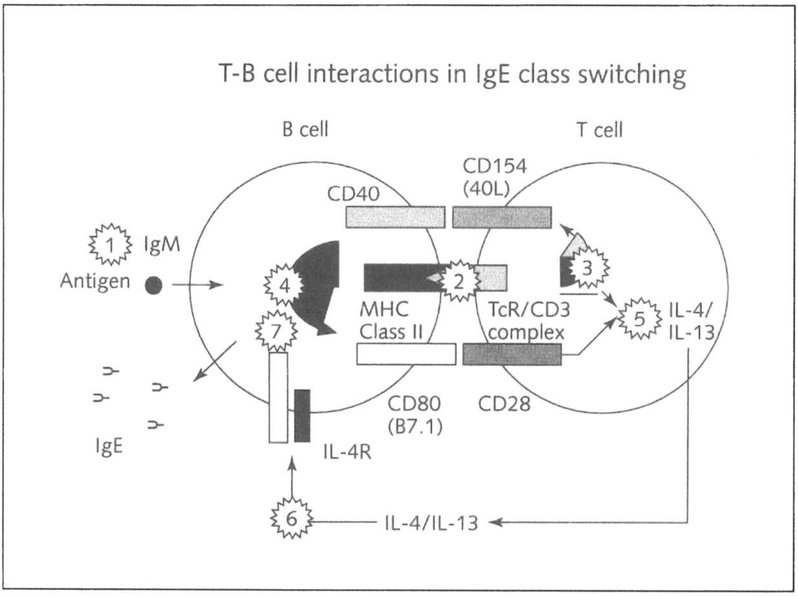

Figure 4
Regulation of immunoglobulin class switching to IgE. Step: 1 Antigen is taken up by B cells which express IgM (primary immune response) or IgE, IgA or IgG (secondary immune response) on their surface. Step 2: The antigen is processed as shown in Figure 1 which results in increased expression of MHC class II-peptide on the surface of the B cell. Increased MHC class II-peptide expression recruits CD4 T cells whose T-cell receptors (TcRs) recognise the specific peptide and signals to the T cell, step 3, to express CD40L. Step 4: Engagement of CD40 by CD40L induced the B cell to express CD80 or CD86 which engages CD28 on the CD4 T cell. Step 5: A combination of CD28 and TcR engagement stimulates Th2 CD4 T cells to produce IL-4 and IL-13. Step 6: IL-4 or IL-13 signal to the B cell to make IgE. Step 7: The B cell secretes IgE.

produces an inflammatory response around small and large airways containing eosinophils and macrophages, Charcot-Leyden-like crystals, and subepithelial airway fibrosis [87]. Other cytokines made by both Th1 and Th2 cells, such as GM-CSF, contribute to lung inflammation by promoting monocyte activation and survival [88–90].

Th1 cells are associated with certain autoimmune disorders such as diabetes [91], rheumatoid arthritis [92, 93] and multiple sclerosis [94]. Th1 cells induce macrophage infiltration and granuloma formation. In the lung Th1 responses are associated with infection with pathogenic organisms such as *Mycobacterium tuberculosis* [95, 96]. An over active Th1 response leads to destruction of the lung architecture and extensive granuloma formation in patients with Sarcoidosis, a disease of unknown etiology [97].

Can T cells alone cause asthma

In most atopic asthmatic patients allergen specific Th2 cells will coexist with IgE antibodies to the same allergens. CD4 Th2 cells are required for IgE production. It is, therefore, very difficult to separate the relative contribution of T cell and IgE mediated mechanisms to allergic inflammation. One way of doing so is to use an animal model. Passive transfer of allergen-specific IgE and IgG1 followed by inhalation of nebulised ovalbumin causes immediate hypersensitivity and airway hyperresponsiveness in mice [98]. Mice and rats sensitized with ovalbumin have increased airway responses to acetylcholine following ovalbumin aerosol challenge [99–102]. Airway bronchial hyperresponsiveness (BHR) is associated with increased Th2 cytokines and reduced Th1 cytokines [103]. BHR can be induced by passive transfer of antigen-primed CD4 T cells [104]. The degree of hyperresponsiveness depends on the strength of the Th2 response. Umetsu and colleagues too showed that Th2 cells alone can cause airway inflammation and BHR [105]. It will require further research to evaluate the contribution that IgE makes to this process but IL-4 and CD40 knockout mice (no IgE or IgG) still exhibit eosinophilia and increased airway hyperresponsiveness [106].

The role of CD8 T cells in the lung

For a number of years it was felt that the Th1/Th2 paradigm did not apply to CD8 T cells. Most CD8 T-cell clones had a Th1 cytokine profile and these cells rarely seemed to produce IL-4. Indeed the most common phenotype for CD8 T cells in humans, mice and rats is the IFNγ secreting Tc1 type [22, 50, 107]. CD8 T cells are negatively associated with the late phase asthmatic response [108]. It is not clear what the cytokine profile of such protective CD8 T cells was. In our experimental animal model Tc1 CD8 and Th1 CD4 T cells can inhibit Th2 cell mediated bronchial hyperresponsiveness (BHR) (Fig. 3). Both Tc1 and Tc2 CD8 T cells can stimulate IL-12 and so promote Th1 cells and inhibit Th2 cells.

It is also possible that Tc2 CD8 T cells can cause disease (Fig. 6). Seder and colleagues showed that mouse CD8 T cells cultured with IL-2 and IL-4 made significant amounts of IL-4 [109]. In Leprosy patients, Salgame et al. [110] showed that CD8 T cells that made IL-4 were associated with the more severe lepromatous form of the disease and could inhibit *M. leprae* specific cytotoxic CD4 T cells. Our own studies of rat T cells showed that CD8 T cells from naïve animals could make more IL-4 than CD4 T cells when stimulated with PMA and ionomycin [50]. Indeed in

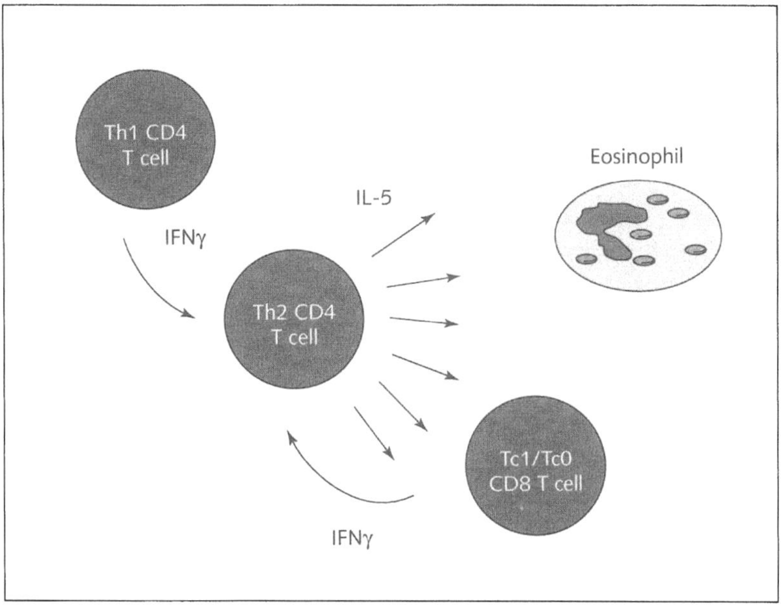

Figure 5
As well as killing virus infected cells, Tc2 CD8 T cells have reduced killing capacity as compared with Tc1 cells and secrete molecules like IL-5 and eotaxin that recruit eosinophils.

thymectomised and CD8-depleted mice, IgE responses were normal but: (i) there was a failure to produce IL-5 from lymph node T cells, (ii) there was no eosinophil infiltration of the lung parenchyma and (iii) they were unable to develop BHR [111]. Furthermore, in mice making a strong Th2 response, the subsequent CD8 T cell response to viral infection can result in an increase in virus-specific CD8 T cells that make IL-5 and subsequent viral infection can cause lung eosinophilia [112]. There is evidence for such a phenomenon in allergic asthmatics where viral infections may contribute to asthma.

Regulation of T-cell function in the lung

In the lung it is clear that T-cell subsets have the potential to co-regulate each other's function. Early on, small numbers of Th1/Tc1 or Th2/Tc2 cells can deviate the inflammatory response in one direction or another. Once a pattern is established, Th1/Tc1 or Th2/Tc2 responses are very hard to alter because groups of polarised cells keep each other in line. Th1 cells make IFNγ, which inhibits the growth and function of Th2 cells; Th2 cells make IL-4 that similarly inhibits Th1 cells. IL-4 and

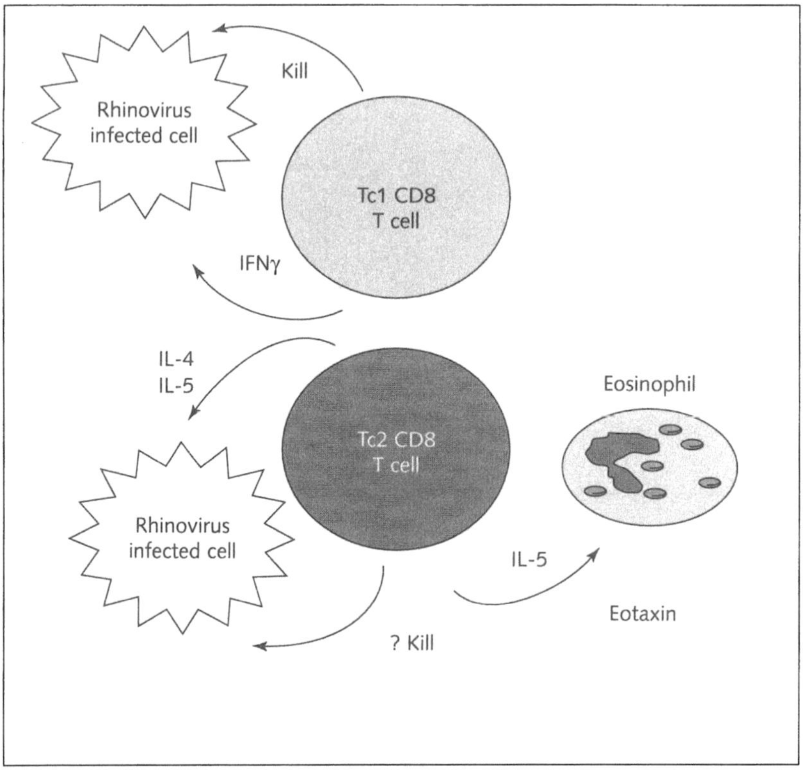

Figure 6
Th1 cells make IFNγ, which inhibits the growth and function of Th2 cells, Th2 cells make IL-4 that similarly inhibits Th1 cells. Thus these cells will grow in small exclusive groups, making it possible for the same individual to have both Th1 and Th2 immune responses simultaneously. When the wrong cell (shown in white) arrives at the wrong cluster it will be inhibited. Th0 cells have the option of surviving in both Th1 and Th2 environments.

IFNγ exert similar effects on the expansion of Th1 and Th2 human T-cell clones [113, 114]. Thus these cells will grow in small exclusive groups making it possible for the same individual to make both Th1 and Th2 immune responses simultaneously. When the wrong cell (shown in white) arrives at the wrong cluster it will be inhibited. Th0 cells have the option of surviving in both Th1 and Th2 environments. Th2 not Th1 cells cause asthma [115]. New arrivals will find it very difficult to change the behaviour of established cells (Fig. 7). There are two potential avenues to altering established lung Th2/Tc2 responses. Inhalation of peptides can anergise CD4 T cells *in vivo* [116]. IFNγ blocks eosinophilia and mucus production [117]. IL-12 targeted to the lung can inhibit BHR [118].

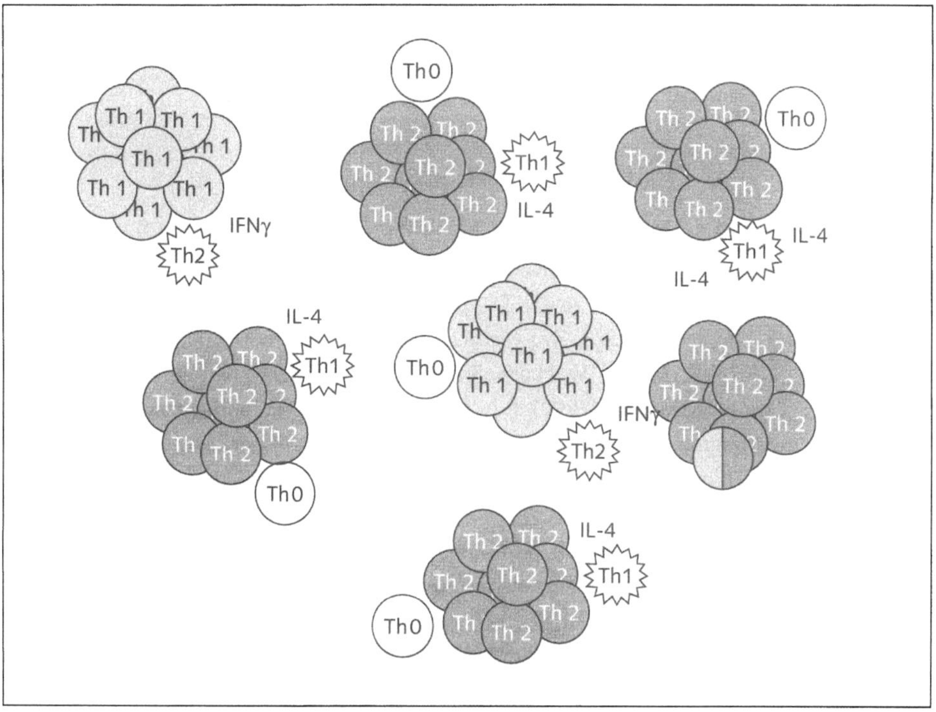

Figure 7
In the lung Th2 CD4 T cells secrete IL-4 and 5 that promote the recruitment and survival of eosinophils that secrete inflammatory molecules. The effects of Th2 cells are antagonized by Th1 CD4 T cells.

T-cell targeted drug therapy

A number of drugs that inhibit T cell function have been effective in treating asthma. In immunotherapy IFNγ goes up [119]. IFNγ reduces airway inflammation and improves lung function [120] but is expensive and may have other side-effects. Cyclosporin A and FK506 have both been shown to reduce Th2 cells in the lung and improve lung function in asthmatic patients [121]. However, the drug of choice is corticosteroid. At the low doses given to asthmatic patients using inhalers it is well tolerated. Interestingly it has comparable effects on Th1 and Th2 cells. In asthmatic patients it reduces Th2 cytokine production [122] while in Sarcoid patients it reduces Th1 cytokine levels and increases IgE and IL-4 concentrations in the BAL [97]. More selective Th2 and Th1 antagonists may yet prove more effective but the long-term safety of corticosteroids and their broad spectrum of anti-inflammatory action make it likely that they will remain the drugs of choice in asthma for many years to come. In mice inhalation of peptide can induce tolerance [116]. Therapy with Allervax Cat (cat peptide) improves tolerance to cats and improves pulmonary function in cat allergic patients with reduced FEV1 [123].

References

1 Gonzalez MC, Diaz P, Galleguillos FR, Ancic P, Cromwell O, Kay AB (1987) Allergen-induced recruitment of bronchoalveolar helper (OKT4) and suppressor (OKT8) T-cells in asthma. Relative increases in OKT8 cells in single early responders compared with those in late-phase responders. *Am Rev Respir Dis* 136 (3): 600–604

2 Frew AJ, Moqbel R, Azzawi M, Hartnell A, Barkans J, Jeffery PK, Kay AB, Scheper RJ, Varley J, Church MK et al (1990) T lymphocytes and eosinophils in allergen-induced late-phase asthmatic reactions in the guinea pig. *Am Rev Respir Dis* 141(2): 407–413

3 Corrigan CJ, Hartnell A, Kay AB (1988) T lymphocyte activation in acute severe asthma. Lancet 1 (8595): 1129–1132

4 Jeffery PK, Wardlaw AJ, Nelson FC, Collins JV, Kay AB (1989) Bronchial biopsies in asthma. An ultrastructural, quantitative study and correlation with hyperreactivity. *Am Rev Respir Dis* 140 (6): 1745–1753

5 Frew AJ, Kay AB (1988) The relationship between infiltrating $CD4^+$ lymphocytes, activated eosinophils, and the magnitude of the allergen-induced late phase cutaneous reaction in man. *J Immunol* 141 (12): 4158–4164

6 Haczku A, Macary P, Huang TJ, Tsukagoshi H, Barnes PJ, Kay AB, Kemeny DM, Chung KF, Moqbel R (1997) Adoptive transfer of allergen-specific $CD4^+$ T cells induces airway inflammation and hyperresponsiveness in brown-Norway rats. *Immunology* 91 (2): 176–185

7 Huang TJ, MacAry PA, Wilke T, Kemeny DM, Chung KF (1999) Inhibitory effects of endogenous and exogenous interferon-gamma on bronchial hyperresponsiveness, allergic inflammation and T-helper 2 cytokines in Brown-Norway rats. *Immunology* 98 (2): 280–288

8 Morel S, Lévy F, Burlet-Schiltz O, Brasseur F, Probst-Kepper M, Peitrequin A-L, Monsarrat B, Van Velthoven R, Cerottini J-C, Boon T, Gairin JE, Van den Eynde BJ (2000) Processing of some antigens by the standard proteasome but not by the immunoproteasome results in poor presentation by dendritic cells. *Immunity* 12: 107–117

9 Kleijmeer MJ, Kelly A, Geuze HJ, Slot JW, Townsend A, Trowsdale J (1992) Location of MHC-encoded transporters in the endoplasmic reticulum and cis-Golgi. *Nature* 357 (6376): 342–344

10 Trowsdale J, Hanson I, Mockridge I, Beck S, Townsend A, Kelly A (1990) Sequences encoded in the class II region of the MHC related to the 'ABC' superfamily of transporters [see comments]. *Nature* 348 (6303): 741–744

11 Powis SJ, Townsend AR, Deverson EV, Bastin J, Butcher GW, Howard JC (1991) Restoration of antigen presentation to the mutant cell line RMA-S by an MHC-linked transporter. *Nature* 354 (6354): 528–531

12 Spies T, Cerundolo V, Colonna M, Cresswell P, Townsend A, DeMars R (1992) Presentation of viral antigen by MHC class I molecules is dependent on a putative peptide transporter heterodimer. *Nature* 355 (6361): 644–646

13 Kelly A, Powis SH, Kerr LA, Mockridge I, Elliott T, Bastin J, Uchanska-Ziegler B, Ziegler A, Trowsdale J, Townsend A (1992) Assembly and function of the two ABC transporter proteins encoded in the human major histocompatibility complex. *Nature* 355 (6361): 641–644

14 Mosmann TR, Cherwinski H, Bond MW, Giedlin MA, Coffman RL (1986) Two types of murine helper T cell clones. 1. Definition according to profiles of lymphokine activities and secreted proteins. *J Immunol* 135: 2348–2357

15 Paliard X, de Waal Malefijt R, Yssel H, Blanchard D, Chretien I, Abrams J, de Vries J, Spits H (1988) Simultaneous production of IL-2, IL-4, and IFN-gamma by activated human CD4+ and CD8+ T cell clones. *J Immunol* 141 (3): 849–855

16 Castro AG, Hauser TM, Cocks BG, Abrams J, Zurawski S, Churakova T, Zonin F, Robinson D, Tangye SG, Aversa G, Nichols KE, de Vries JE, Lanier LL, O'Garra A (1999) Molecular and functional characterization of mouse signaling lymphocytic activation molecule (SLAM): differential expression and responsiveness in Th1 and Th2 cells. *J Immunol* 163 (11): 5860–5870

17 Annunziato F, Manetti R, Tomasevic I, Guidizi MG, Biagiotti R, Gianno V, Germano P, Mavilia C, Maggi E, Romagnani S (1996) Expression and release of LAG-3-encoded protein by human CD4+ T cells are associated with IFN-gamma production. *FASEB J* 10 (7): 769–776

18 Annunziato F, Manetti R, Cosmi L, Galli G, Heusser CH, Romagnani S, Maggi E (1997) Opposite role for interleukin-4 and interferon-γ on CD30 and lymphocyte activation gene-3 (LAG-3) expression by activated naïve T cells. *Eur J Immunol* 27 (9): 2239–2244

19 Xu D, Chan WL, Leung BP, Huang F, Wheeler R, Piedrafita D, Robinson JH, Liew FY (1998) Selective expression of a stable cell surface molecule on type 2 but not type 1 helper T cells. *J Exp Med* 187 (5): 787–794

20 Nakamura T, Lee RK, Nam SY, Al-Ramadi BK, Koni PA, Bottomly K, Podack ER, Flavell RA (1997) Reciprocal regulation of CD30 expression on CD4+ T cells by IL-4 and IFN-γ. *J Immunol* 158 (5): 2090–2098

21 Del Prete G, De Carli M, D'Elios MM, Daniel KC, Almerigogna F, Alderson M, Smith CA, Thomas E, Romagnani S (1995) CD30-mediated signaling promotes the development of human T helper type 2-like T cells. *J Exp Med* 182 (6): 1655–1661

22 Vukmanovic-Stejic M, Vyas B, Gorak-Stolinska P, Noble A, Kemeny DM (2000) Human Tc1 and Tc2/Tc0 CD8 T-cell clones display distinct cell surface and functional phenotypes. *Blood* 95 (1): 231–240

23 Pernis A, Gupta S, Gollob KJ, Garfein E, Coffman RL, Schindler C, Rothman P (1995) Lack of interferon gamma receptor beta chain and the prevention of interferon gamma signaling in TH1 cells [see comments]. *Science* 269 (5221): 245–247

24 Lu B, Ebensperger C, Dembic Z, Wang Y, Kvatyuk M, Lu T, Coffman RL, Pestka S,

Rothman PB (1998) Targeted disruption of the interferon-gamma receptor 2 gene results in severe immune defects in mice. *Proc Natl Acad Sci USA* 95 (14): 8233–8238

25 MacAry PA, Holmes BJ, Kemeny DM (1997) Generation of rat MHC class-I-restricted ovalbumin-specific IgE inhibitory CD8+ T cell clones. *Int Arch Allergy Immunol* 113 (1–3): 279–280

26 MacAry PA, Holmes BJ, Kemeny DM (1998) Ovalbumin-specific, MHC class I-restricted, alpha beta-positive, Tc1 and Tc0 $CD8^+$ T cell clones mediate the *in vivo* inhibition of rat IgE. *J Immunol* 160 (2): 580–587

27 McMenamin C, Holt PG (1993) The natural immune response to inhaled soluble protein antigens involves major histocompatibility complex (MHC) class I-restricted $CD8^+$ T cell-mediated but MHC class II-restricted $CD4^+$ T cell-dependent immune deviation resulting in selective suppression of immunoglobulin E production. *J Exp Med* 178 (3): 889–899

28 McMenamin C, McKersey M, Kuhnlein P, Hunig T, Holt PG (1995) Gamma delta T cells down-regulate primary IgE responses in rats to inhaled soluble protein antigens. *J Immunol* 154 (9): 4390–4394

29 Miller A, Lider O, Roberts AB, Sporn MB, Weiner HL (1992) Suppressor T cells generated by oral tolerization to myelin basic protein suppress both *in vitro* and *in vivo* immune responses by the release of transforming growth factor beta after antigen-specific triggering. *Proc Natl Acad Sci USA* 89(1): 421–425

30 Fukaura H, Kent SC, Pietrusewicz MJ, Khoury SJ, Weiner HL, Hafler DA (1996) Induction of circulating myelin basic protein and proteolipid protein-specific transforming growth factor-β 1-secreting Th3 T cells by oral administration of myelin in multiple sclerosis patients. *J Clin Invest* 98(1): 70–77

31 Strober W, Kelsall B, Fuss I, Marth T, Ludviksson B, Ehrhardt R, Neurath M (1997) Reciprocal IFN-γ and TGF-β responses regulate the occurrence of mucosal inflammation. *Immunol Today* 18 (2): 61–64

32 Marth T, Strober W, Kelsall BL (1996) High dose oral tolerance in ovalbumin TCR-transgenic mice: systemic neutralization of IL-12 augments TGF-β secretion and T cell apoptosis. *J Immunol* 157 (6): 2348–2357

33 Groux H, O'Garra A, Bigler M, Rouleau M, Antonenko S, de Vries JE, Roncarolo MG (1997) A $CD4^+$ T-cell subset inhibits antigen-specific T-cell responses and prevents colitis. *Nature* 389: 737–742

34 Cavani A, Nasorri F, Prezzi C, Sebastiani S, Albanesi C, Girolomoni G (2000) Human $CD4^+$ T lymphocytes with remarkable regulatory functions on dendritic cells and nickel-specific Th1 immune responses. *J Invest Dermatol* 114 (2): 295–302

35 Powrie F, Leach MW, Mauze S, Menon S, Caddle LB, Coffman RL (1994) Inhibition of Th1 responses prevents inflammatory bowel disease in scid mice reconstituted with CD45RBhi $CD4^+$ T cells. *Immunity* 1 (7): 553–562

36 Asseman C, Mauze S, Leach MW, Coffman RL, Powrie F (1999) An essential role for interleukin 10 in the function of regulatory T cells that inhibit intestinal inflammation. *J Exp Med* 190 (7): 995–1004

37 Powrie F, Correa-Oliveira R, Mauze S, Coffman RL (1994) Regulatory interactions between CD45RB^{high} and CD45RB^{low} CD4^{+} T cells are important for the balance between protective and pathogenic cell-mediated immunity. *J Exp Med* 179 (2): 589–600
38 Leach MW, Bean AG, Mauze S, Coffman RL, Powrie F (1996) Inflammatory bowel disease in C.B-17 scid mice reconstituted with the CD45RB^{high} subset of CD4^{+} T cells. *Am J Pathol* 148(5): 1503–1515
39 Read S, Mauze S, Asseman C, Bean A, Coffman R, Powrie F (1998) CD38^{+} CD45RB(low) CD4^{+} T cells: a population of T cells with immune regulatory activities *in vitro*. *Eur J Immunol* 28 (11): 3435–3447
40 Neurath MF, Fuss I, Kelsall BL, Presky DH, Waegell W, Strober W (1996) Experimental granulomatous colitis in mice is abrogated by induction of TGF-β-mediated oral tolerance. *J Exp Med* 183 (6): 2605–2616
41 Lepault F, Gagnerault MC (2000) Characterization of peripheral regulatory CD4+ T cells that prevent diabetes onset in nonobese diabetic mice. *J Immunol* 164 (1): 240–247
42 Maggi E, Del Prete G, Macchia D, Parronchi P, Tiri A, Chretien I, Ricci M, Romagnani S (1988) Profiles of lymphokine activities and helper function for IgE in human T cell clones. *Eur J Immunol* 18 (7): 1045–1050
43 Del Prete G, Tiri A, Maggi E, De Carli M, Macchia D, Parronchi P, Rossi ME, Pietrogrande MC, Ricci M, Romagnani S (1989) Defective *in vitro* production of gamma-interferon and tumor necrosis factor-alpha by circulating T cells from patients with the hyper-immunoglobulin E syndrome. *J Clin Invest* 84(6): 1830–1835
44 Wierenga EA, Snoek M, De Groot C, Chretien I, Bos JD, Jansen HM, Kapsenberg ML (1990) Evidence for compartmentalization of functional subsets of CD4(+) T lymphocytes in atopic patients. *J Immunol* 144 (12): 4651–4656
45 Parronchi P, Macchia D, Piccinni MP, Biswas P, Simonelli C, Maggi E, Ricci M, Ansari AA, Romagnani S (1991) Allergen- and bacterial antigen-specific T-cell clones established from atopic donors show a different profile of cytokine production. *Proc Natl Acad Sci USA* 88 (10): 4538–4542
46 Del Prete GF, De Carli M, Ricci M, Romagnani S (1991) Helper activity for immunoglobulin synthesis of T helper type 1 (Th1) and Th2 human T cell clones: the help of Th1 clones is limited by their cytolytic capacity. *J Exp Med* 174 (4): 809–813
47 Parronchi P, De Carli M, Manetti R, Simonelli C, Piccinni MP, Macchia D, Maggi E, Del Prete G, Ricci M, Romagnani S (1992) Aberrant interleukin (IL)-4 and IL-5 production *in vitro* by CD4^{+} helper T cells from atopic subjects. *Eur J Immunol* 22 (6): 1615–1620
48 Wierenga EA, Snoek M, Jansen HM, Bos JD, Van Lier RAW, Kapsenberg ML (1991) Human atopen-specific types 1 and 2 T helper cell clones. *J Immunol* 147 (9): 2942–2949
49 Swain SL, Weinberg AD, English M, Huston G (1990) IL-4 directs the development of Th2-like helper effectors. *J Immunol* 145 (11): 3796–3806
50 Noble A, Macary PA, Kemeny DM (1995) IFN-gamma and IL-4 regulate the growth

and differentiation of CD8+ T cells into subpopulations with distinct cytokine profiles. *J Immunol* 155 (6): 2928–2937

51 Maggi E, Del Prete G, Macchia D, Parronchi P, Tiri A, Chretien I, Ricci M, Romagnani S (1988) Profiles of lymphokine activities and helper function for IgE in human T cell clones. *Eur J Immunol* 18 (7): 1045–1050

52 Gajewski TF, Joyce J, Fitch FW (1989) Antiproliferative effect of IFN-gamma in immune regulation. III. Differential selection of TH1 and TH2 murine helper T lymphocyte clones using recombinant IL-2 and recombinant IFN-γ. *J Immunol* 143 (1): 15–22

53 Swain SL, Huston G, Tonkonogy S, Weinberg A (1991) Transforming growth factor-β and IL-4 cause helper T cell precursors to develop into distinct effector helper cells that differ in lymphokine secretion pattern and cell surface phenotype. *J Immunol* 147 (9): 2991–3000

54 Powrie F, Menon S, Coffman RL (1993) Interleukin-4 and interleukin-10 synergize to inhibit cell-mediated immunity *in vivo*. *Eur J Immunol* 23 (11): 3043–3049

55 Kamogawa Y, Minasi LA, Carding SR, Bottomly K, Flavell RA (1993) The relationship of IL-4- and IFN-γ-producing T cells studied by lineage ablation of IL-4-producing cells. *Cell* 75 (5): 985–995

56 Manetti R, Gerosa F, Giudizi MG, Biagiotti R, Parronchi P, Piccinni MP, Sampognaro S, Maggi E, Romagnani S, Trinchieri G et al (1994) Interleukin-12 induces stable priming for interferon gamma (IFN-γ) production during differentiation of human T helper (Th) cells and transient IFN-γ production in established Th2 cell clones. *J Exp Med* 179 (4): 1273–1283

57 Hosken NA, Shibuya K, Heath AW, Murphy KM, O'Garra A (1995) The effect of antigen dose on CD4+ T helper cell phenotype development in a T cell receptor-alpha beta-transgenic model. *J Exp Med* 182 (5): 1579–1584

58 Diaz-Sanchez D, Kemeny DM (1990) The sensitivity of rat CD8+ and CD4+ T cells to ricin *in vivo* and *in vitro* and their relationship to IgE regulation. *Immunology* 69 (1): 71–77

59 Jarrett EEE, Hall E (1984) The development of IgE-suppressive immunocompetence in young animals: Influence of exposure to antigen in the presence or absence of maternal immunity. *Immunology* 53 (2): 365–373

60 Holt PG, Rose AH, Batty JE, Turner KJ (1981) Induction of adjuvant-independent IgE responses in inbred mice: primary, secondary, and persistent IgE responses to ovalbumin and ovomucoid. *Int Arch Allergy Appl Immunol* 65 (1): 42–50

61 Vaz EM, Vaz NM, Levine BB (1971) Persistent formation of reagins in mice injected with low doses of ovalbumin. *Immunology* 21: 11–15

62 Constant S, Pfeiffer C, Woodard A, Pasqualini T, Bottomly K (1995) Extent of T cell receptor ligation can determine the functional differentiation of naive CD4+ T cells. *J Exp Med* 182 (5): 1591–1596

63 Tao X, Grant C, Constant S, Bottomly K (1997) Induction of IL-4-producing CD4+ T cells by antigenic peptides altered for TCR binding. *J Immunol* 158 (9): 4237–4244

64 Tao X, Constant S, Jorritsma P, Bottomly K (1997) Strength of TCR signal determines

the costimulatory requirements for Th1 and Th2 CD4+ T cell differentiation. *J Immunol* 159 (12): 5956–5963

65 Leitenberg D, Boutin Y, Constant S, Bottomly K (1998) CD4 regulation of TCR signaling and T cell differentiation following stimulation with peptides of different affinities for the TCR. *J Immunol* 161 (3): 1194–1203

66 Noble A, Vyas B, Vuckmanovic-Stejic M, Kemeny DM (2000) The balance of calcium and protein kinase c signalling directs T cell subset development. *J Immunol* 164: 1807–1813

67 Boutin Y, Leitenberg D, Tao X, Bottomly K (1997) Distinct biochemical signals characterize agonist- and altered peptide ligand-induced differentiation of naïve CD4+ T cells into Th1 and Th2 subsets. *J Immunol* 159 (12): 5802–5809

68 Croft M, Carter L, Swain SL, Dutton RW (1994) Generation of polarized antigen-specific CD8 effector populations: reciprocal action of IL-4 and IL-12 in promoting type 2 versus type 1 cytokine profiles. *J Exp Med* 180 (5): 1715–1728

69 Cronin DN, Stack R, Fitch FW (1995) IL-4-producing CD8+ T cell clones can provide B cell help. *J Immunol* 154 (7): 3118–3127

70 Sad S, Marcotte R, Mosmann TR (1995) Cytokine-induced differentiation of precursor mouse CD8+ T cells into cytotoxic CD8+ T cells secreting Th1 or Th2 cytokines. *Immunity* 2 (3): 271–279

71 Gerosa F, Paganin C, Peritt D, Paiola F, Scupoli MT, Aste-Amezaga M, Frank I, Trinchieri G (1996) Interleukin-12 primes human CD4 and CD8 T cell clones for high production of both interferon-gamma and interleukin-10. *J Exp Med* 183 (6): 2559–2569

72 Cerwenka A, Carter LL, Reome JB, Swain SL, Dutton RW (1998) *In vivo* persistence of CD8 polarized T cell subsets producing type 1 or type 2 cytokines. *J Immunol* 161 (1): 97–105

73 Okumura K, Takemori T, Tokuhisa T, Tada T (1977) Specific enrichment of the suppressor T cell bearing I-J determinants: parallel functional and serological characterizations. *J Exp Med* 146 (5): 1234–1245

74 Okumura KO, Tada T (1971) Regulation of homocytotrophic antibody formation in the rat. III. effect of thymectomy and splenectomy. *J Immunol* 106: 1019–1026

75 Okumura KO, Tada T (1971) Regulation of homocytotrophic antibody formation in the rat. IV. Inhibitory effect of thymocytes on the homocytotrophic antibody response. *J Immunol* 107: 1682–1689

76 Katz DH, Bargatze RF, Bogowitz CA, Katz LR (1980) Regulation of IgE antibody production by serum molecules. VII. The IgE-selective damping activity of suppressive factor of allergy (SFA) is exerted across both strain and species restriction barriers. *J Immunol* 124 (2): 819–824

77 Ishizaka K (1988) IgE-binding factors and regulation of the IgE antibody response. *Ann Rev Immunol* 6: 513–534

78 Coffman RL, Ohara J, Bond MW, Carty J, Zlotnik A, Paul WE (1986) B cell stimulato-

ry factor-1 enhances the IgE response of lipopolysaccharide-activated B cells. *J Immunol* 136 (12): 4538–4541
79 Snapper CM, Paul WE (1987) Interferon-γ and B cell stimulatory factor-1 reciprocally regulate Ig isotype production. *Science* 236: 944–947
80 Punnonen J, Aversa G, Cocks BG, McKenzie ANJ, Menon S, Zurawski G, De Waal-Malefyt R, De Vries JE (1993) Interleukin 13 induces interleukin 4-independent IgG4 and IgE synthesis and CD23 expression by human B cells. *Proc Natl Acad Sci USA* 90 (8): 3730–3734
81 Corrigan CJ, Kay AB (1990) CD4 T-lymphocyte activation in acute severe asthma. Relationship to disease severity and atopic status. *Am Rev Respir Dis* 141 (4 Pt 1): 970–977
82 Robinson DS, Hamid Q, Ying S, Tsicopoulos A, Barkans J, Bentley AM, Corrigan C, Durham SR, Kay AB (1992) Predominant TH2-like bronchoalveolar T-lymphocyte population in atopic asthma. *N Engl J Med* 326 (5): 298–304
83 Moser R, Fehr J, Bruijnzeel PL (1992) IL-4 controls the selective endothelium-driven transmigration of eosinophils from allergic individuals. *J Immunol* 149 (4): 1432–1438
84 Foster PS, Hogan SP, Ramsay AJ, Matthaei KI, Young IG (1996) Interleukin 5 deficiency abolishes eosinophilia, airways hyperreactivity, and lung damage in a mouse asthma model [see comments]. *J Exp Med* 183 (1): 195–201
85 DiCosmo BF, Geba GP, Picarella D, Elias JA, Rankin JA, Stripp BR, Whitsett JA, Flavell RA (1994) Airway epithelial cell expression of interleukin-6 in transgenic mice. Uncoupling of airway inflammation and bronchial hyperreactivity. *J Clin Invest* 94 (5): 2028–2035
86 Ray P, Tang W, Wang P, Homer R, Kuhn C, 3rd, Flavell RA, Elias JA (1997) Regulated overexpression of interleukin 11 in the lung. Use to dissociate development-dependent and -independent phenotypes. *J Clin Invest* 100 (10): 2501–2511
87 Zhu Z, Homer RJ, Wang Z, Chen Q, Geba GP, Wang J, Zhang Y, Elias JA (1999) Pulmonary expression of interleukin-13 causes inflammation, mucus hypersecretion, subepithelial fibrosis, physiologic abnormalities, and eotaxin production. *J Clin Invest* 103 (6): 779–788
88 Hallsworth MP, Soh CP, Lane SJ, Arm JP, Lee TH (1994) Selective enhancement of GM-CSF, TNF-alpha, IL-1 beta and IL-8 production by monocytes and macrophages of asthmatic subjects. *Eur Respir J* 7 (6): 1096–1102
89 Sousa AR, Lams BE, Pfister R, Christie PE, Schmitz M, Lee TH (1997) Expression of interleukin-5 and granulocyte-macrophage colony-stimulating factor in aspirin-sensitive and non-aspirin-sensitive asthmatic airways. *Am J Respir Crit Care Med* 156 (5): 1384–1389
90 Caulfield JJ, Hawrylowicz CM, Kemeny DM, Lee TH (1997) GM-CSF increases the ability of cultured macrophages to support autologous $CD4^+$ T-cell proliferation in response to *Dermatophagoides pteronyssinus* and PPD antigen. *Immunology* 92 (1): 123–130
91 Wilson SB, Kent SC, Patton KT, Orban T, Jackson RA, Exley M, Porcelli S, Schatz DA,

Atkinson MA, Balk SP, Strominger JL, Hafler DA (1998) Extreme Th1 bias of invariant Valpha24JalphaQ T cells in type 1 diabetes. *Nature* 391 (6663): 177–181
92 Gattorno M, Facchetti P, Ghiotto F, Vignola S, Buoncompagni A, Prigione I, Picco P, Pistoia V (1997) Synovial fluid T cell clones from oligoarticular juvenile arthritis patients display a prevalent Th1/Th0-type pattern of cytokine secretion irrespective of immunophenotype. *Clin Exp Immunol* 109 (1): 4–11
93 Mauri C, Chu CQ, Woodrow D, Mori L, Londei M (1997) Treatment of a newly established transgenic model of chronic arthritis with nondepleting anti-CD4 monoclonal antibody. *J Immunol* 159 (10): 5032–5041
94 Pearson CI, van Ewijk W, McDevitt HO (1997) Induction of apoptosis and T helper 2 (Th2) responses correlates with peptide affinity for the major histocompatibility complex in self-reactive T cell receptor transgenic mice. *J Exp Med* 185 (4): 583–599
95 Lai CK, Ho S, Chan CH, Chan J, Choy D, Leung R, Lai KN (1997) Cytokine gene expression profile of circulating CD4+ T cells in active pulmonary tuberculosis. *Chest* 111 (3): 606–611
96 Zhu X, Venkataprasad N, Thangaraj HS, Hill M, Singh M, Ivanyi J, Vordermeier HM (1997) Functions and specificity of T cells following nucleic acid vaccination of mice against Mycobacterium tuberculosis infection. *J Immunol* 158 (12): 5921–5926
97 Milburn HJ, Poulter LW, Dilmec A, Cochrane GM, Kemeny DM (1997) Corticosteroids restore the balance between locally produced Th1 and Th2 cytokines and immunoglobulin isotypes to normal in sarcoid lung. *Clin Exp Immunol* 108 (1): 105–113
98 Oshiba A, Hamelmann E, Takeda K, Bradley KL, Loader JE, Larsen GL, Gelfand EW (1996) Passive transfer of immediate hypersensitivity and airway hyperresponsiveness by allergen-specific immunoglobulin (Ig) E and IgG1 in mice. *J Clin Invest* 97 (6): 1398–1408
99 Xu LJ, Eidelman DH, Bates JH, Martin JG (1990) Late response of the upper airway of the rat to inhaled antigen. *J Appl Physiol* 69 (4): 1360–1365
100 Du T, Sapienza S, Eidelman DH, Wang NS, Martin JG (1991) Morphometry of the airways during late responses to antigen challenge in the rat. *Am Rev Respir Dis* 143 (1): 132–137
101 Elwood W, Sakamoto T, Barnes PJ, Chung KF (1993) Allergen-induced airway hyperresponsiveness in Brown-Norway rat: role of parasympathetic mechanisms. *J Appl Physiol* 75(1): 279–284
102 Renz H, Smith HR, Henson JE, Ray BS, Irvin CG, Gelfand EW (1992) Aerosolized antigen exposure without adjuvant causes increased IgE production and increased airway responsiveness in the mouse. *J Allergy Clin Immunol* 89(6): 1127–1138
103 Haczku A, Macary P, Haddad EB, Huang TJ, Kemeny DM, Moqbel R, Chung KF (1996) Expression of Th-2 cytokines interleukin-4 and -5 and of Th-1 cytokine interferon-gamma in ovalbumin-exposed sensitized Brown-Norway rats. *Immunology* 88 (2): 247–251
104 Haczku A, Macary P, Haddad EB, Huang T-J, Kemeny DM, Chung KF, Moqbel R

(1997) Adoptive transfer of airway hyperresponsiveness with CD4+ and CD8+ T cells in Brown-Norway rats sensitised and exposed to ovalbumin. *Immunology* 91: 176–185
105 Hansen G, Berry G, DeKruyff RH, Umetsu DT (1999) Allergen-specific Th1 cells fail to counterbalance Th2 cell-induced airway hyperreactivity but cause severe airway inflammation. *J Clin Invest* 103 (2): 175–183
106 Hogan SP, Mould A, Kikutani H, Ramsay AJ, Foster PS (1997) Aeroallergen-induced eosinophilic inflammation, lung damage, and airways hyperreactivity in mice can occur independently of IL-4 and allergen-specific immunoglobulins. *J Clin Invest* 99 (6): 1329–1339
107 Carter LL, Dutton RW (1995) Relative perforin- and Fas-mediated lysis in T1 and T2 CD8 effector populations. *J Immunol* 155 (3): 1028–1031
108 Gonzalez MC, Diaz P, Galleguillos FR, Ancic P, Cromwell O, Kay AB (1987) Allergen-induced recruitment of bronchoalveolar helper (OKT4) and suppressor (OKT8) T-cells in asthma. Relative increases in OKT8 cells in single early responders compared with those in late-phase responders. *Am Rev Respir Dis* 136 (3): 600–604
109 Seder RA, Boulay JL, Finkelman F, Barbier S, Ben-Sasson SZ, Le Gros G, Paul WE (1992) CD8+ T cells can be primed *in vitro* to produce IL-4. *J Immunol* 148 (6): 1652–1656
110 Salgame P, Abrams JS, Clayberger C, Goldstein H, Convit J, Modlin RL, Bloom BR (1991) Differing lymphokine profiles of functional subsets of human CD4 and CD8 T cell clones. *Science* 254 (5029): 279–282
111 Hamelmann E, Oshiba A, Paluh J, Bradley K, Loader J, Potter TA, Larsen GL, Gelfand EW (1996) Requirement for CD8+ T cells in the development of airway hyperresponsiveness in a marine model of airway sensitization. *J Exp Med* 183 (4): 1719–1729
112 Coyle AJ, Erard F, Bertrand C, Walti S, Pircher H, Le Gros G (1995) Virus-specific CD8+ cells can switch to interleukin 5 production and induce airway eosinophilia. *J Exp Med* 181 (3): 1229–1233
113 Maggi E, Parronchi P, Manetti R, Simonelli C, Piccinni MP, Rugiu FS, De Carli M, Ricci M, Romagnani S (1992) Reciprocal regulatory effects of IFN-γ and IL-4 on the *in vitro* development of human Th1 and Th2 clones. *J Immunol* 148 (7): 2142–2147
114 Parronchi P, De Carli M, Manetti R, Simonelli C, Sampognaro S, Piccinni MP, Macchia D, Maggi E, Del Prete G, Romagnani S (1992) IL-4 and IFN (alpha and gamma) exert opposite regulatory effects on the development of cytolytic potential by Th1 or Th2 human T cell clones. *J Immunol* 149 (9): 2977–2983
115 Cohn L, Tepper JS, Bottomly K (1998) IL-4-independent induction of airway hyperresponsiveness by Th2, but not Th1, cells. *J Immunol* 161 (8): 3813–3816
116 Tsitoura DC, DeKruyff RH, Lamb JR, Umetsu DT (1999) Intranasal exposure to protein antigen induces immunological tolerance mediated by functionally disabled CD4+ T cells. *J Immunol* 163 (5): 2592–2600
117 Cohn L, Homer RJ, Niu N, Bottomly K (1999) T helper 1 cells and interferon gamma regulate allergic airway inflammation and mucus production. *J Exp Med* 190 (9): 1309–1318

118 Hogan SP, Foster PS, Tan X, Ramsay AJ (1998) Mucosal IL-12 gene delivery inhibits allergic airways disease and restores local antiviral immunity. *Eur J Immunol* 28 (2): 413–423
119 Durham SR, Ying S, Varney VA, Jacobson MR, Sudderick RM, Mackay IS, Kay AB, Hamid QA (1996) Grass pollen immunotherapy inhibits allergen-induced infiltration of $CD4^+$ T lymphocytes and eosinophils in the nasal mucosa and increases the number of cells expressing messenger RNA for interferon-gamma. *J Allergy Clin Immunol* 97 (6): 1356–1365
120 Lack G, Renz H, Saloga J, Bradley KL, Loader J, Leung DY, Larsen G, Gelfand EW (1994) Nebulized but not parenteral IFN-γ decreases IgE production and normalizes airways function in a murine model of allergen sensitization. *J Immunol* 152 (5): 2546–2554
121 Sihra BS, Kon OM, Durham SR, Walker S, Barnes NC, Kay AB (1997) Effect of cyclosporin A on the allergen-induced late asthmatic reaction. *Thorax* 52 (5): 447–452
122 Kay AB (1994) Immunosuppressive agents in chronic severe asthma. *Allergy Proc* 15 (3): 147–150
123 Maguire P, Nicodemus C, Robinson D, Aaronson D, Umetsu DT (1999) The safety and efficacy of ALLERVAX CAT in cat allergic patients. *Clin Immunol* 93 (3): 222–231

Index

actin 267
activation, biomechanical 228
adenosine 91, 278
adenylate cyclase 102
adhesion 138
adhesion, firm 232
adhesion, neutrophil 133
adhesion-dependent activation 229
adhesion molecule 254, 313
adhesion molecule, endothelial 223, 230
adhesion molecule-1 (sICAM-1), soluble intercellular 251
ADP 89
β-adrenoceptor 274, 279, 282
β-agonist 273
airway epithelial cell 245
airway epithelium 245
airway hyperresponsiveness 247, 283
airways inflammation 79, 135, 247
airway smooth muscle hyperplasia 286
airway wall remodelling 284
airway, structure of 159
allergic inflammation, basophil, role in 65
allergic rhinitis 250
angiotensin-converting enzyme (ACE) 254
antigen, HLA class II 255
antigen, HLA-DR 255
antigen, MHC II 255
antigen presentation, dendritic cell 208, 212
antigen presenting cell, fibroblast 172
anti-inflammatory agent, modulation of fibroblast function by 177
anti-inflammatory and relaxing mediator 247
antiplatelet agent 110
anti-protease 137, 140
apoptosis 126, 134
arachidonic acid metabolism 87, 249
asthma 12, 135, 168, 249, 250
asthma, airway remodelling in 168

basal cell 245
basement membrane 3, 16, 161
basophil, activation of 57
basophil, adhesion molecule 54–57
basophil, chemokine release 63
basophil, cytokine release 63
basophil, detection in airway mucosa 53
basophil, granule content 60
basophil, growth factor 54
basophil, heparin release 61
basophil, histamine release 58, 60
basophil, immunoglobulin 57, 65
basophil, lipid metabolism 61, 62
basophil, release product 61–64
basophil, role in allergic inflammation 65
basophil, role in viral and bacterial immunity 66
biglycan 165
biomechanical activation 228
bradykinin 283
bronchial epithelial cell 248
bronchial hyperresponsiveness, effect of PDE inhibitors 309

bronchial hyperresponsiveness, major basic protein 149
bronchial smooth muscle 17
bronchiole, structure of 159
bronchiolitis 33
bronchitis 26

calcium ($Ca^{2+}{}_i$), intracellular free, smooth muscle tone 271
carboxypeptidase N (CPN) 254
cell activation, endothelial 223
cell activation inhibitor 316
cetirizine 314
CD44, basophil function 56
CD4T cell 333
CD8T cell 333
CDP840 308
chemoattractant for eosinophil 249
chemokinesis, macrophage 202
chemotaxin 132
chemotaxis of fibroblasts 171
chronic obstructive pulmonary disease (COPD) 31, 135, 173
cilia 246
ciliated columnar epithelium 245
cNOS 248
coagulation cascade product 168
collagen 163
collagen, type I 161
collagen, type III 161
collagen, type IV 161
cuboidal epithelium 245
cyclic AMP (cAMP) 271, 272
cyclic AMP, dendritic cell 214
cyclic AMP, macrophage 207
cyclic GMP (cGMP) 271
cyclin D1 288
cyclin-dependent kinase 4 (CdK4) 288
cyclooxygenase 80, 280
cyclooxygenase inhibitor 282
cysteinyl leukotriene 310
cytokine 279, 336
cytokine, fibroblast activation by 168
cytokine, basophil function 59
cytokine, endothelial-activating 226
cytokine, inflammatory 250
cytokine release, eosinophil 149

decorin 165
degradation, extracellular collagen 167
degradation, intracellular collagen 167
dendritic cell, accessory molecule 209
dendritic cell, antigen presentation 208, 212
dendritic cell, cyclic AMP 214
dendritic cell, glucocorticosteroid 213
dendritic cell, immunoglobulin 211
dendritic cell, major histocompatibility complex 212, 213
dendritic cell, neuropeptide 214
dendritic cell, recruitment 211
development, role of fibroblast in airway 166
disodium cromoglycate (DSCG) 305

elastic recoil, of lung tissue 174
elastin 163
emphysema 35
endothelial, activation 223, 226
endothelial adhesion molecule 223, 230
endothelial cell, structure 223
endothelial P- and E-selectin 230
endothelial permeability 223, 235
endothelial-activating cytokine 226
endothelial-derived vasodilator 223
endothelin 49
eosinophil, bronchial hyperresponsiveness 153
eosinophil, cell recruitment 152
eosinophil, chemokine 152
eosinophil, chemoattractant for 249
eosinophil, cytokine release 149
eosinophil, eotaxin 152
eosinophil, granule product 147
eosinophil, IL-5 151, 154
eosinophil, immune function 150

eosinophilia, effect of PDE4 inhibitors 308
eotaxin 152, 312
eotaxin, eosinophil 152
epinephrine 90
epithelial cell, bronchial 248
epithelium 2, 3, 14, 279
epithelium, ciliated columnar 245
excitatory non-adrenergic, non-choligergic nerve (eNANC) 275
extracellular collagen, degradation 167
extracellular matrix (ECM), structural components of 263, 282
extracellular matrix production, by fibroblasts and myofibroblasts 168
extracellular-regulated protein kinase 272, 287

FcεRI 311
FcεRII (CD23) 311
fibrinopeptide 171
fibroblast 159
fibroblast activation, polypeptide growth factor 168
fibroblast, airways morphogenesis 166
fibroblast, airway remodelling 159
fibroblast, as antigen presenting cell 172
fibroblast, chemotaxis of 171
fibroblast, development, role of in airway 166
fibroblast, proliferation of 171
fibronectin 161
fibrosing alveolitis (FA) 40
fibrosis 168

G protein 100
G protein-coupled receptor 86
G-CSF 250
glucocorticoid 281
glucocorticosteroid, dendritic cell 213
glucocorticosteroid, effects in asthma 303
glucocorticosteroid, macrophage 207
glucocorticosteroid, mechanism of action 304
glypican 165
GM-CSF 250, 341
GM-CSF, dendritic cell function 211–213
GM-CSF, macrophage function 203
goblet cell 246
granulocyte macrophage-colony stimulating factor (GM-CSF) 170
growth factor 286
growth factor, basophil 54
GTP-binding protein 100

H_1 receptor antagonist 314
haemostasis 79
heparin, effect on inflammation 312
histamine 271, 275
histamine receptor 278
histamine, release from basophil 58, 60
hyperplasia, airway smooth muscle 286
hyperresponsiveness, airway 247, 283
hyperresponsiveness, bronchial, effect of PDE inhibitors 309
hyperresponsiveness bronchial, eosinophil 153
hypoxia, activation of fibroblasts by 172

IFNγ 344
IgE 311, 339
IgE-mediated inflammation 333
IL-1, macrophage function 202, 206
IL-1β 250, 273
IL-3 250
IL-3, basophil function 54, 58
IL-4, dendritic cell function 211, 213
IL-4, macrophage function 203
IL-4, synthesis in basophil 64
IL-4, synthesis in mast cell 64
IL-5 151, 154
IL-5, eosinophil 151, 154
IL-6 250
IL-8 250
IL-10, dendritic cell function 210, 211
IL-10, macrophage function 203, 206
IL-12, dendritic cell function 210
IL-13, macrophage function 203

IL-13, release from basophil 64
IL-13, release from mast cells 64
IL-16 250
immune T cell 333
immunoglobulin 81
immunoglobulin, basophil 57, 65
immunoglobulin, dendritic cell 211
immunoglobulin superfamily 254
immunoproteosome 333
immunotherapy 344
inducible nitric oxide synthase (iNOS) 248, 277
inflammation, lung 341
inflammation, neurogenic 279
inflammation, platelet 105
inflammatory cell 6, 21
inflammatory cytokine 250
inflammatory mediator 247
inhibition, phosphodiesterase, macrophage 207
inhibition, PDE4 308
inhibitor, cell activation 316
inhibitor, cyclooxygenase 282
inhibitory non-adrenergic, non-cholinergic nerve (iNANC) 275
inositol 1,4,5-triphosphate (IP_3) 271
insulin-like growth factor (IGF) 287
integrin 81, 254
integrin, β_1 254
integrin, $\beta_1\alpha_{2-6}$ 254
integrin β_2, basophil function 55, 56
intercellular adhesion molecule-1 (ICAM-1) 227, 232, 255, 313
intercellular adhesion molecule-2 (ICAM-2) 232
intercellular adhesion molecule, basophil 56
interdependence 174
inter-endothelial junction 225
interferon, dendritic cell function 210
interferon, macrophage function 202
intracellular free calcium ($Ca^{2+}{}_i$), smooth muscle tone 271
intracellular collagen, degradation 167
ischemic cardiovascular disorder 79

ketotifen 315
kinase, extracellular-regulated protein 272, 287

lamina reticularis 159
laminin 161
leukocyte chemoattractant 223, 233
leukocyte emigration 223
leukotriene (LT) 277
leukotriene (Cys LT) receptor antagonist 280
leukotriene, cysteinyl 310
LFA-1 313
lipid mediator 168
lipid metabolism, basophil 61, 62
LTB_4 249
LTC_4 249
LTD_4 249
LTE_4 249
lung inflammation 341
lung tissue, elastic recoil of 174
lysosome 93

macrophage, activation 202
macrophage, antigen presentation 206
macrophage, arachidonic acid metabolite 204
macrophage, chemokinesis 202
macrophage, cyclic AMP 207
macrophage, cytokine release 202, 203
macrophage, glucocorticosteroid 207
macrophage, migration 204
macrophage, oxygen radical 205
macrophage, phagocytosis 205
macrophage, phosphodiesterase inhibition 207
macrophage, turnover 201
major basic protein, bronchial hyper-responsiveness 149
major basic protein, pharmacology 148, 149
mast cell 170
mast cell deficient 66
major histocompatibility complex, dendritic cell 212, 213
matrix metalloproteinase 287
MCP-1 250

mechanical load, airway 171
metalloproteinase 167
metalloproteinase, matrix 287
methacholine 283
microvilli 246
MIP-1α, expression in basophil 64
mitogen-activated protein kinase (MAPK) 272
mucociliary clearance 246
mucosa 1
mucus 17
muscarinic cholinoceptor 273
myofibroblast 159
myosin light-chain kinase (MLCK) 267
myosin 267

NADPH oxidase 130
nedocromil sodium 305
nerve 23
neurogenic inflammation 279
neurokinin A 278
neurokinin-1 (NK1) receptor 276
neurokinin-2 (NK2) receptor 276
neurokinin-1 (NK1) receptor antagonist 276
neurokinin-2 (NK2) receptor antagonist 276
neuropeptide Y (NPY) 273
neuropeptide, dendritic cell 214
neutral endopeptidase (NEP) 254
neutrophil adhesion 133
neutrophil granule content 127
neutrophil migration 132
neutrophil priming 132
nidogen (entactin) 161
nitric oxide (NO) 248, 271, 273, 275
nitric oxide synthase (NOS) 248
non-asthmatic subject 250

oxygen radical, macrophage 205

PDE4 inhibitor, rolipram 308
peptide 333
perennial allergic rhinitis 255
perlecan 161
PGD_2 249
$PGF_{2\alpha}$ 249
phagocytosis, macrophage 205
phenotype 337
phosphodiesterase (PDE), inhibition of 272
phosphoinositol-3-kinase 288
phospholipase A_2, basophil 62
phospholipase 89
phospholipase C 271
phospholipid-derived mediator 276
platelet 79
platelet activating factor (PAF) 86, 277
platelet activating factor, basophil 56
platelet adhesion 93
platelet aggregation 96
platelet, airways 107
platelet, inflammation 105
platelet migration 99
platelet, shape change 95
polypeptide growth factor, fibroblast activator by 168
potassium channel, ATP-sensitive 272
potassium channel, calcium-activated 272, 273
priming, neutrophil 132
proliferation, of fibroblasts 171
prostacyclin 277
prostaglandin (and sub-types) 276
prostaglandin E_2 (PGE_2) 271
prostaglandin E_2 (PGE_2), dendritic cell function 271
protease-activated receptor (PAR) 286
protective mediator 252
protein kinase A (PKA) 271, 272
protein kinase C (PKC) 272
proteosome 333

RANTES 152, 250
receptor, G protein-coupled 86
retinoblastoma protein (pRb) 287
rhinitic subject 250
rhinitis 8, 250
rhinitis, allergic 250

Ro201724 308
rolipram, PDE4 inhibitor 308
RP73401 308

secreted protein, acidic and rich in cysteine (SPARC) 161, 162
selectin 81
selectin, E- 227, 232, 255, 313
selectin, L- 230
serotonin 91
sialyl Lewis^X, basophil function 55, 56
signal transduction mechanism 88
smooth muscle cell, contraction 267
smooth muscle cell, heterogeneity 270
smooth muscle cell, structure in culture 265
soluble intercellular adhesion molecule-1 (sICAM-1) 251
squamous epithelium 245
substance P 278
suplatast tosilate 315
syndecan 163

tachykinin 276
T-cell receptor (TcR) 338
tenascin 165
Th3 cell 337
T-helper 1 (Th1) 336
T-helper 2 (Th2) 336
theophylline 306
thrombin 88, 171
thrombosis 79
thromboxane (TX)A_2 86, 277, 310
thromboxane (TX)A_2 receptor 87
thromboxane (TX)A_2 receptor antagonist and synthesis inhibitor 280
thymocyte-1 antigen 172
tight junction 246
Tr1 337
transforming growth factor β (TGFβ) 165
transforming growth factor β, macrophage function 203, 206
transmigration 233
tryptase 170, 314
tumour necrosis factor-α (TNFα) 250, 273
tumour necrosis factor-α, dendritic cell function 211
tumour necrosis factor-α, macrophage function 202, 206

vascular cell adhesion molecule 1 (VCAM-1) 227, 232
vascular cell adhesion molecule 1 (VCAM-1), basophil 56
vasoactive intestinal peptide (VIP) 271, 273, 275
vasodilator 237
vasodilator, endothelial-derived 223
versican 165
vessel 20
viral and bacterial immunity, basophil, role in 66
VLA-4 313

FSC
www.fsc.org
MIX
Papier aus verantwortungsvollen Quellen
Paper from responsible sources
FSC® C105338

If you have any concerns about our products,
you can contact us on
ProductSafety@springernature.com

In case Publisher is established outside the EU,
the EU authorized representative is:
Springer Nature Customer Service Center GmbH
Europaplatz 3, 69115 Heidelberg, Germany

Printed by Libri Plureos GmbH
in Hamburg, Germany